# www.wadsworth.com

*wadsworth.com* is the World Wide Web site for Wadsworth and is your direct source to dozens of online resources.

At *wadsworth.com* you can find out about supplements, demonstration software, and student resources. You can also send email to many of our authors and preview new publications and exciting new technologies.

**wadsworth.com**
Changing the way the world learns®

# PRINCIPLES

*of*

# HEALTH EDUCATION

*and*

# HEALTH PROMOTION

### Third Edition

J. Thomas Butler
*Delaware State University*

**WADSWORTH**

™

**THOMSON LEARNING**

Australia • Canada • Mexico • Singapore • Spain
United Kingdom • United States

**WADSWORTH**

**THOMSON LEARNING**

Publisher: Peter Marshall
Associate Editor: April Lemons
Assistant Editor: John Boyd
Editorial Assistant: Andrea Kesterke
Marketing Manager: Joanne Terhaar
Project Editor: Sandra Craig
Print Buyer: Robert King

Permissions Editor: Joohee Lee
Production and Composition: Ash Street Typecrafters, Inc.
Text and Cover Designer: Liz Harasymczuk
Photo Researcher: Myrna Engler
Copy Editor: Carol Lombardi
Printer: Von Hoffmann Graphics

Printed in the United States of America
2  3  4  5  6  7  04  03

For permission to use material from this text, contact us by
Web: http://www.thomsonrights.com
Fax: 1-800-730-2215
Phone: 1-800-730-2214

**Wadsworth/Thomson Learning**
**10 Davis Drive**
**Belmont, CA 94002-3098**
**USA**

For more information about our products, contact us:
**Thomson Learning Academic Resource Center**
**1-800-423-0563**
http://www.wadsworth.com

**International Headquarters**
Thomson Learning
International Division
290 Harbor Drive, 2nd Floor
Stamford, CT 06902-7477
USA

**UK/Europe/Middle East/South Africa**
Thomson Learning
Berkshire House
168-173 High Holborn
London WC1V 7AA
United Kingdom

**Asia**
Thomson Learning
60 Albert Street, #15-01
Albert Complex
Singapore 189969

**Canada**
Nelson Thomson Learning
1120 Birchmount Road
Toronto, Ontario M1K 5G4
Canada

**Library of Congress Cataloging-in-Publication Data**
Butler, J. Thomas.
    Principles of health education and health promotion / J. Thomas Butler.—3rd ed.
        p. cm.
    Includes bibliographical references and index.
    ISBN 0-534-52374-9
    1. Health education.  2. Health promotion.  I. Title.

RA440.5.B88 2000
613—dc21

*For my students, past, present, and future. Thanks.*
*And*
*for the patience, tolerance, and love of Lily and Charlene.*

# Contents

## Chapter 4    History of Health Education and Health Promotion    61

## Chapter 5    Health Education and Promotion as a Profession    97

## Chapter 6    Settings for Health Education and Health Promotion    121

## Chapter 7    Coordinated School Health Programs    139

# Preface

Because we believe that readers are the best source of criticism and recommendations, this text has been revised to reflect the comments and needs expressed by users of the second edition. Further, every effort has been made to base changes on the most current points of view in the field. It is the sincere wish of the author that the changes included in this revision serve students who are preparing to embark on careers in health education and health promotion.

The discipline of health education and the practice of health promotion are continually evolving. Many forces within the profession as well as pressures and demands from the society at large affect that evolution. Professionals must be aware of elements that affect their work and be capable of adjusting to them. Many of those factors are similar to those that affect our health: heredity, lifestyle, health care services, and environment. Practitioners have the potential to influence the impact of these factors on the health of individuals and groups.

## NEW TO THE THIRD EDITION

This edition takes a slightly different view of the relationship between health promotion and health education. Rather than present health promotion as an outgrowth of health education, we conceptualize health promotion as a larger entity, comprising many intervention components, the core of which is health education. Perhaps the clearest portrayal of health promotion is seen in the health promotion triad of health education, prevention, and health protection.

This edition also addresses a number of special themes in health promotion, including empowerment and community organization. Health education continues to be a unique discipline with enormous potential to improve the health of communities and the lives of the individuals that constitute them. Other new features of this edition include the following:

**Chapter 5** is new to the text. It presents a list of nine characteristics of a profession, (borrowed from Simons-Morton and colleagues) to which the features of health education/promotion are applied to determine if they truly form a full-fledged profession. Although the profession is described as emerging, sufficient room for discussion and argument is left for students to consider the current professional status of our discipline and practice. This chapter encourages students to consider, among other things, the ethics of practice within the profession and the roles of many professional associations within the profession.

**Chapter 6** now includes the faith community and the military in its discussion of the various practice settings of health education/promotion. It also describes several effective programs in various communities.

**Chapter 8** contains much greater detail about specific federal initiatives to improve the health of Americans.

**Chapter 9's** presentation of successful programs have been updated to include the most recent innovations and results.

**Chapter 10**, which explores the theories and models that explain the processes of establishing and altering human behavior, now emphasizes the Theory of Reasoned Action and Theory of Planned Behavior. In addition, fresh and more thorough explanations of the Transtheoretical Model, Health Belief Model, Health Promotion Model, and Social Cognitive Theory are incorporated into this chapter.

**Chapter 11** explores the updated processes of needs assessment, planning, and program development and implementation. The planning models utilized here are the PRECEDE-PROCEED Model, Mico's Model for Health-Education Planning, the Planned Approach to Community Health (PATCH), and Multilevel Approach to Community Health (MATCH). PATCH and MATCH are new to this edition.

**Chapter 13** considers the current and future issues relating to the profession of health education/ promotion as it continually changes in response to social and political environments. For instance, in just a few short years it has become evident that the demographics of the United States has shifted dramatically, and even more substantial changes are predicted. Demands upon health educators are growing because of education reform and the accountability movement. These and other issues are presented in the context of their impact on the future of professionals' practice.

We believe that this text is enhanced by the substantial revisions that contributed to this new edition. Its usefulness to students and their instructors has been the driving force behind the changes you will encounter.

# ACKNOWLEDGMENTS

I wish to acknowledge and thank Dr. Joanne S. Chopak of Georgia Southern University, Dr. Michael Peterson of the University of Delaware, and Dr. Stephen Bohnenblust of the University of Minnesota at Mankato for their careful and valuable chapter reviews.

# The Meaning of Health and Wellness

The practice of health education and health promotion has evolved from a poorly defined, disconnected field into an emerging profession based upon a considerable theoretical and historical foundation. Fully certified and appropriately educated workers in many states practice health education as a specialty. School health education, once viewed as a rainy-day activity conducted by physical education teachers or coaches, is now taught by health promoters/educators with degrees equivalent to those in English, mathematics, and social studies. The level of their expertise and practice should be regarded as equivalent to those of other disciplines. To understand the nature of their work, we first will examine the nature of health.

## WHAT IS HEALTH?

Having health or feeling healthy has different meanings for different people at different times. We also experience it in different ways. For most of us, health includes emotions, beliefs, temperaments, experiences, and situations. The word "health" has nearly as many definitions as authors on the subject. The definitions in Box 1.1 illustrate differences—and similarities—in perspectives on health.

By far, the most quoted and frequently used definition is that of the World Health Organization—but this definition is inherently flawed if it is used to define a condition. The state of "complete well-being" is probably unattainable. In fact, it may be argued that health is not a state, but more a dynamic process (as suggested in Noack's definition). In addition, a person may have a high level in one of the dimensions identified, say the social, yet be only moderately satisfactory in the physical dimension. The WHO definition does, however, include the valuable implication of health as a holistic concept in which each dimension is interdependent with the others. Perhaps it is best to view that popular 1947 definition as a standard toward which we, as individuals and health promoters, can strive.

Several definitions of health utilize the notions of adaptation and function. Rene Dubos (1965) wrote, "The states of health or disease are the expressions of the success or failure experienced by the organism in its efforts to respond adaptively to environmental challenges." When a person's functional capacity becomes limited, health is changed and adaptation is required to adjust to the environment. "However, adaptive behavior has a wider scope. It may involve not only a modification of the individual organism but also a more or less extensive transformation of its environment" (Smith, 1983). From this perspective, disability is viewed as "different" ability requiring altering the environment in order to achieve vital life functions.

A primary theme common to all of these definitions of health is that of an explicitly positive element: a state of well-being, balance, or quality. They make no reference at all to bad health or the common description of ill people, "They are in poor health." Health, by definition, is good; the lack of it is bad.

Terris (1975) stated:

> Disease may occur without illness. Health and illness are mutually exclusive, but health and disease are not . . . Since health and disease may coexist, one cannot construct a continuum to show their relationship.

Shirreffs (1984) modified this theme only slightly by asserting that health and illness are separate and can exist together. **Illness** in this context is the presentation of visible symptoms, whereas **disease** is the underlying defect or malfunction within the organism. According to this point of view, you can be ill and still be quite healthy. You may be socially, mentally, and emotionally well, with a temporary physical malfunction to which the immune system has the ability to adapt.

Hoyman (1975) stated, "Health is a multidimensional unity, involving the whole person in his total environment." This reinforces the common theme of most definitions of the term "health"— that physical well-being is only a part of being healthy. Physical illness may seriously affect the physical body, while the mental, social, spiritual, and emotional dimensions may be less affected, equally affected, or even unaffected. Further, because health is a dynamic entity, it requires ongoing maintenance. The total person is a multidimensional creature, and his or her health also has many dimensions.

How would you measure your own health? Would it be in terms of years in your lifespan or the quality of those years? Would it be the quality of

---

**Box 1.1**   Definitions of "Health"

Health

. . . is a state of complete physical, mental, and social well-being and not merely the absence of disease or infirmity. (World Health Organization, 1947)

. . . is the condition of the organism which measures the degree to which its aggregate powers are able to function. (Oberteuffer, 1960)

. . . is the quality of life involving dynamic interaction and interdependence among the individual's physical well being, his mental and emotional reactions and the social complex in which he exists. (Sliepcevich, 1967)

. . . [is] an integrated method of functioning which is oriented toward maximizing the potential of which the individual is capable. It requires that the individual maintain a continuum of balance and purposeful direction with the environment where he is functioning. (Dunn, 1967)

. . . is a quality of life, involving social, emotional, mental, spiritual and biological fitness on the part of the individual, which results from adaptations to the environment. (Dubos, 1968)

. . . is a state of well-being sufficient to perform at adequate levels of physical, mental and social activity, taking age into account. (Lalonde, 1974)

. . . is a relational concept . . . not an entity that can be directly promoted but a relationship between capacities and demands. (Baranowski, 1981)

. . . [is] the capacity to cope with or adapt to disruptions among the organic, social, and personal components of the individual's health system. (Bates & Winder, 1984)

. . . is a state of dynamic balance—or more appropriately is a process maintaining such a state— within any given subsystem, such as an organ, an individual, a social group, or a community. (Noack, 1987)

. . . [is] an integrated method of functioning which is oriented toward maximizing the potential of which the individual is capable. It requires that the individual maintain a continuum of balance and purposeful direction with the environment where he (she) is functioning. (1990 Joint Committee on Health Education Terminology, 1991)

. . . can be defined as the quality of people's physical, psychological, and sociological functioning that enables them to deal adequately with the self and others in a variety of personal and social situations. (Bedworth & Bedworth, 1992)

. . . [is] a reflection of your ability to use the intrinsic and extrinsic resources within each dimension of health in order to participate fully in the activities that contribute to growth and development during each stage of the life cycle. (Payne & Hahn, 1998)

your relationships, your lack of debilitating illnesses, your ability to work? These are questions for each individual to consider. Perhaps more important questions would be: How can you improve your own health? What are you willing to do to make yourself healthier? Do some factors over which you have no control affect your health?

# DIMENSIONS OF HEALTH

The word "health" originally meant "wholeth," or "wholeness" (Dolfman, 1973). The state of being called health, as viewed through the origin of the word, implies involvement of the entire individual, a unique entity, albeit constituted of several dimensions. This is what the World Health Organization meant in 1947 when it defined health as including "physical, mental, and social well-being." A few authors (Donatelle & Davis, 1998; Insel & Roth, 2000) have advocated the inclusion of an environmental dimension in the overall scheme of health. Many authors (e.g., Levy, Dignan, & Shirreffs, 1992; Bensley, 1991; Osman & Russell, 1979) have proposed emotional and spiritual dimensions.

With the current emphasis on recognizing one's cultural heritage and on multicultural appreciation, one could argue that a cultural dimension of health is indicated. Certainly, examples such as the Asian belief that illness is an imbalance of the yin and yang forces and the ancient practice of Ayurveda, originating in India, which holds that imbalances in *doshas* (physiologic principles) can cause specific diseases, argue for a cultural dimension. These arguments sometimes are countered by contentions that cultural development is an element of the social dimension. Similarly, some have argued that the spiritual realm is linked inexorably to the emotional and mental dimensions. This text takes the position that all of the dimensions have undeniable links. Nevertheless, our discussion will focus on the dimensions of physical, emotional, social, mental (also referred to as intellectual), and spiritual health because these are addressed most frequently in the health education/promotion literature and programming.

No dimension of health functions in isolation. When an individual has a high level of health, all dimensions function in an integrated, coordinated way. Overemphasizing one dimension may sacrifice another. The interactions of the dimensions contribute to the richness of a person's life and help determine that individual's uniqueness.

## Physical Health

**Physical health** can be defined as "the absence of disease and disability; functioning adequately from the perspective of physical and physiological abilities; the biological integrity of the individual" (Goodstadt, Simpson, & Loranger, 1987). It also includes such characteristics as body size and shape, sensory acuity, susceptibility to disease and disorders, and recuperative ability. The physical condition of the body is reflected in a number of ways. Measurements of blood pressure, heart rate, body composition, flexibility, agility, muscular strength and endurance, vital capacity, and strength provide some insight into physical health. Response to injuries and recovery from disease can be indicative of physical health. People can behave in ways that enhance physical health, such as exercising regularly, maintaining proper weight, and adequate nutrition; similarly, they might avoid behaviors that erode physical health, such as cigarette smoking and excessive alcohol consumption.

Our bodies frequently send messages to us— "Please let me get a good night's sleep." "Allow my sprained ankle to heal." "Send down some vegetables tonight." "My muscles are tense."—that can guide us toward physical health. Getting regular medical checkups and practicing appropriate self-care for minor health problems can head off medical problems before they become serious.

In many ways, physical health serves as a foundation for achieving wellness in the other dimensions of health. Progressing toward higher levels of health in other dimensions is difficult until basic

**illness** the presentation of visible symptoms

**disease** the underlying defect or malfunction within the organism

**physical health** the absence of disease and disability; functioning adequately from the perspective of physical and physiological abilities; the biological integrity of the individual

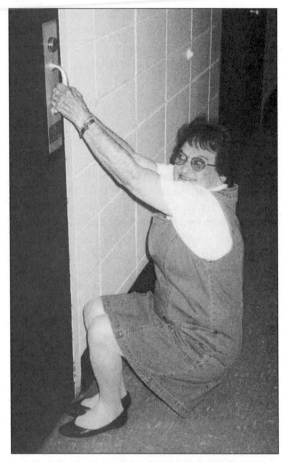

Age is no barrier to receiving the physical, emotional, and mental benefits of exercise—regardless of setting or lack of equipment.

physical needs, such as food, shelter, activity, and protection from environmental dangers, are met.

## Emotional Health

**Emotional health** is generally defined as the ability to feel and express the full range of human emotions, give and receive love, achieve a sense of fulfillment and purpose in life, and develop psychological hardiness (discussed below). Expressing emotions when appropriate and controlling such expressions at other times is a sign of emotional health. It requires understanding one's emotions and knowing how to cope with problems that arise and the stress we all endure in everyday life. It means being able to

work and study, love and be loved, pursue the activities that define our being, and enjoy those activities. Emotional health encompasses self-esteem, self-acceptance, self-control, and the ability to share one's feelings. The quality of a person's life is reflected largely in his or her emotions.

Emotions can affect our physical health. For example, people with high-level emotional health have low rates of stress-related symptoms, such as skin problems, stomachaches, asthma and other allergies. Long-term stress or emotional strife can lead to collapse of the immune system (Ornstein & Sobel, 1987; Squires, 1987), increasing the risk of developing other diseases. The ability to manage stress is an important part of emotional health.

Considerable evidence suggests that long-term stress can also increase the risk of heart disease. Beginning in the 1950s, cardiologists Rosenman and Friedman (1966) conducted a series of investigations into the relationship between coronary heart disease and personal life stress. Although their work is now controversial, it is the basis for much current research. They identified a personality type, which they labeled **Type A**, that seemed to be a significant risk factor in coronary heart disease when found in combination with elevated blood pressure and blood fats. Coronary-prone Type A individuals are supposedly hard-driving, competitive, subject to vocational deadlines, restless, impatient, frequently in a hurry, self-centered, perfectionistic, and oblivious to the environment (Friedman & Rosenman, 1974), whereas Type B individuals are relaxed and noncompetitive. As a group, Type C personalities appear to succeed more than Type B personalities and sometimes more than Type A personalities, yet suffer few of the cardiovascular effects—even while displaying Type A patterns of behavior.

In recent years, a personality trait called "**hardiness**" has been credited with strengthening the immune system against the destructive effects of stress (Kobasa, 1979). Hardy people see change as a challenge instead of a threat and develop strong levels of personal commitment and coping skills (Hawks, 1994). Hardiness is an optimistic and committed approach to life, viewing problems, including disease, as challenges that can be handled. Hardiness, or something akin to it, can be developed through stress management techniques and reassessment of one's own goals and priorities.

Many of the things that cause our stress, such as our families and work, also give us joy. One of the keys to emotional health is to realize that we usually can manage stressful situations and can reduce the effects of stress on our bodies and minds.

## Social Health

We all occupy roles in a number of groups or institutions, including son or daughter, friend, student or teacher, neighbor, co-worker, and mate. Each role

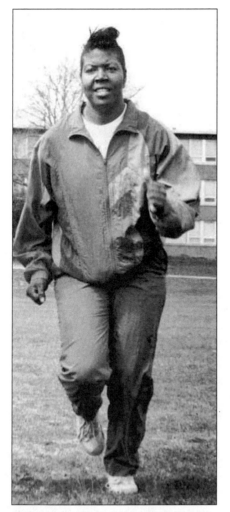

Regular exercise can enhance emotional health.

has expectations. **Social health** refers to the ability to perform the expectations of our roles effectively, comfortably, with pleasure, without harming other people (Levy, Dignan, & Shirreffs, 1992); to interact effectively with other people and the social environment (Goodstadt, Simpson, & Loranger, 1987); to "connect" with other people; to maintain intimacy; and to demonstrate respect and tolerance toward others. It is characterized by a concern and fondness for others, the ability to show respect, a sense of belonging within a larger social unit, the ability to communicate effectively, and efforts to make a positive contribution to family and community.

Performing role expectations sometimes means taking risks. It means having responsibilities that frequently affect other people and involve meeting others' needs. These include the needs for love, intimacy, safety, companionship, and cooperation—all important to social health. When people are deprived of these needs, they at times act in ways that threaten their overall health and well-being (Moss, 1973; Gore, 1978).

The social dimension is a good example of how dimensions of health merge to facilitate one another. Sociologists and epidemiologists have demonstrated health implications for social support and connectedness to others (House, Landis, & Umberson, 1988; Kaplan et al., 1988) that emphasize the association of the social, physical, and spiritual dimensions.

**emotional health**   the ability to feel and express the full range of human emotions, give and receive love, achieve a sense of fulfillment and purpose in life, and develop psychological hardiness

**Type A**   an action-emotion complex observed in a person aggressively involved in a long-term, ceaseless struggle to achieve more and more in less and less time, even against opposition by other things or persons

**hardiness**   an optimistic and committed approach to life, viewing problems as challenges that can be handled

**social health**   ability to perform the expectations of our roles effectively, comfortably, with pleasure, without harming other people; the ability to interact effectively with others and the social environment

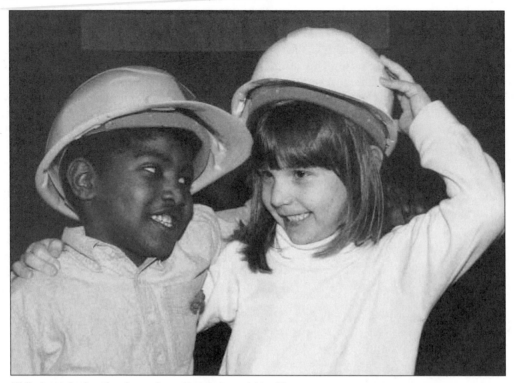

Well-planned educational experiences promote social health.

## Mental Health

**Mental (or intellectual) health** encompasses the intellectual processes of reasoning, analysis, evaluation, curiosity, humor, alertness, creativity, logic, learning, and memory. Therefore, it includes the ability to make sound decisions and to think critically. It also includes striving for continued personal growth and willingness to learn and use new information effectively for personal, family, and career development (Anspaugh, Dignan, & Anspaugh, 2000). Emotional health sometimes is considered a part of mental health, because emotions can act to the detriment of intellectual decision making.

Conforming to social demands is not necessarily a mark of mental health. Questioning what goes on around you indeed may be a sign of mental health. Actions and reactions alone do not automatically classify us as mentally healthy or mentally ill. A situation that may produce anxiety for some people may not cause anxiety for others because of basic personality differences or different experiences.

Showing no anxiety in a given circumstance, however, may be a sign that the person is not facing a problem or trying to resolve it. In actuality, anxiety may lead to solving problems.

Looking at a group of people he thought had fulfilled a good measure of their potential, Abraham Maslow (1968) identified qualities that he believed characterized, in his phrase, self-actualized people. The same qualities also may be applied to people who are mentally healthy. According to Maslow, these people

- are able to deal with the world as it is and do not demand that it should be otherwise,

- are able to largely accept themselves, others, and nature,

- experience profound interpersonal relations,

- have a continuing fresh appreciation for what goes on around them,

- are able to direct themselves rather independently of culture and environment,

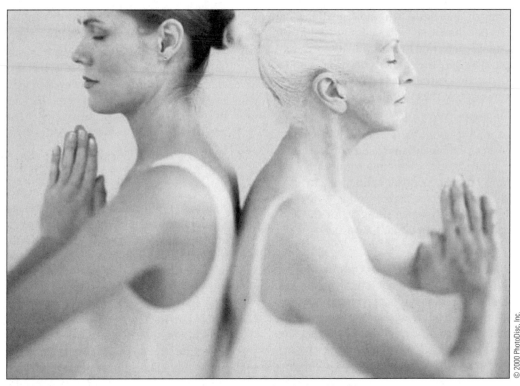

© 2000 PhotoDisc, Inc.

Meditation can help reduce stress and enhance emotional and mental health.

- trust their own senses and feelings,
- are creative, and
- are democratic in their attitudes.

## Spiritual Health

Defining **spiritual health** has been impaired by a lack of clear structure or measurable outcomes and by controversy over the relationship of spirituality and religion. An example of the nebulous nature of the task is the U.S. Office of Alternative Medicine's (1994) definition of spirituality as "one's inward sense of something greater than the individual self or the meaning one perceives that transcends the immediate circumstances." Fortunately, Hawks (1994) overcame these problems by formulating the following definition:

A high level of faith, hope and commitment in relation to a well-defined worldview or belief system that provides a sense of meaning and purpose to existence in general, and that offers an ethical path to personal fulfillment which includes connectedness with self, others, and a higher power or larger reality.

Banks (1980) found that the spiritual dimension of health contains four aspects: a unifying force within individuals, meaning in life, a common bond between individuals, and individual perceptions of faith. These are defined as follows:

1. The unifying aspect of the spiritual dimension is the force that integrates all the other dimensions (physical, mental, social, and emotional).

**mental (or intellectual) health**  ability to make sound decisions and think critically

**spiritual health**  a high level of faith, hope, and commitment in relation to a well-defined worldview or belief system that provides a sense of meaning and purpose to existence in general, and that offers an ethical path to personal fulfillment that includes connectedness with self, others, and a higher power or larger reality (Hawks, 1994)

Viewing the individual as a whole, anything that affects one dimension will act upon all the others, thereby affecting the individual's total well-being. The spiritual dimension, then, can be viewed as the central core that bonds and serves as a support for the other dimensions.

2. An individual's spiritual dimension identifies what that person finds meaningful in life. People can express meaning and purpose to life in many ways, such as through nature, art, meditation, religion, political action, or altruism. This is highly personal and specific to the person. It may be the main stimulus for the individual's successes in life and the criterion he or she interprets as life failure.

3. The spiritual dimension transcends the individual to create a common bond between individuals, a trait unique to this dimension. This capacity could be manifested in various ways: perhaps as a set of principles or ethics that govern our conduct, a sense of selflessness and empathy for others, or a commitment to a higher power. Banks and associates (1984) reviewed three studies of how health education practitioners viewed the spiritual dimension of health. Significant numbers identified selflessness as a major component of this dimension.

4. This component of the spiritual dimension has to do with perceptions of what causes the universe to work the way it does: recognition of powers beyond the natural and rational; survival; and pleasure (Banks, 1980). Each individual has a unique sense of his or her own perception of the cosmos.

Pilch (1988) took a slightly different approach to spirituality, identifying five elements of human spiritual life—freedom, purpose in life, life's fulfillment, motivation, and conversion—and defining them as follows:

1. Spirituality must be freely chosen, including religious aspects.

2. Purpose in life corresponds roughly to meaning in life in Banks' system, above, although Pilch ascribed a distinctly more religious meaning to this element than did Banks.

3. Life's fulfillment is defined as discovering how to make the best of bad situations.

4. Motivation is a way of getting things started and keeping them going while remaining in charge of the process or development. Two powerful motivating factors are a strong sense of self-esteem and a critical assessment and appreciation of one's values.

5. Conversion, seen more as a process than a state, is a broadening of one's horizons, a widening of perspective.

Seaward (1991) added a different facet, a strong personal value system, to the construct of human spirit. He noted that values forge a framework for self-validation, moral development in judgment of right and wrong, good and bad, and pain and pleasure.

The spiritual dimension may or may not involve religion. In view of the doctrine of separation of church and state that we enjoy in the United States, educators, especially those practicing in public schools, should distinguish between religion and spirituality. Although religion is an integral part of the notion of spirituality for some, one does not have to profess any particular religion to be spiritual. Spirituality neither excludes nor is exclusive to the religious (Diaz, 1993).

A growing body of research (National Institute for Healthcare Research, 1999) suggests that people who are more spiritually committed tend to cope better with and recover more quickly from serious illness. Recent research has suggested that religious and spiritual considerations can play important roles in helping people live longer and in reducing mortality.

# MAJOR FACTORS INFLUENCING HEALTH

The Health Field Concept is commonly used to identify causes of morbidity and mortality. It holds that disease and death are attributable to four main factors: heredity, environment, health care services, and behavior. It is estimated that heredity is responsible for 16 percent of the years of life lost before age 65 by Americans, environment for 22 percent, health care services (or lack of them) for 8 percent, and lifestyle for 54 percent (McGinnis & Foege, 1993).

## Heredity

A number of factors affecting our health are inherited and therefore beyond our control. Some of these traits may contribute to effective functioning; others may interfere with it. Disorders such as Down syndrome, Marfan's syndrome, sickle cell anemia, thalassemia, and Tay-Sachs disease are inherited. Almost daily, scientists discover links between certain defective genes or gene combinations and specific diseases. Recent research has targeted a gene responsible for familial breast cancer and genes that make a person susceptible to colon cancer.

Tendencies toward disorders such as hypertension have been shown to be genetic and more likely to appear in certain ethnic groups. **Heredity** is a contributing but not defining factor in heart disease, cancer, diabetes, obesity, alcoholism, and schizophrenia.

Our gender, and possibly our size, can make us susceptible to certain influences on our health. Percentage of body fat, weight, and obesity can be partially inherited. Just as a genetic propensity toward high levels of body fat may influence an individual's health negatively, the propensity toward a low or moderate level of body fat is a positive influence on health. However, it is often difficult to separate these propensities from aspects of culture, such as recreational patterns and food preparation habits.

As part of any reproductive planning, individuals at risk for such disorders should consider genetic screening and counseling, including prenatal diagnosis and screening of newborns. Health educators/promoters should serve a role in encouraging these procedures.

## Environment

Our awareness of the environment's importance to our health and the deterioration of health is increasing. As the ozone layer is being depleted, we humans are exposed to more ultraviolet radiation.

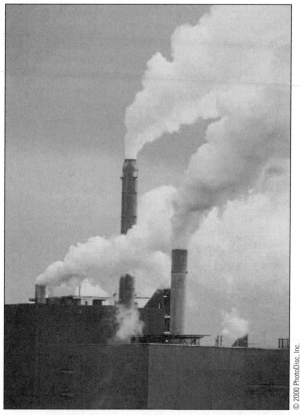

© 2000 PhotoDisc, Inc.

Air pollution is a threat to health in many parts of the United States.

The risk of eye damage and skin cancer is greater with exposure to the sun. Sunburn is really radiation burn, and skin cancer can develop even without sunburn.

Our water and food supplies have long been polluted by agricultural runoff and some irresponsible industries. Certain forms of cancer and even fetal damage have been traced to polluted water. If water is contaminated, the food we eat also is likely to be contaminated.

The air we breathe is a health hazard to many of us. For years, several large urban areas have exceeded acceptable levels of pollutants, such as ozone and carbon monoxide. Winds, offending industries,

**heredity**  genetic background that programs each of us in some ways

and automobiles have spread dense pollutants to many rural areas as well. Pollutants in the air may fall to the earth in the form of acid rain, further damaging the soil, water, and food. Fortunately, levels of many air pollutants (smog, carbon monoxide, sulfur dioxide emissions, soot) have improved measurably, though it remains to be seen if any long-range positive environmental impact will occur.

The U.S. Congress and governmental agencies such as the Environmental Protection Agency have wrestled for years with the problem of air pollution. The lobbying power of big business has hampered the effectiveness of many initiatives to clean up the air because implementation of the regulations carries tremendous financial burdens. In recent years,

stricter regulations mandated by the federal Clean Air Act have been implemented. These have been successful in reducing air pollution in some places.

Millions of people are susceptible to allergic reactions to substances in the environment. The presence of these substances may be increased by climactic conditions.

Noise has been identified as an environmental hazard. Some exposures to noise, such as listening to music played at high volume through headphones and at rock concerts, are voluntary. Many people, however, are exposed to high decibel levels in their workplace and at home. Besides the noise of appliances, televisions, and stereos, many Americans live close to airports, highways, highly congested areas, and construction sites. Indeed, areas of high population density are a source of almost constant exposure to excessive noise levels. In some areas, noise has been reduced as a result of enforcement of nuisance laws and judicious placement of airports and roads.

Many Americans consider themselves and their children subject to social and cultural pollution via television, radio, and the Internet. Depictions of violence and sexuality are offensive to many people and certainly present an unhealthy and unrealistic picture of sex. Advertisements for foods, alcohol, and tobacco depict inaccurate and misleading situations regarding these products. Young children and teens do not have the maturity to decipher advertising messages accurately. Saying that parents can turn off the television or throw out the magazine is missing the point. Children cannot avoid these images in today's world.

The modern network of society may not provide an environment conducive to individual growth. Instead it may impinge on the individual's freedom to function adequately. Overcrowding is an example. Failure of the family, the school, and the church to provide opportunities for children to develop self-esteem may contribute to experimentation with alcohol or other drugs (Butler, 1982).

Our social environment is increasingly seen as a contributor to our health—or the lack of it. For example, poor people suffer health problems disproportionately. Certain behaviors or customs in different communities may influence the health of that community and its individual members. For

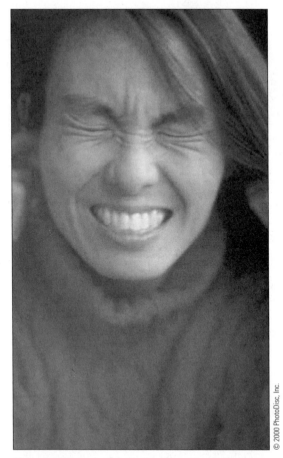

© 2000 PhotoDisc, Inc.

Noise can have physiological and emotional effects on human health.

example, the degree of acceptance of unwed pregnancies in different ethnic groups or the acceptance of the community's responsibility for all of its children in some populations may affect the health of the social group. The social environment may also affect an individual's access to the health care delivery system. Poverty, distrust of the medical establishment or of government, or a preference for traditional, yet-unproven, remedies may act to lessen access to or use of the health care system.

## Health Care Services

The cost and availability of health care services have an obvious effect on people's health. The rise in cost of health care over the past several years has far outdistanced inflation. An ever-increasing percentage of the U.S. gross national product is devoted to the delivery of health care. In 1950, health care expenditures totaled about 4.4 percent of the gross national product. That percentage rose to 11.1 in 1988 and, after stabilizing from 1993–1998 at around 13.6 percent, is expected to reach 16.2 percent of the GNP by 2008 (Health Care Financing Administration, 1999). The total projected expenditures of $2.2 trillion in 2008 would represent about $7500 per person per year. Even as expenditures increase, insurance companies have become more selective in the procedures they cover and the clients they will insure. All this has made health care too expensive for many Americans.

For those who can afford health care—whether it be through their own resources, private or group health insurance, or government-sponsored programs such as Medicaid—the primary emphasis of care traditionally has been on diagnosis and treatment rather than on prevention. The emphasis on expensive treatment is a major cause of the higher costs and lack of availability. We know how to prevent many illnesses and disorders, but the medical community could do more in stressing prevention to its patients. Of course, the medical community cannot bear the full blame, because we, the consumers, must put prevention into practice by making decisions that affect our lifestyles and daily lives. We will thereby gain the full benefit of preventive medicine and lessen the costs of treatment.

In 1972, the Health Maintenance Organization Assistance Act was passed with the hope of setting up a new system for delivering health care. As defined in this act, HMOs have an education component. In practice, HMOs and other forms of managed care differ widely in delivery of services, costs, and health education.

Effectiveness of health care frequently depends upon the quality of communication between practitioner and patient. Communication may be weakened by physicians who fail to bridge the gap between medical jargon and the patient's ability to understand and comprehend. Physicians should consider each patient's strengths and weaknesses and try to overcome weaknesses that impede good communication.

Patients, too, may impede communication. They may be reluctant to describe their symptoms or talk about issues that are embarrassing to them. Health educators can assume a role in this area. Students and clients should understand the importance of taking an active part in their own health and complying with physicians' advice. They cannot do this unless they make a special effort to provide all the information a physician needs to render an accurate diagnosis and unless they understand fully the advice they receive. Patients have to feel comfortable and be assertive enough to ask questions and to leave the appointment only after they have all the information necessary to comply with the physician's advice. Fostering patient assertiveness is one role of health educators.

A debate once arose as to whether health care was a right or a privilege. With the advent of insurance companies, most Americans gained access to health care. In recent years, however, health care costs have driven insurance premiums beyond the reach of many citizens. Approximately 44.3 million Americans (16.3 percent), including 11.1 million children (15.4 percent), were without health insurance for the entire year 1998 (U.S. Bureau of the Census, 1999). Put in perspective, the number of uninsured Americans exceeds the entire population of Canada by about 50 percent. In addition, 31 million people have health insurance but are underinsured (Consumers Union, 1998).

Insurers now determine the cost of health care in most cases, which gives an enormous amount of power to a third party in the delivery relationship. This is most apparent in the Medicaid system of establishing diagnosis-related groups (DRGs). DRGs establish payment schedules for specific diagnoses, which means that Medicaid will pay only so much for a medical procedure. In managed care plans, nonphysicians often decide which procedures to approve and the allowable cost of those procedures. It means the insurer, rather than the physician, influences the choice of treatment procedures or even whether to treat the patient at all. As this power is concentrated in the hands of for-profit insurers, the implications for health care are frightening.

The traditional practice wherein a single physician maintains and operates an office is rapidly becoming a part of history in most areas. Grouping several physicians in one office enables reduction of overhead and staff salaries. An example of this trend is the HMO, one form of which is a single company that employs physicians of many specialties and pays each a salary. This is a powerful contrast to individual physicians who charge each patient for each service.

Undoubtedly, the health care delivery system must be changed in substantial ways. Opposition to comprehensive health care reform has been effective as powerful lobbies and interest groups wage campaigns to defeat major proposals in Congress. Several states, however, have begun to conduct statewide demonstrations that they hope will reduce costs, provide more coverage, and furnish models for other states and the federal government.

The most potentially powerful force in health care is the consumer. Once totally dependent on physicians and passive recipients of health care, more people are becoming active in their own care. They are demanding that physicians regard them as partners in the support of their own health, realizing that their greatest health ally is the self. The Surgeon General's 1979 report (U.S. Department of Health, Education, and Welfare, 1979) stated that "you the individual can do more for your own health and well-being than any doctor, any hospital, any drug, any exotic medical device."

The historical importance of medical care may be overestimated. Free access to health care has

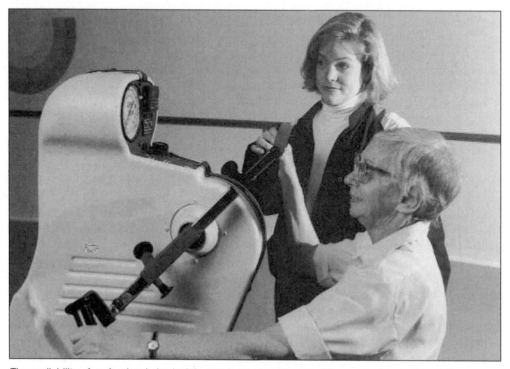

The availability of professional physical therapy is an example of health care services to the public.

failed to reduce the gap in status between higher-income and lower-income patients in Great Britain (Marmot, Kogevinas, & Elston, 1987) or Canada (Terris, 1990). This would indicate that the roles of the health-care delivery system and the individual are both subject to economic and social duress.

## Behavior

To maximize the health of the population, individuals must take responsibility for their own actions and the status of their own health. Although many causes of illness and deteriorating health are linked to heredity and to environmental pollutants, lifestyle is a determining factor in the state of one's health. Lifestyle should be viewed as a consistent complex of related practices and behavioral patterns in a person or group, usually based on some combination of cultural heritage, social relationships, geographic and socioeconomic circumstances, and personality. Although we must surely acknowledge the role of the social environment, the individual makes many decisions that affect his or her health. What we do is the major influence on our health. The implications of behavior change, habit formation, and lifestyle development form a significant foundation for the role of health promotion and education.

Consider that

- Cancer is the second leading cause of death in the United States, and lung cancer causes more deaths than any other form of cancer. The American Cancer Society (2000) estimated that cigarette smoking is responsible for 87 percent of the lung cancers.

- The use of smokeless tobacco is a major risk factor for oral cancer (American Cancer Society, 2000).

- A diet high in fat or low in fiber, or both, may be associated with colon and rectum cancer (American Cancer Society, 2000).

- Diet, cigarette smoking, and lack of exercise are closely related to heart disease, the leading cause of death in the United States (Insel & Roth, 2000).

- Even though HIV is not contracted readily, many people engage in the precise acts (unprotected sex and injectable drug use) that transmit the disease.

- Even though the U.S. Public Health Service identified cigarette smoking as "clearly the largest single preventable cause of illness and premature death in the United States" (U.S. Department of Health, Education and Welfare, 1979), about one-fourth of adults and 36 percent of adolescents are current smokers (U.S. Dept. of Health and Human Services, 2000).

- Although immunizations are inexpensive and have been available for decades, many parents are not having their children immunized. The number of fully immunized American children ages 19–35 months was at a record high in 1998; still, about 20 percent of the nation's preschoolers were not fully immunized against mumps, measles, polio, and other common childhood diseases (Centers for Disease Control and Prevention [CDC], 1999).

- Although regular exercise reduces the risk of premature death (U.S. Department of Health and Human Services, 1996); heart disease (National Institutes of Health Consensus Development Panel, 1996); diabetes (Helmrich et al., 1991); breast cancer (Bernstein et al., 1994; Thune et al., 1997); colon cancer (Colditz, Cannuscio, & Frazier, 1997); depression (Pappas, Golin, & Meyer, 1990); obesity (Bar-Or, 1993); and increases longevity (Paffenbarger et al., 1994) and immune system functioning (Nieman, 1994), only about half of U.S. youths regularly participate in vigorous physical activity and about one-fourth participate in no vigorous physical activity (U.S. Department of Health and Human Services, 1996).

- Although using lap and shoulder safety belts in vehicles reduces the risk of serious injuries and fatalities significantly, many adults fail to use the restraints and more than 19 percent of high school students rarely or never use safety belts when riding in a vehicle driven by someone else (CDC, 1995).

The recognition that behavior is related to health is not new. Belloc and Breslow (1972) followed nearly 7,000 adults for 5½ years. Their research showed that life expectancy and better health are related significantly to simple health habits. Among the findings were that 80 percent of deaths caused by cancer and cardiovascular disease are premature and can be prevented by altering health practices.

A former Surgeon General (U.S. Department of Health, Education and Welfare, 1979) pointed out that individuals can improve their health by taking actions for themselves, including the following:

- eliminating cigarette smoking
- decreasing alcohol use
- making moderate dietary changes, including reducing the intake of calories, fat, salt, and sugar
- doing moderate regular exercise
- periodically being screened for disorders such as high blood pressure and certain cancers
- adhering to speed laws and using seat belts

Kolbe (1993) stated that only six types of behaviors cause the major health problems that face the nation. If looked upon as behaviors that could be changed or eliminated, they bear remarkable resemblance to the former Surgeon General's list of actions to improve individual health. They are

- behaviors that result in unintentional or intentional injuries
- drug and alcohol abuse
- sexual behaviors that result in pregnancy or sexually transmitted diseases, including HIV infection
- tobacco use
- excessive consumption of fat and calories
- insufficient physical activity

Kann et al. (1995) found that the same behaviors (including the more general description of "dietary patterns that cause disease") are responsible for 70 percent of morbidity and mortality in adolescents.

Both studies indicated that these behaviors are usually established in youth; are interrelated; persist into adulthood; contribute simultaneously to diminished levels of health, education, and social outcomes; and are preventable. Moreover, health-compromising behaviors tend to occur in clusters—that is, individuals engaging in one type of high-risk behavior also tend to engage in others (Donovan, Jessor, & Costa 1988; National Research Council, 1995; Resnicow, Ross, & Vaughn, 1995).

The obvious question becomes: If we know how to reduce health risks, why do so many people behave in ways that put them at greater risk? Although the answers to this question are not easy to come by, let us postulate a few:

- They do not value health.
- They enjoy the thrill of risk-taking.

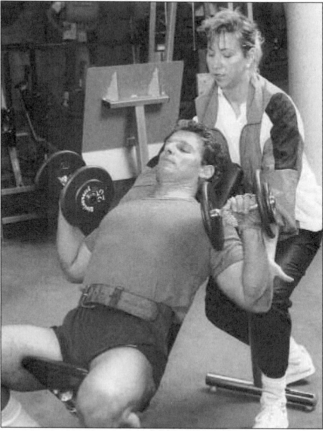

The Surgeon General and other health experts encourage regular exercise as a means of improving health.

- They are unable to balance the risk versus the benefits of the action.
- The immediate benefit gained from the action is worth the future risk of shorter lifespan, disease, or injury.
- They are unaware of the risks.
- People take unnecessary risks because risk-taking behaviors, habits, and addictions are established early in life before developing sufficient maturity.
- Choices are influenced by the social environment.

Whatever the reasons, they relate to factors that influence all behavior and which can be grouped into three categories

1. **Predisposing factors** are present before the behavior occurs; they are things we bring to the decision point, including life experiences, values, knowledge, attitudes, beliefs, and demographic variables such as age, gender, ethnicity, education, and income. For example, a person may avoid environmental tobacco smoke because he has knowledge of the risk it poses and he values his health. On the other hand, such predisposing factors as teens' erroneous belief that most peers smoke and their inability to appreciate the long-term health effects of smoking may contribute to experimenting with smoking.

2. **Enabling factors** are also present before the behavior; they are the arsenal of weapons we use to decide whether to pursue or not pursue an action. They include skills and abilities (such as the ability to evaluate health information); the availability of health resources; access to affordable health care; and physical, emotional, and mental faculties. For a person interested in avoiding environmental tobacco smoke, laws and regulations restricting smoking in the workplace and public places enables her to more easily avoid others' smoke. For teens, the easy availability of cigarettes and their own lack of ability to evaluate advertising targeting them are enabling factors toward health-risk behavior.

3. **Reinforcing factors** appear after the behavior has occurred. They can serve to encourage us to repeat the behavior or to abandon it. They include support from family and friends, feedback and encouragement from teachers, rewards given by employers, and the good feeling that one may experience from engaging in a healthy activity. A reinforcing factor that could prove disastrous is the thrill of risk-taking associated with some recreational activities. The person who avoids environmental tobacco smoke may find reinforcement in favorable comments from others, the fact that his clothing no longer smells like smoke at the end of the day, and reduction in coughing. Teen smoking may be reinforced by support from friends; images of musicians, actors, and athletes who smoke; and the pleasure derived from smoking.

## WHAT IS "WELLNESS"?

Another way of describing the quality of life of an individual is through the concept of **wellness**. According to Meeks, Heit, and Page (1996), wellness is the quality of life that includes physical, mental-emotional, and family-social health. This text takes the position that spiritual health also is included in personal wellness, thus creating the following five dimensions.

Physical health is the condition of a person's body, influenced by eating nutritious meals, exercising regularly, and getting adequate sleep. Mental-emotional health is the condition of the individual's mind and the way he or she expresses feelings. Acquiring and assessing information, engaging in

---

**predisposing factors**    factors that are present before a behavior occurs that provide a rationale or motivation for the behavior

**enabling factors**    factors that are present before a behavior occurs that allow the behavior to be carried out by providing the necessary ability, skills, opportunity, or resources

**reinforcing factors**    factors that are present after the behavior has occurred that can encourage repetition or abandonment of it

**wellness**    the quality of life that includes physical, mental-emotional, family-social, and spiritual health

intellectually challenging conversation, and synthesizing concepts from different arenas are examples of ways the mind achieves healthy condition. Emotional health is nurtured by taking time to understand feelings and by expressing them in healthful ways, as well as meeting one's own needs without interfering with others' rights. Family-social health is the condition of the person's relationships with others. Maintaining family-social health requires listening carefully when others are speaking, expressing oneself clearly, and learning to give and receive affection in appropriate ways. Spiritual health is characterized by selfless behavior, finding meaning in life, and comfort with one's perceptions of faith. Anspaugh and colleagues (1997) state that wellness means engaging in attitudes and behaviors that enhance quality of life and maximize personal potential.

Figure 1.1 depicts the wellness scale, indicating a range in quality of life from optimal well-being to premature death. In between are high-level wellness, average wellness, minor illness or injury, and major illness or injury. The individual exercises control over nine factors that influence wellness. Health status is the sum total of the positive and negative influences of the following:

- the level of health knowledge a person has, meaning the information needed to develop health literacy, maintain and improve health, prevent disease, and reduce health-related risk behaviors

- the wellness behaviors a person chooses that promote health; prevent disease, injury, and premature death; and improve the quality of the environment versus the risk behaviors that increase the likelihood of illness or premature death and destroy the quality of the environment (this may include the social as well as the physical environment)

**Figure 1.1**  The Wellness Scale

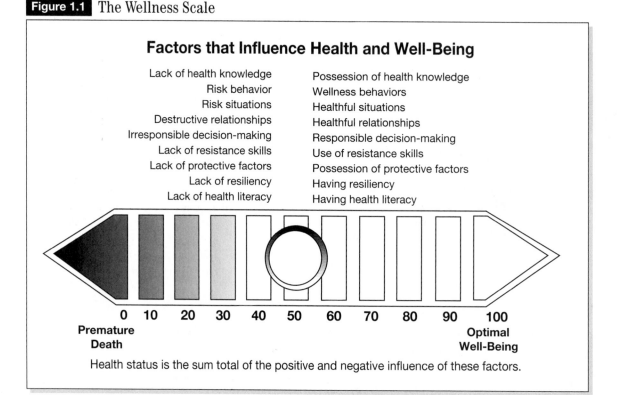

### Factors that Influence Health and Well-Being

| Lack of health knowledge | Possession of health knowledge |
| Risk behavior | Wellness behaviors |
| Risk situations | Healthful situations |
| Destructive relationships | Healthful relationships |
| Irresponsible decision-making | Responsible decision-making |
| Lack of resistance skills | Use of resistance skills |
| Lack of protective factors | Possession of protective factors |
| Lack of resiliency | Having resiliency |
| Lack of health literacy | Having health literacy |

0  10  20  30  40  50  60  70  80  90  100

**Premature Death**                    **Optimal Well-Being**

Health status is the sum total of the positive and negative influence of these factors.

- the situations in which a person participates that promote health versus risky or harmful situations that threaten health

- the relationships in which a person engages: Healthful relationships promote self-esteem and productivity, encourage health-enhancing behavior, and are free of violence and drug abuse. Destructive relationships destroy self-esteem, interfere with productivity and health, and may include violence and drug abuse.

- the decisions a person makes: Healthful decisions promote health and safety, observe laws, show respect for self and others, follow guidelines set by responsible adults, and demonstrate good character.

- the skills that help a person resist pressure to engage in actions that threaten health or safety, violate laws, exhibit lack of respect for self and others, disobey guidelines set by responsible adults, and demonstrate lack of character

- the protective factors either in a person's behavior or environment that promote safety, health, and well-being versus risk factors that threaten safety, health, and well-being

- the extent to which a person is resilient or able to prevent, recover from, and learn from adversity, change, and pressure

- the degree of health literacy, or competence in critical thinking and problem solving, responsible and productive citizenship, self-directed learning, and effective communication (Joint Committee on Health Education Standards, 1995) a person has achieved

The more positive factors present (shown on the right in Figure 1.1) at any given time, the greater the likelihood of health and well-being.

## WHAT IS OPTIMAL HEALTH?

Everybody does not have the same capacity for health. Each person is defined by his or her own set of conditions that may affect health. **Optimal health** is the highest level of health possible given the current set of environmental conditions and capacity of the organism, a balance among the five dimensions of health mentioned above.

An individual's optimal level of health varies according to environmental constraints, capacity to deal with those constraints, and permanent or temporary disabilities. A person who adapts to stressful environmental changes has a higher level of optimal health than a person who cannot. A person who labors under enormous environmental constraints has a lower level of optimal health than a person with fewer constraints. Certainly, people with severe physical or mental disabilities might be less able to adapt to their environments and have a lower optimal health level. However, many people with severe physical handicaps have attained extremely high levels of overall health despite their limitations. Factors that may explain achievement of optimal health in the face of disabilities and chronic illness are the development of strong spiritual health, emotional strength, social supports, and hardiness.

One's level of optimal health combines each of the complementary dimensions of health—physical, emotional, social, mental, and spiritual. Although some components may be more prominent, none should be overlooked. Individuals and health educators may be most likely to neglect the spiritual dimension. As Richardson and Nolan (1984) concluded, optimum health cannot be achieved without consideration of spiritual values, given that so many health issues now have spiritual overtones, including assisted suicide, sex education, and lifestyle concerns. Figure 1.2 depicts the shared contributions of the five components of optimal health.

Achieving or even approaching optimal health carries many benefits. A few of these benefits are

- reduction in risk of major diseases
- improved quality of life
- potential for greater longevity
- improved self-image, self-esteem, and self-confidence

**optimal health** the highest level of health possible under the current set of environmental conditions and the individual's capacity

**Figure 1.2** The Dimensions of Optimal Health

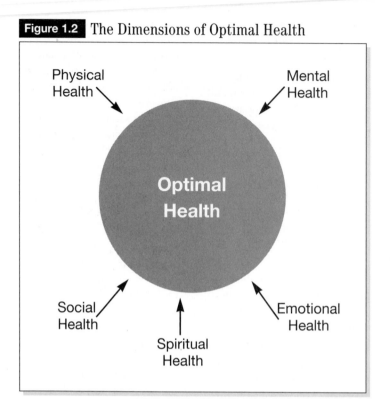

- improved physical appearance
- higher energy levels resulting in increased productivity
- more satisfying sex life
- improved ability to resist infectious diseases
- greater ability to manage and control stress
- greater ability to concentrate and learn
- improved cardiorespiratory function
- more personal control of your life
- increased muscle tone, flexibility, and endurance
- increased levels of spiritual health, including feelings of oneness with self and nature
- improved social relationships

The challenge for each individual is to gain the highest level of health possible. Health care deliverers and educators, perhaps more than any other group, must assist others to attain optimal health. This is what health education is really all about.

## SO HOW ARE WE DOING?

A country as diverse as the United States will always exhibit positive and negative indicators of health. A few examples may give a snapshot of the national health situation:

- The life expectancy at birth increased to 76.5 years in 1997, an all-time high, primarily because of decreases in mortality from HIV/AIDS, heart disease, cancer, stroke, and homicide (National Center for Health Statistics, 1999).
- Infant mortality rates reached a record low of 7.2 infants deaths per 1,000 live births in 1997 (National Center for Health Statistics, 1999). One of the most important factors in increasing life expectancy is the reduction in infant death. Still, the U.S. ranks 22nd among industrialized nations (Children's Defense Fund, 2000).
- The percentage of high school students who reported ever having sex dropped from 54 percent

in 1990 to 48 percent in 1997 (The Annie E. Casey Foundation, 1998).

- The 1995 rate of pregnancies for young women aged 15 to 19 dropped to a twenty-year low of 101 per 1,000, and the teen birth rate dropped from 62 for every 1,000 young women in 1991 to 54 per 1,000 in 1996. The U.S. teen birth rate is still about twice that of any other developed country (The Annie E. Casey Foundation, 1998).

- The teen birth rate in the U.S. is about 5.3 percent, compared to 0.6 percent in the Netherlands, 0.9 percent in Denmark, 1.3 percent in Sweden, 2.3 percent in Austria, and 3.2 percent in Great Britain (Moore et al., 1995; Ventura et al., 1998).

- Each year about 12 million Americans, about one-fourth teens, contract a sexually transmitted disease (The Annie E. Casey Foundation, 1998).

- The majority of high school students, and particularly seniors (66 percent), have engaged in sexual intercourse, many clearly at too early an age and with too many partners (CDC, 1996a).

- More than half of high school students reported having at least one drink of alcohol during the preceding 30 days and a third reported having five or more drinks on at least one occasion during the past 30 days (CDC, 1998a).

- More than 36 percent of high school students reported smoking cigarettes on at least one of the preceding 30 days (CDC, 1998b) and more than 3,000 young people in the U.S. become daily smokers each day (CDC, 1997).

- In 1995 an estimated 61 million Americans were current smokers. This represents a smoking rate of 29 percent for the population age 12 and older (CDC, 1996b).

These few examples point out that, although some progress is being made in altering behaviors that put individuals' health at risk, much work remains to be done if the health and lives of Americans are to improve.

## KEY POINTS

1. Whereas the term "health" is defined in many ways, a primary theme is that of a positive element.

2. Health is a changing, dynamic entity requiring ongoing maintenance.

3. Individual health is composed of at least five interrelated dimensions: physical, emotional, social, mental, and spiritual.

4. The Health Field Concept identifies four causes of morbidity and mortality: heredity, environment, health care services, and behavior.

5. Wellness is the quality of life dependent on the individual's status in the five dimensions of health.

6. Optimal health is dependent on the current set of environmental conditions and the capacity of the organism. It represents the highest level of health possible for the individual at any given time and depends on a balance among the dimensions of health.

# REFERENCES

American Cancer Society. (2000). *Cancer facts & figures—2000.* Atlanta, GA.

The Annie E. Casey Foundation. (1998). *When teens have sex: Issues and trends.* Baltimore, MD.

Anspaugh, D.J., Dignan, M.B., & Anspaugh, S.L. (2000). *Developing health promotion programs.* Boston: McGraw-Hill.

Anspaugh, D.J., Hamrick, M.H., & Rosato, F.D. (1997). *Wellness: Concepts and applications.* St. Louis: Mosby.

Banks, R. (1980). Health and the spiritual dimension: Relationships and implications for professional preparation programs. *Journal of School Health, 50*(4), 195–202.

Banks, R.L, Poehler, D.L., & Russell, R.D. (1984). Spirit and human-spiritual interaction as a factor in health and in health education. *Health Education, 15*(5), 16–19.

Baranowski, T. (1981). Toward the definition of concepts of health and disease, wellness and illness. *Health Values, 5*(6), 246–256.

Bar-Or, O. (1993). Physical activity and physical training in childhood obesity. *Journal of Sports Medicine and Physical Fitness, 33*(4), 323–329.

Bates, I.J., & Winder, A.E. (1984). *Introduction to health education.* Palo Alto, CA: Mayfield.

Bedworth, D.A., & Bedworth, A.E. (1992). *The profession and practice of health education.* Dubuque, IA: Wm. C. Brown.

Belloc, N.B., & Breslow, L. (1972). Relationship of physical health status and health practices. *Preventive Medicine, 1*(3), 415–521.

Bensley, R.J. (1991). Spiritual health as a component of worksite health promotion/wellness programming: A review of the literature. *Journal of Health Education, 22*(6), 352–353+.

Bernstein, L., Henderson, B.E., Hanisch, R., Sullivan-Halley, J., & Ross, R.K. (1994). Physical exercise and reduced risk of breast cancer in young women. *Journal of the National Cancer Institute, 86*(18), 1403–1408.

Butler, J.T. (1982). Early adolescent alcohol consumption and self-concept, social class and knowledge of alcohol. *Journal of Studies on Alcohol, 43*(5), 603–607.

Centers for Disease Control and Prevention. (1995). CDC surveillance summaries, March 24, 1995. *Morbidity and Mortality Weekly Report, 44*(No. SS-1), 4.

Centers for Disease Control and Prevention. (1996a). CDC surveillance summaries. *Morbidity and Mortality Weekly Report, 45*(No. SS-4), 16–19.

Centers for Disease Control and Prevention. (1996b). *1995 national household survey on drug abuse, tobacco related statistics, SAMHSA, August 1996* [On-line]. Available: http://cdc.gov.nccdphp/osh/samhsa.htm

Centers for Disease Control and Prevention. (1997). *Preventing tobacco use and addiction.* Atlanta, GA.

Centers for Disease Control and Prevention. (1998a). *1997 Youth risk behavior surveillance system (YRBSS): Summary* [On-line]. Available: http://cdc.gov/nccdphp/dash/yrbs/natsum97/sual97.htm

Centers for Disease Control and Prevention. (1998b). *1997 Youth risk behavior surveillance system (YRBSS): Summary* [On-line]. Available: http://cdc.gov/nccdphp/dash/yrbs/natsum97/suto97.htm

Centers for Disease Control and Prevention. (1999). National vaccination coverage levels among children aged 18–35 months—United States, 1998. *Morbidity and Mortality Weekly Report, 48*(37), 829–830.

Children's Defense Fund. (2000). *The state of America's children yearbook: 2000.* Washington, DC.

Colditz, G.A., Cannuscio, C.C., & Frazier, A.L. (1997). Physical activity and reduced risk of colon cancer: Implications for prevention. *Cancer Causes and Control, 8,* 649–667.

Consumers Union. (1998). *Hidden from view: The growing burden of health care costs* [On-line]. Available: http://igc.org/consunion/health/0122exec.htm

Diaz, D.P. (1993). Foundations of spirituality: Establishing the viability of spirituality within the health disciplines. *Journal of Health Education, 24*(6), 324–326.

Dolfman, M.L. (1973). The concept of health: An historic and analytic examination. *Journal of School Health, 43*(8), 491–497.

Donatelle, R.J., & Davis, L.G. (1998). *Access to health* (5th ed.). Boston: Allyn & Bacon.

Donovan, J., Jessor, R., & Costa, F.M. (1988). Syndrome of problem behavior in adolescence: A replication. *Journal of Consulting and Clinical Psychology, 56*(5), 762–765.

Dubos, R. (1965). *Man adapting.* New Haven, CT: Yale University Press.

Dubos, R. (1968). *So human an animal.* New York: Charles Scribner's.

Dunn, H. (1967). *High level wellness.* Arlington, VA: R.W. Beatty.

Friedman, M., & Rosenman, R.H. (1974). *Type A behavior and your heart.* Greenwich, CT: Fawcett.

Goodstadt, M.S., Simpson, R.I., & Loranger, P.O. (1987). Health promotion: A conceptual integration. *American Journal of Health Promotion, 1*(3), 158–165.

Gore, S. (1978). The effect of social support in moderating health. *Journal of Personality and Social Behavior, 19*(1), 157–165.

Hawks, S. (1994). Spiritual health: Definition and theory. *Wellness Perspectives: Research, Theory, and Practice, 10*(4), 3–13.

Health Care Financing Administration, U.S. Department of Health and Human Services. (1999). *National health expenditures projections: 1998–2008* [On-line]. Available: http://www.hcfa.gov/stats/NHE-Proj1998/hilites.htm

Helmrich, S.P., Ragland, D.R., Leung, R.W., & Paffenbarger Jr., R.S. (1991). Physical activity and reduced occurrence of noninsulin-dependent diabetes mellitus. *New England Journal of Medicine, 325*(3), 147–152.

House, J., Landis, K., & Umberson, D. (1988). Social relationships and health. *Science, 241*(4865), 540–545.

Hoyman, H. (1975). Rethinking an ecologic system model of man's health, disease, aging, death. *Journal of School Health, 45*(9), 509–518.

Insel, P.M., & Roth, W.T. (2000). *Core concepts in health* (8th ed.). Mountain View, CA: Mayfield.

Joint Committee on Health Education Standards. (1995). *National health education standards: Achieving health literacy.* Atlanta: American Cancer Society.

Kann, L., Collins, J.L., Pateman, B.C., Small, M.L., Russ, J.G., & Kolbe, L.J. (1995). The school health policies and programs study (SHPPS): Rationale for a nationwide status report on school health programs. *Journal of School Health, 65*(8), 291–294.

Kaplan, G., Salonen, J., Cohen, R., Cohen, R.J., Brand, R.J., Syme, S.L., & Pusker, P. (1988). Social connections and mortality from all causes and from cardiovascular disease: Prospective evidence from Eastern Finland. *American Journal of Epidemiology, 128*(2), 370–380.

Kobasa, S.C. (1979). Stressful life events, personality, and health: An inquiry into hardiness. *Journal of Personality and Social Psychology, 37*(1), 1–11.

Kolbe, L.J. (1993). Developing a plan of action to institutionalize comprehensive school health education programs in the United States. *Journal of School Health, 63*(1), 12–13.

Lalonde, M.A (1974). *New perspective on the health of Canadians.* Ottawa: Information Canada.

Levy, M.R., Dignan, M., & Shirreffs, J.H. (1992). *Life and health: Targeting wellness.* New York: McGraw-Hill.

Marmot, M.G., Kogevinas, M., & Elston, M.A. (1987). Social economic status and disease. *Annual Review of Public Health, 8*, 111–135.

Maslow, A.H. (1968). *Toward a psychology of being* (2d ed.). Princeton, NJ: Van Nostrand Reinhold.

McGinnis, J.M. & Foege, W.H. (1993). Actual causes of death in the United States. *Journal of the American Medical Association, 270*(18), 2207–2212.

Meeks, L., Heit, P., & Page, R. (1996). *Comprehensive school health education: Totally awesome strategies for teaching health* (2d ed.). Blacklick, OH: Meeks Heit.

Moore, K.A., Sugland, B.W., Blumenthal, C., Glei, D., & Snyder, N. (1995). *Adolescent pregnancy prevention programs: Interventions and evaluations.* Washington, DC: Child Trends.

Moss, G.M. (1973). *Illness, immunity and social interaction.* New York: John Wiley.

National Center for Health Statistics, Centers for Disease Control and Prevention. (1999). *Latest final mortality statistics available* [On-line]. Available: http://www.cdc.gov/nchswww/releases/99facts/99sheets/97mortal.htm

National Institute for Healthcare Research. (1999). *Spirituality and health: What's the connection? NIHR media fact sheet* [On-line]. Available: http://nihr.org/media2/mediafactsheet.html

National Institutes of Health Consensus Development Panel on Physical Activity and Cardiovascular Health. (1996). Physical activity and cardiovascular health. *Journal of the American Medical Association, 276*(3), 241–246.

National Research Council. (1995). *Measuring poverty: A new approach.* Washington, DC.

Nieman, D.C. (1994). Exercise, upper respiratory infection, and the immune system. *Medicine and Science in Sports and Medicine, 26*(2), 128–139.

1990 Joint Committee on Health Education Terminology. (1991). Report of the 1990 Joint Committee on Health Education Terminology. *Journal of Health Education, 22*(2), 97–108.

Noack, H. (1987). Concepts of health and health promotion. In T. Abeline, Z.J. Brzezinski, & V.D.L. Carstairs (Eds.), *Measurement in health promotion and protection.* Geneva, Switzerland: World Health Organization.

Oberteuffer, D. (1960). *School health education: A textbook for teachers, nurses, and other professional personnel.* New York: Harper and Brothers.

Ornstein, R., & Sobel, D. (1987). *The healing brain: A new perspective on the brain and health.* New York: Simon & Schuster.

Osman, J., & Russell, R. (1979). The spiritual aspects of health. *Journal of School Health, 49*(6), 359.

Paffenbarger Jr., R.S., Hyde, R.T., Wing, A.L., Lee, I-M., & Kampert, J.B. (1994). Some interrelations of physical activity, physiological fitness, health, and longevity. In C. Bouchard, R.J. Shephard, & T. Stephens (Eds.), *Physical activity, fitness, and health: International proceedings and consensus statement.* Champaign, IL: Human Kinetics.

Pappas, G.P., Golin, S., & Meyer, D.L. (1990). Reducing symptoms of depression with exercise. *Psychosomatics, 31*(1), 112–113.

Payne, W.A., & Hahn, D.B. (1998). *Understanding your health* (5th ed.). Boston: WCB McGraw-Hill.

Pilch, J.J. (1988). Wellness spirituality. *Health Values, 12*(3), 28–31.

Resnicow, K., Ross, D., & Vaughn, R. (1995). The structure of problem and conventional behaviors in African American youth. *Journal of Clinical and Consulting Psychology, 63*(4), 594–603.

Richardson, G.E., & Nolan, M.P. (1984). Treating the spiritual dimension through educational imagery. *Health Values, 8*(6), 25–30.

Rosenman, R. H., & Friedman, M. (1966). Coronary heart disease in Western collaborative group study. *Journal of the American Medical Association, 195*(2), 86–92.

Sliepcevich, E.M. (1967). Health education: A conceptual approach to curriculum design. In E.M. Sliepcevich. *School health education study.* St. Paul: 3M Education Press.

Seaward, B.L. (1991). Spiritual wellbeing: A health education model. *Journal of Health Education, 22*(3), 166–169.

Shirreffs, J. (1984). The nature and meaning of health education. In L. Rubinson & W.F. Alles (Eds.), *Health education: Foundations for the future.* Prospect Heights, IL: Waveland.

Smith, J.A. (1983). *The idea of health: Implications for the nursing profession.* New York: Teachers College.

Squires, S. (1987). The power of positive imagery: Visions to boost immunity. *American Health, 6*(6), 56–61.

Terris, M. (1975). Approach to an epidemiology of health. *American Journal of Public Health, 65* (10), 1037–1041.

Terris, M. (1990). Public health policy for the 1990s. *Annual Review of Public Health, 11*, 39–51.

Thune, I., Brenn, T., Lund, E., & Gaard, M. (1997). Physical activity and the risk of breast cancer. *New England Journal of Medicine, 336*(18), 1269–1275.

U.S. Bureau of the Census. (1999). *Health insurance coverage—1997* [On-line]. Available: http://www.census.gov/hhes/hlthins/hlthin97/hi97t2.html

U.S. Bureau of the Census. (1999). *Health insurance coverage: 1998* [On-line]. Available: http://census.gov/hhes/hlthins/hlthin97/hi97t2.html

U.S. Department of Health and Human Services. (1996). *Physical activity and health: A report to the Surgeon General.* Atlanta: Department of Health and Human Services, Centers for Disease Control and Prevention, National Center for Chronic Disease Prevention and Health Promotion.

U.S. Department of Health and Human Services. (2000). *Healthy people 2010* (Conference ed.). Washington, DC.

U.S. Department of Health, Education and Welfare. (1979). *Healthy people: The Surgeon General's report on health promotion and disease prevention* (Publication No. 79-55071). Washington, DC: U.S. Public Health Service.

U.S. Office of Alternative Medicine, National Institutes of Health. (1994). *Alternative medicine: Expanding medical horizons. A report to the National Institutes of Health on alternative medical systems and practices in the U.S.* Washington, DC.

Ventura, S.F., Anderson, R.N., Martin, J.A., & Smith, B.L. (1998). *Births and deaths: Preliminary data for 1997.* National Vital Statistics Reports. Hyattsville, MD: National Center for Health Statistics.

World Health Organization. (1947). Constitution of the World Health Organization. *Chronicle of the World Health Organization, 1.* Geneva, Switzerland.

# Health Promotion

## WHAT IS HEALTH PROMOTION?

Health promotion is a broad field encompassing educational, social, economic, and political efforts to improve the health of a population. Health education, **health protection**, and disease prevention form the essential triad of health promotion. Health promotion is practiced in a variety of settings—schools, churches, worksites, health care facilities, voluntary health agencies, health maintenance organizations, correctional institutions, private clubs, and self-help groups—by practitioners of varied backgrounds and occupations—physicians, nurses, exercise scientists, nutritionists, social workers, physical therapists, and health educators. Health promotion workers put health on the agenda of policy makers, directing them to be aware of the health consequences of their decisions and to accept their responsibilities for public health (Monash Health Promotion Unit, 1999). It has unified a number of separate, even disparate, fields of study under one umbrella and now forms an important part of the health services of most industrially developed countries (Macdonald & Bunton, 1992). *Healthy People 2000* (U.S. Department of Health and Human Services, 1991), a publication that guided the nation's health promotion efforts for nearly a decade, contained the words, "Health promotion and disease prevention comprise perhaps our best opportunity to reduce the ever-increasing portion of our resources which we spend to treat preventable illness and functional impairment."

Two of the most commonly quoted definitions of health promotion are

> A planned combination of educational, political, regulatory, and organizational supports for actions and conditions of living conducive to the health of individuals, groups, or communities (Green & Kreuter, 1999).

> The process of enabling people to increase control over and to improve their health . . . a commitment to dealing with the challenges of reducing inequities, extending the scope of prevention, and helping people to cope with their circumstances . . . creating environments conducive to health, in which people are better able to take care of themselves (World Health Organization, 1986).

The definitions imply a broad spectrum of interventions. Health promotion attempts to promote adaptations and adjustments in individuals and communities to encourage maintenance and improvement of the health of whole populations, usually by applying wellness principles to organizations and institutions. These adaptations and adjustments may be attitudinal, environmental, or behavioral, but all are directed toward sustaining or increasing the level of well-being, self-actualization,

**health protection**   legal or fiscal controls, other regulations and policies, and voluntary codes of practice aimed at the enhancement of health and the prevention of illness

and fulfillment (Teague & McGhee, 1992). It is also appropriate for health promotion to function on an economic level, given that larger gaps between the haves and have nots correlate strikingly with increased mortality rates among the have nots. The gap between rich and poor children is greater in the United States than in any other industrialized country (Seffrin, 1997)—one reason that reducing health disparities has become a national goal (U.S. Department of Health and Human Services, 2000).

The Working Group on Concepts and Principles in Health Promotion (1987) listed the basic characteristics of health promotion as

1. Enabling people to take control over, and responsibility for, their health as an important component of everyday life—both as spontaneous and as organized action for health

2. Requiring the close cooperation of sectors beyond the health services, reflecting the diversity of conditions that influence health

3. Combining diverse, but complementary, methods or approaches, including communication, education, legislation, fiscal measures, organizational changes, community development, and spontaneous local activities against health hazards

4. Encouraging effective and concrete public participation, encompassing the development of individual and collective problem-solving and decision-making skills and involving health professionals in education and health advocacy, particularly those in primary care

Health promotion is arena-based in the sense that it seeks to deal with whole populations and their needs and strengths. Health promotion is less effective when it attempts to lessen the effects of a specific disease or condition. Rather than take the "disease of the month" approach, health promoters seek to improve health by improving the overall condition of the target population.

## THE TRIAD OF HEALTH PROMOTION

The three facets of health promotion are prevention, health education, and health protection. Each

plays a vital role in the achievement of individual and community health, but none is independent of the others.

## Prevention

Prevention contributes mightily to health promotion, and the aspiring health education/promotion professional needs a clear understanding of its practice. Prevention occurs on three levels—primary, secondary, and tertiary. Each has different implications for health promoters/educators, and each requires a different set of objectives and interventions.

### Primary Prevention
**Primary prevention** emphasizes interventions to avert disease, illness, injury, or deterioration of health before it occurs. It may include interventions to avoid an unwanted situation, including pregnancy. Strategies usually

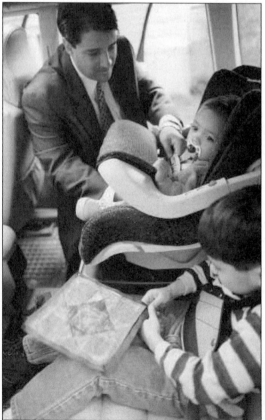

© 2000 PhotoDisc, Inc.

Using child restraint devices is primary prevention.

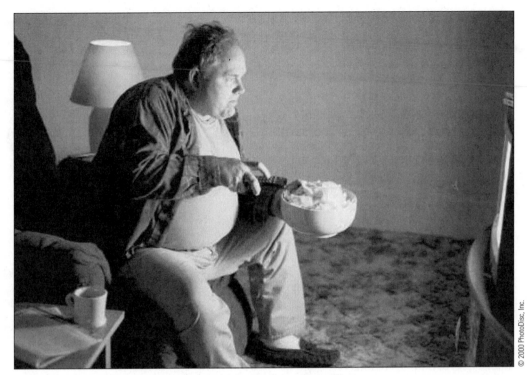

Lack of exercise, poor diet, and obesity are risk factors for health problems.

incorporate health promotion in medical, societal, and educational arenas. They also involve behaviors that decrease the probability of illness or injury by actively protecting the body against risks and stressors.

Medical examples of primary prevention—including scheduled immunizations, regular dental prophylaxis, and genetic screening—do exist. However, history reveals that medicine has concentrated its resources on diagnosis and treatment, thus relegating primary prevention to a subordinate position. Medicine's reputation has been built on its concentration on treatment at the expense of real preventive medicine. The medical care system offers some preventive services through its technology and medications, but it does little in primary prevention in comparison to the individual and the community.

Legislative interventions are found in laws requiring mandatory use of safety belts and child restraint devices in cars, prohibition of tobacco sales to minors, stipulations that food handlers undergo periodic tests for certain infectious diseases, and requirements that children be immunized before attending school. This illustrates an overlap with health protection.

Societal interventions are exemplified by provision of adequate housing and recreation, fluoridation of water, environmental sanitation, and vector surveillance and eradication. In addition, primary prevention embodies a societal principle that exhorts individuals to assume responsibility for the health of the community.

Educational examples include promoting skills that enable young people to cope with peer pressure; imparting knowledge of the relationships between weight control and heart disease; establishing nutrition programs based on a variety of healthy foods; and encouraging sexual abstinence or monogamous relationships to prevent transmission of sexually transmissible infections.

**primary prevention**   action taken to avert the occurrence of disease

The more directly a behavior is linked to a health problem as a risk factor, the better candidate it is for primary prevention efforts (Simons-Morton, Greene, & Gottlieb, 1995). For example, people who are overweight and smoke cigarettes run a greater risk of diseases of the cardiovascular system. These individuals are excellent candidates for primary prevention activities aimed at reducing these risk factors.

Individual primary prevention efforts against major health threats are familiar to most people. Cardiovascular disease is the leading recorded cause of death in the United States. Individuals can decide to lower their risk of cardiovascular disease by not smoking, by eating nutritious foods with low saturated fat, by learning how to deal with stress, and by exercising regularly. The second leading recorded cause of death in the United States is cancer. People can reduce the risk of developing cancer by not smoking cigarettes, by adhering to a diet high in fiber and low in fat, and by avoiding excessive exposure to ultraviolet light. Anyone can practice primary prevention to reduce the risk of accidental injury or death: People can wear safety belts and shoulder harnesses each time they ride in a motor vehicle, forgo alcohol when driving an automobile, wear safety equipment when working with machinery, and avoid three-wheeled, all-terrain vehicles. Health education and health promotion have played an important role in establishing these practices.

## Secondary Prevention

**Secondary prevention is** identifying diseases at their earliest stages and applying treatments to limit the consequences, severity, and prevalence of the disease. Secondary prevention thus entails early detection and treatment; it is curative. Medicine has long focused much of its resources on secondary prevention, which attempts to limit the course and destruction of conditions that already have occurred.

Medical examples of secondary prevention are numerous. Women are encouraged to have regular mammograms to detect breast cancer and Pap tests to detect cervical cancer while they are treatable. Men are advised to examine their testicles regularly to expedite treatment of testicular cancer by its early detection. People with high blood pressure are

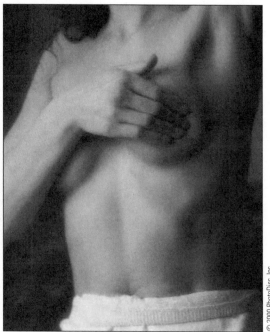

© 2000 PhotoDisc, Inc.

Breast self-examination is an excellent example of secondary prevention against breast cancer.

advised to take their medication as prescribed. Doctors advise checking our cholesterol level periodically and using diet and exercise to reduce high cholesterol levels. When dealing with infectious diseases, mass case-finding measures (surveillance efforts that locate cases) also can be employed as secondary prevention. When cases are detected, secondary prevention can include early treatment to interrupt the disease process and to prevent the further transmission of the disease.

The health educator, or frequently the patient educator, has a crucial role in secondary prevention. Education may be the key to motivating people to schedule mammograms or do testicular self-examination. Effective educators often spell the difference between minor consequences of a health problem and its development into a debilitating or life-threatening occurrence.

Schools sometimes are agents of secondary prevention. For instance, pupils are inspected regularly for the telltale nits that signal the presence of head lice. Another example is the periodic vision screening of school children that most states require.

Unfortunately, the medical community, insurers, and most individuals have relied too heavily upon secondary prevention. Preventing the onset of a disease is obviously more cost-effective than treating it. Gradually, Americans are beginning to realize that primary prevention is more desirable than secondary prevention. This climate offers opportunities to develop comprehensive health education programs in the schools and broad programs of primary prevention at other sites.

### Tertiary Prevention

**Tertiary prevention** prescribes specific interventions to help people with disabilities or diseases limit the effects of those conditions. Tertiary prevention also may include activities to prevent recurrence of a disease.

This level of prevention relies heavily upon the medical care system. Rehabilitation services and physical and occupational therapy are crucial components of tertiary prevention. It may also include surgery, administering medications, or counseling in lifestyle changes (for example, for patients recovering from cardiac events).

Patient education plays an important role in tertiary prevention. Clients can be trained and educated after surgery to take actions to reduce negative effects. Those diagnosed with diabetes may learn to monitor their conditions and take corrective actions. Too often, patients fail to follow through on their physicians' recommendations—one of the main reasons for relapses. Thorough patient education can help patients understand why making lifestyle changes or following a consistent program of rehabilitation is beneficial and can help them keep track of their own compliance and progress. Tertiary prevention also may involve educating the public and industry to use rehabilitated persons to the fullest possible extent.

Although we have relied heavily on secondary prevention, the high cost of treatment has resulted in the majority of resources of the health care delivery system being directed toward tertiary prevention. Through redefinition of priorities and development of more effective health promotion programs, a shift in resources to primary and secondary prevention could reduce the need for much treatment and rehabilitation now practiced. Every provider-client encounter has the potential to provide multiple

levels of prevention. If this potential is developed, the health care professional becomes a health promotion agent.

Potter and Perry (1993) neatly summed up the three main purposes of health promotion/education in terms applicable to the three levels of prevention: promotion of health and illness prevention, restoration of health when one becomes ill, and maintenance of health while coping with chronic, long-term conditions.

Both humanitarianism and cost-effectiveness suggest that a better approach is to enhance and preserve the health of individuals rather than wait and treat disease and injury. Herein lies a major role for health promoters, who must aim for more than just the "absence of disease or infirmity" mentioned in the World Health Organization definition of health (see page 2). They must aim for overall improvement in wellness of the individual and community. Adequately prepared professionals have an important role in achieving this end at all three levels of prevention.

## Role of Health Education

An integral piece of a total health promotion program, health education

— is a planned process,

— usually combines a variety of educational experiences, and

— facilitates voluntary adaptations or establishment of behavior conducive to health.

Figure 2.1 depicts it at the core of the health promotion environment. It can play an important role in all three levels of disease and injury prevention, often reminding clients of the reasons for their participation and pursuit of behavior change. The

---

**secondary prevention**   action taken to identify diseases at their earliest stages and to apply appropriate treatments to limit their consequences and severity

**tertiary prevention**   specific interventions to assist diseased or disabled persons in limiting the effects of their diseases or disabilities; also may include activities to prevent recurrence of a disease

## Figure 2.1    Health Education and Environmental Components of Health Promotion

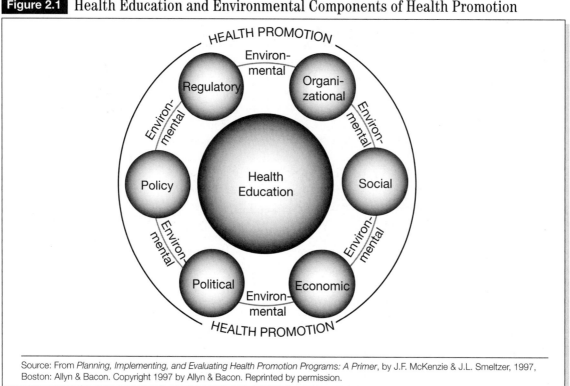

distinction between health promotion and health education is described by Sharkey and associates (1995) as one of ethics. Health promoters advance a position; they promote a point of view, often a paternalistic one. Health educators provide information, often value-laden, that helps clients understand all the relevant alternatives—and their implications and consequences—in an effort to encourage voluntary behavior choices. They also help people to acquire the skills necessary to carry out their chosen behaviors. Green and Kreuter (1999) stated that

> health education aims primarily at the voluntary actions people can take on their own part, individually or collectively, for their own health or the health of others and the common good of the community. Health promotion encompasses health education . . . and is aimed at the complementary social and political actions that will facilitate the necessary organizational, economic, and other environmental supports for the conversion of individual actions into health enhancements and quality-of-life gains.

The distinction clarifies that health education is considered one of the mechanisms of health promotion. (We will examine the nature of health education in detail in Chapter 3.)

Whereas other professions are involved in health promotion, health education is the only profession specifically devoted to health promotion and whose practitioners are trained in a range of health promotion change processes (Simons-Morton, Greene, & Gottlieb, 1995). The health educator has the skills to help clients develop attainable objectives and organize activities around those objectives. More and more, the health educator, in the role of health promoter, must also assume a broader perspective on how we help to shape not only individuals' lifestyles but also to foster change within institutions and communities. In this broader context, Labonte (1986) would have us ask ourselves

> How can we, as health educators, inspire the changes necessary to ensure that health in its broadest sense becomes a

central concern of all political, economic and personal decisions? How can we, as health educators, cooperate with the many groups lobbying for these changes to occur? Most poignantly, how can we, as health educators, assist in empowering those people in society—the poor, the unemployed, the economically marginal or exploited whose social situation places them at highest risk of disease and premature death?

Many health promotion interventions at the community, state or provincial, or national level are legal, regulatory, political, or economic. These include health protection measures such as fines for illegal dumping, penalties for school districts that allow children who are not immunized to attend, increased insurance premiums for people who routinely engage in high-risk behaviors, laws restricting placement of bars and liquor stores near schools and churches, and requiring that billboards advertising tobacco be a certain distance from schools. These are necessarily coercive in nature. Nevertheless, as Green and Ottoson (1999) pointed out, such interventions to be successful must be supported by consent from an informed public. Informed consent requires health education. These coercive measures may be directed at people whose actions may affect the health of others, such as manufacturers, distributors, and advertisers of hazardous products. Health education can help develop action groups to apply pressure to other targets of coercive interventions, including schools, government officials, law enforcement, or commercial interests. This illustrates the relationship of health education to health protection.

Our society may not be ready or able to attempt the broad changes implied in Labonte's query. Considering the realities of social conditions, economic inequities, and political whim, this is a daunting task. The future of Medicare is in doubt, the price of treating illness continues to escalate, and the reformation of the health care delivery system is perpetually on hold, despite years of political wrangling. Although these forces are discouraging, they offer added opportunities for our profession to promote wellness for social and economic reasons.

Many determinants affect an individual's decisions regarding health practices. Knowledge, self-concept, religious beliefs, peer pressure, educational level, economic conditions, cultural variables, personal values, and family models are some of these factors. The role of the health educator—in concert with other members of the health promotion team—is to identify factors that affect the individual's personal characteristics, environment, and behavior and plan a program that will elicit change that is conducive to a high level of health.

Health educators need expertise in many different forms of communication and insight into which medium to use in each situation. The range of problems, the levels of prevention, the size of the client group (from one to thousands), and the sensitivity of the issue demand sensible choices in methods and approaches, from one-on-one dialogue to advertising on highway billboards to Internet courses.

Frequently, health educators assist health care providers in planning the delivery of services. Health care providers may need to be informed about the community, how individuals feel about health, or certain practices and treatments. For instance, Amish women are not likely to take routine secondary prevention measures such as mammography, Pap smears, and breast self-examination because they are not comfortable displaying their bodies. Many African Americans distrust the medical system because of past maltreatment. Elderly persons may fear new technology. Native Americans, including Native Alaskans, may prefer traditional remedies, regardless of their lack of scientific efficacy. Health educators can often serve as the liaison between community members and the provider to resolve such conflicts.

Health educators facilitate, coordinate, or carry out evaluation of behavioral determinants; assist people in their own self-care; and evaluate possible alternative actions. These tasks require the health educator's knowledge of behaviors that affect health and of what determines behavior plus the skills to assist individuals in taking control of their own lives and actions. To put this knowledge and skill to work, the health educator implements strategies dealing with any feature of health-related behavior. He or she then must be able to evaluate effectiveness of the strategy, including its planning and implementation, in an unbiased way.

On the more global level, "to create social and health conditions that are premised on health promotion and which allow all the world's citizens to achieve a state of health" (Labonte, 1986), the health educator may be involved in programs that publicize the role of social and economic inequalities in health issues. Beyond educating individuals about their own health, professionals may educate the media, elected officials, and community leaders via relentless advocacy for healthier environments. Health educators may contribute by encouraging community participation and involvement in decision making, which may include promoting environments that reinforce social support, community development, mutual assistance, and collective and intersectoral cooperation.

## Health Protection

"Health protection comprises legal or fiscal controls, other regulations and policies, and voluntary codes of practice, aimed at the enhancement of positive health and the prevention of ill-health" (Downie, Tannahill, & Tannahill, 1996). With origins in the old regulatory public health measures, current health protection focuses on the political, legislative, and social parts of the environment—often controlling the physical portion. Its mission is to reduce the likelihood that people will encounter environmental hazards or behave in unsafe or unhealthy ways. Health protection makes healthy choices easier.

Legislation mandating the use of seat belts in automobiles, restricting the sale of alcohol to minors, decreeing that school children be vaccinated, and holding employers responsible for the physical safety of the workplace are examples of legal protections. Increasing the tax on cigarettes to reduce use by minors is an example of using fiscal control as a form of health protection. Policies and regulations such as those imposed by an employer to require drug testing or to forbid smoking in the workplace are also protective of health.

However, barriers to health protection are abundant. Greed may be at the heart of much opposition. Many people feel that certain video games or the manufacture of candy cigarettes provide opportunities for children to practice unhealthy behaviors. Yet, because of the popularity and profit

associated with these products, only weak, voluntary steps are taken to control their use. In some cases, the enormous power of vested interests exerts influence over public policy.

Lobbying and political contributions from big business have frequently worked against pro-health policies and legislation. A notable example is the tobacco industry's efforts to reduce appropriations for anti-tobacco education and block increased taxation on tobacco products in state government and the Congress.

## Relationships Among the Triad

The triad—prevention, health education, and health protection—should be viewed as interlocking spheres of activity. Tannahill (1985) depicted the three spheres and the seven domains of each as shown in Figure 2.2.

The seven domains (numbered in the figure) are as follows:

1. Prevention: This domain includes primary preventive measures, such as immunization and exercise programs, and secondary preventive measures, such as Pap smears, hypertension case-finding, and smoking cessation programs.

2. Lifestyle: This includes educational efforts to influence lifestyle to prevent health-related problems and to encourage the uptake of preventive services.

3. Preventive policies: This sphere represents preventive health protection, including fluoridation of public water supplies and inspections of restaurants. It can be viewed as a policy commitment to the provision of preventive services such as those described under domain 1.

4. Policy maker education: Given that health protection measures do not emerge spontaneously, education of policy makers is important. An example of this is the lobbying by safety-conscious groups to encourage mandated use of automobile seat belts in the face of much public apathy. Efforts to stimulate a social environment that demands or accepts preventive health protection measures are also part of this domain (Downie, Tannahill, & Tannahill, 1996), as

is a policy commitment to preventive health education.

5. Health education: This domain comprises all aspects of positive health education, including influencing behavior by helping individuals, groups, or whole communities develop positive health attributes, such as life skills and self-esteem.

6. Health protection: This domain includes implementation of a workplace policy forbidding smoking, graduated drivers' licenses, and commitment of public funds to provide safe walking areas and bicycle paths.

7. Policy support: This domain embraces raising awareness of, and securing support for, positive health protection measures among the public and policy makers. It includes a policy commitment to positive health.

# FRAMEWORK FOR HEALTH PROMOTION

The World Health Organization (1984) stated that health promotion represents "a mediating strategy between people and their environments, synthesizing personal choice and social responsibility in health." Building upon the Lalonde Report—a pioneering document in the health promotion field published in 1974 (see page 40)—and incorporating the 1984 WHO document, the Canadian government developed and implemented a framework for health promotion that has come to be known as "the Epp Report" (Epp, 1986). The framework, presented in Figure 2.3, delineated three levels of concern and action: health challenges, health promotion mechanisms, and implementation strategies.

The Epp Report framework explores the complex biopsychosocial processes that motivate

**Figure 2.2**  The Triad of Health Promotion

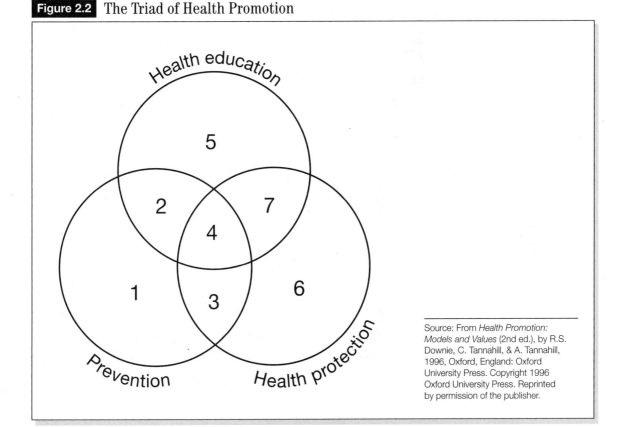

Source: From *Health Promotion: Models and Values* (2nd ed.), by R.S. Downie, C. Tannahill, & A. Tannahill, 1996, Oxford, England: Oxford University Press. Copyright 1996 Oxford University Press. Reprinted by permission of the publisher.

individuals to engage in health-enhancing behaviors. It makes three points that are particularly noteworthy: First, it uses the protection-education-prevention triad throughout the framework. Second, the report states that the most important challenge for health promotion is reducing health inequities between low- and high-income populations. Third,

it emphasizes large-scale institutional or environmental change.

## Health Inequities

In the U. S. and Canada, discrepancies, major health problems, frequently presented by contrasting rates

**Figure 2.3**  A Framework for Health Promotion

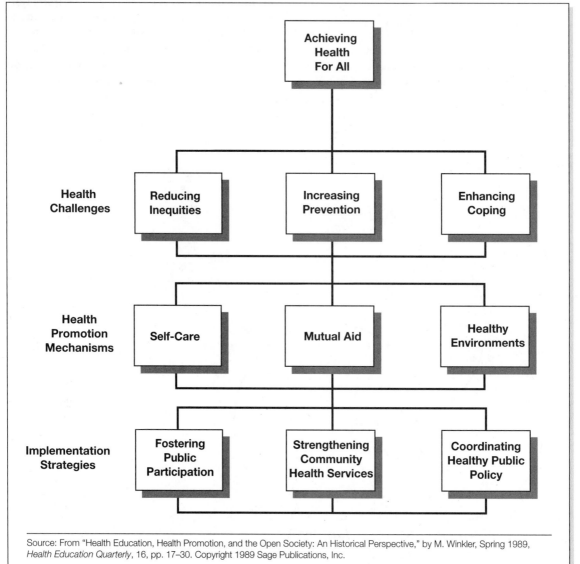

Source: From "Health Education, Health Promotion, and the Open Society: An Historical Perspective," by M. Winkler, Spring 1989, *Health Education Quarterly*, 16, pp. 17–30. Copyright 1989 Sage Publications, Inc.

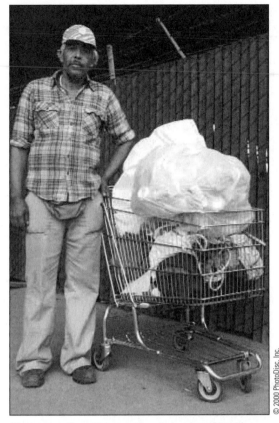

The poor suffer a disproportionate burden of health problems.

among ethnic groups, are more likely a result of poverty than ethnicity. In its *Kids Count Data Book,* the Annie E. Casey Foundation (1999) stated the following:

> The percent of children in poverty is perhaps the most global and widely used indicator of child well-being. This is due, in part, to the fact that poverty is closely linked to a number of undesirable outcomes in areas such as health, education, emotional well-being, and delinquency.

In addition, the World Health Organization (2000) reported that some groups in the United States—such as Native Americans, rural African Americans, and the inner-city poor—have extremely low levels of health more characteristic of a poor developing country than a rich industrialized one. In the Epp Report, the challenge of reducing inequities was presented more in terms of societal responsibility than of individual responsibility. Recent analyses (Iannantuono & Eyles, 1997) of the Epp Report also demonstrated its attention to broad health determinants and a more cost containment–oriented health care delivery system. Therefore, the attack on health inequities will utilize cost-saving strategies directed toward the far-reaching factors that produce the inequities. These strategies include primary and secondary prevention, fostering public participation, and strengthening services within communities.

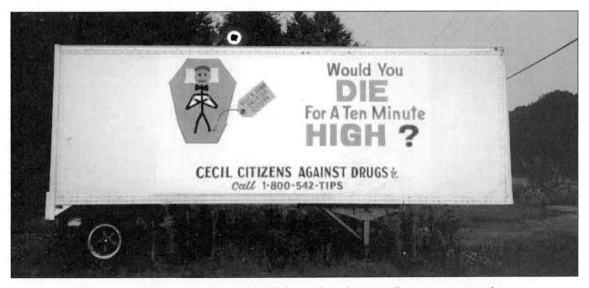

Would You **DIE** For A Ten Minute **HIGH?**

CECIL CITIZENS AGAINST DRUGS
Call 1-800-542-TIPS

Citizen groups often organize to target health issues through community awareness campaigns.

# Large-Scale Change

The Epp Report's emphasis on sweeping institutional or environmental change suggests many possibilities: For example, when a government promotes self-care by encouraging smoking cessation, it can also promote healthy environments by changing policies on tobacco marketing and advertising, restricting access to tobacco products to minors, and requiring smoke-free workplaces. Fiscal/ecological strategies also could include safety belt and bicycle helmet legislation, alcohol and tobacco legislation, and ecological and environmental measures. A number of options are available for institutional and community implementation strategies—many of them are listed in Box 2.1. As Sigerist (1946) wrote more than a half century ago:

> Health is promoted by providing a decent standard of living, good labor conditions, education, physical culture, means of rest and recreation. The coordinated efforts of large groups are needed to this end, of the statesman, labor, industry, of the educator and of the physician.

## Box 2.1    Examples of Health Promotion Strategies

**Educational interventions**

- stress management classes for middle-management employees in a corporation
- mailouts to the public describing positive steps a person can take to reduce exposure to HIV
- educational programs designed to reduce personal vulnerability to crime
- classes for elementary school children to develop the skills to cope with peer pressure

**Organizational interventions**

- annual hearing and vision screening in schools
- automobile, bicycle, and firearm safety programs conducted by law enforcement agencies
- identification of designated smoking areas and development of a smoking policy in a worksite
- official recognition by business management of alcoholism as a disease and not a weakness in character
- development of support groups by nonprofit organizations and health care facilities that provide services to people with epilepsy, muscular dystrophy, cancer, and other chronic diseases and disorders

**Political/legislative interventions**

- passage of laws requiring use of helmets while riding motorcycles and bicycles
- a requirement by the state Board of Education to implement a comprehensive family life curriculum in grades K–12 or a science-based drug prevention curriculum
- legislation requiring environmental polluters to measure their pollution and implement effective plans to reduce the pollution

- regulations requiring agencies and companies to monitor air pollution and governmental actions to reduce it
- regulations aimed at reducing youth access to tobacco products and alcohol
- a requirement that sports venues provide a smoke- and alcohol-free section

**Community and social interventions**

- organization and training of college students to reduce vulnerability to sex crimes
- formation of neighborhood walking clubs
- fluoridation of the water supply
- creation of wellness centers in health maintenance organizations, hospitals, and colleges; employing health educators to encourage positive health behaviors through programs that appeal to the community
- establishment of a school health council made up of members of the community to encourage healthy lifestyles in children and a healthy environment in the school
- health fairs at shopping malls

**Economic interventions**

- tax incentives to landlords of low-income housing to encourage maintenance of property and reduction of pest infestation
- incentives from insurance companies to those who practice healthy lifestyles
- incentives from employers to employees who stay healthy and do not miss work

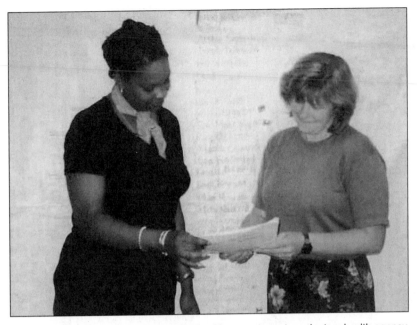

With lists of supporters and opponents, health promoters at a voluntary health agency plan strategy to pass tobacco control legislation.

Box 2.1 shows the breadth of activities that can be included under the mantle of health promotion. Consistent with the Framework for Health Promotion and analysis of the Epp Report, examples of interventions cover both the micro and macro levels.

## SPECIAL THEMES IN HEALTH PROMOTION

### Empowerment

Individuals' physical and emotional well-being are enhanced when their environments are personally controllable and predictable (Karasek & Thorell, 1990). The ecological perspective focuses on adjusting one's environment so that the individual and the community have control over variables that affect them; this is the substance of empowerment.

> In its broadest definition, empowerment is a multilevel construct that involves people assuming control and mastery over their lives in the context of their social and political environment; they gain a sense of control and purposefulness to exert political power as they participate in the democratic life of their community for social change (Wallerstein, 1992).

Embedded throughout the Framework for Health Promotion is the concept of empowerment. Reducing inequities; enhancing coping, self-care, and mutual aid; and fostering public participation are conspicuous examples of strategies that promote empowerment.

Power and control, or lack thereof, is a pivotal issue in the health of communities and, therefore, of individuals. When we have power, we can predict, control, and participate in our environment; when we do not, the environment in large measure controls us. Power enables groups to achieve equity. Poverty robs individuals of much control over their own lives and, subsequently, of power. There is a strong link between individuals' and communities' sense of power and the level of health they experience (Robertson & Minkler, 1994). Consequently, empowerment is a central component in the health promotion strategy.

The roots of empowerment are in community psychology, feminist theory, liberation theology, and social activism (Sheinfeld Gorin & Arnold, 1998). Empowerment theory is based on a conflict model that assumes that a society consists of separate groups possessing different levels of power and control over resources (Gutierrez, 1990). People who are impoverished and who lack education have little control over community resources and possess little power. Health promotion efforts are often aimed at assisting these groups to gain power and control over factors that affect their lives and health. They become able to take power and act effectively in transforming their lives and their environments.

Sheinfeld Gorin and Arnold (1998) wrote that the moral values underpinning the empowerment construct in health promotion are

— promoting human diversity (promoting respect and appreciation for diverse social entities)

— self-determination (promoting the ability of clients to pursue their chosen goals without excessive frustration and in consideration of other person's needs) for individuals and marginalized groups

These values can be implemented on personal, community organization, or political action levels. The strength of health promotion is its ability to foster environmental changes that promote diversity and protect the rights of individuals and groups to determine and follow their own course. Health promoters know that self-determination requires individual responsibility.

A major tenet of empowerment that is captured in the Framework for Health Promotion is the belief that individuals possess diverse self-care abilities. In order to practice self-care, individuals must feel in control and able to direct their own lives. These self-care abilities can be developed in individuals and groups and would reflect a commitment to personal responsibility for the health of self and community.

Bracht (1990) summed up the notion of empowerment leading to individual involvement by writing,

> The primary consideration in health promotion is not policy or education, but the ordinary people whose health is at stake. They should not just be "consulted" or "educated." They should be brought actively into the health enterprise in a significant way through the processes encompassed by the term "enabling."

On an individual level, empowerment includes the enhancement of the following three qualities:

**self-efficacy** the perception of having the skills required to accomplish tasks to affect one's own health

**hardiness** the perception of control over one's life and decisions, commitment to something worthwhile, and the capacity to view change as a challenge

**self-esteem** the perception of self-worth

When health education teaches necessary information and skills and healthy self-esteem, clients learn that control resides within them rather than in external forces. The client is then empowered to affect his or her own internal and external environments.

## Ecological Perspective

The ecological perspective of health promotion views health as a product of interdependence between the individual and the ecosystem, whose subsystems include family, culture, and physical and social environments. It attends to the social, institutional, and cultural contexts of human–environment and person–person relations. These primarily include political, economic, and social aspects but may also contain architectural, geographical, and technological features. The ecological perspective

> recognizes that health behaviors are part of the larger social system (or ecology) of behaviors and social influences, much like a river, forest or desert is part of a larger biological system (or ecosystem), and that lasting changes in health behaviors require supportive changes in the whole system, just as the addition of a power plant, the flooding of a reservoir, or the growth of a city in a desert produce changes in the whole ecosystem (O'Donnell, 1996).

The ecological perspective of health promotion is based upon the reciprocal relationship between individuals and their social environments. Behavior is affected by and affects multiple levels of influence (McLeroy et al., 1988). Health-related behaviors and conditions are influenced by intrapersonal or individual factors; interpersonal factors; institutional or organizational factors; community factors; and public factors. Thus, the causes of individual behaviors and conditions in the social environment are reciprocal, that is, the behavior of individuals influences and is influenced by the social environment (Stokols, 1992).

This key idea leads to the conclusion that, because intrapersonal, interpersonal, organizational, social, economic, and public policy factors are interrelated, programs that address one factor are likely to enhance outcomes in others. Green and Kreuter (1999) indicated that, to promote health, the ecosystem must offer economic and social conditions conducive to health and healthful lifestyles.

Many of these influences are addressed by health educators as they provide information and skills so individuals can reduce their health risk behaviors. For example, interpersonal factors are often addressed in education about conflict resolution, recognizing and resisting social pressures, refusal skills, and assertiveness skills.

The ecosystem must contain the resources for healthy choices. Healthful options among goods and services must be available. For example, tax incentives can encourage large supermarkets to locate in low-income neighborhoods so that residents have access to a wider selection of foods at lower prices. Similarly, providing sidewalks, lighting, and police protection encourages people to walk and, therefore, stimulates physical activity. This often requires health advocates to educate members of the political arena.

When addressing issues of health on a broad scale, health promotion workers need to recognize that human environments are complex systems. For example, safety and health in work settings involve many levels of interaction. Federal laws mandating certain environmental protections and personal actions, state and local ordinances aimed at protecting public health and environmental quality, risks inherent in certain occupations, management policies and concern for the welfare of workers, and individuals' relationships with one another form a framework for understanding the ecology of a work setting. Interventions may be strengthened by coordination of individuals and groups acting inside and outside of the actual worksite that may include individual workers, family members, corporate managers, members of the political system, and regulators.

Elbaz (1998), in describing the role of social movements as opportunities for education, noted that modern educators understand education as a process combining learners' experience, self-involvement, and scientific knowledge. Thus a health educator might help learners connect their own personal experiences with, for instance, an inequitable social structure. Ideally, learners' consciousness, broadened by such pedagogy, will translate into action and social change (Friere 1970; Giroux, 1994). In this way health education fulfills its role (number 5 in Figure 2.2) of fostering health promotion and helping communities become empowered.

## Community Organization

A community can be defined geographically or by shared interests or characteristics, such as ethnicity, sexual orientation, or occupation (Fellin, 1995). When a community of people come together, they can act politically and socially to make improvements. *The Ottawa Charter for Health Promotion* (World Health Organization, 1986) emphasized the role of community action with these words:

> Health promotion works through concrete and effective community action in setting priorities, making decisions, planning strategies and implementing them to achieve better health. At the heart of this process is the empowerment of communities, their ownership and control of their own endeavors and destinies.

Health promotion cultivates empowerment through community action.

**Community organization** is a multiphased process by which community groups are helped to produce change and develop their community. The first phase is identifying common problems or goals. Strict definitions of community organization suggest that the needs or problems around which community groups are organized must be identified by the community itself rather than by an outside change agent (Minkler & Wallerstein, 1997). The next phase is mobilizing resources, both

**community organization**   the process by which community groups identify common problems or goals, mobilize resources, and develop and implement strategies for reaching the goals they collectively have set

human and material, in the community to enhance self-help and social support. The final phase is developing and implementing strategies to reach collectively set goals. Community organization is very important in health promotion and health education because it reflects the fundamental principle of "starting where the people are."

Community organization can facilitate interventions that are organizational, political/legislative, economic, educational, or social. Examples include the civil rights movement, the women's movement, the gay rights movement, the antiwar movement during the Vietnam War, the AIDS awareness campaigns, and the New Right's campaign to ban abortions.

Coalitions among organizations, community groups, and interested community members have emerged as prominent contemporary strategies. Power is found in numbers. When groups share their expertise and skills, they multiply their influence and capabilities. Community coalitions have become astute in their understanding and use of the political process in its broadest sense—including judicial, legislative, and regulatory structures and processes—for change. They have provided creative means for the involvement and retention of consumers and citizens in political advocacy and service planning (Sheinfeld Gorin & Arnold, 1998). Examples of successful coalitions are those working in the areas of tobacco control, physical activity, and AIDS awareness.

As more people participate in community organizing, community empowerment outcomes can include increased sense of community; more effective participatory processes and greater community competence; and actual changes in policies, transformed conditions, or increased resources that may reduce inequities (Minkler & Wallerstein, 1997). Such social involvement and participation can improve perceived control, individual coping capacity, health behaviors, and health status (Cohen & Syme, 1985; Eng, Briscoe, & Cunningham, 1990). With increased psychological empowerment, individuals may develop increased political efficacy and motivation to act (Zimmerman, 1990) and enhanced social support. Empowered communities become more effective at collective problem solving, which may be reflected in key health and social indicators,

such as declining rates of teenage pregnancy, divorce, suicide, crime, and other social problems.

## Individual Behavior

Although authoritative documents, including the *Ottawa Charter for Health Promotion*, the *United Kingdom Charter for Health Promotion*, and the *Jakarta Declaration on Health Promotion into the 21st Century*, have emphasized the importance of social and economic factors in health, we must not ignore the personal lifestyle factor. The Lalonde Report (discussed on p. 40) and *Healthy People* recognized the role of individual behavior in health outcomes. This recognition has led to criticisms of "victim blaming" in some quarters, but it would be foolhardy to eliminate the goal of changing and establishing individual lifestyles from health promotion efforts. Indeed, lifestyle is responsible for much of the years lost prematurely in the more developed nations of the world. Most mortality in the United States is related to cigarette smoking, diet, and lack of physical activity.

The Division of Adult and Community Health —a part of the National Center for Chronic Disease Prevention and Health Promotion—administers the Behavioral Risk Factor Surveillance System, a questionnaire with which states collect data about adult health risk behavior. All states, the District of Columbia, and three territories participate in the BRFSS. Examples of results are presented in Box 2.2. Data presented are the medians of the means among the fifty states, the District of Columbia, and Puerto Rico.

Box 2.2 clearly shows that some groups and individuals are more at risk than others. In addition, evidence suggests that men have worse health habits than women. A report from the Centers for Disease Control and Prevention (2000) states that 25.3 percent of men and 21.1 percent of women are smokers; 61.9 percent of men and 74.8 percent of women always wear a seat belt; 22.3 percent of men and 6.7 percent of women are binge drinkers; and 5.4 percent of men and 0.8 percent of women are chronic drinkers. To mitigate vulnerability to low levels of health, health practitioners and legislators must broaden the design of health policy to address social and economic contexts of disease and correlates of risk-taking behaviors.

**Box 2.2**   Surveillance Data: Adults, United States, 1998

- 60.3 percent of whites, 49.8 percent of African Americans, and 53.1 percent of Hispanic Americans described their health as excellent or very good
- 11.9 percent of whites, 17.7 percent of African Americans, and 14.8 percent of Hispanic Americans described their health as fair or poor
- 36.2 percent of adults with incomes less than $15,000; 46.5 percent of adults with incomes $15,000–$24,999; 56.3 percent of adults with incomes $25,000–34,999; 64.7 percent of adults with incomes $35,000-49,999; and 72.9 percent of adults with incomes $50,000 or more described their health as excellent or very good
- 31.8 percent of adults with incomes less than $15,000; 19.8 percent of adults with incomes $15,000–24,999; 12.4 percent of adults with incomes $25,000–34,999; 8.0 percent of adults with incomes $35,000–49,999; and 4.8 percent of adults with incomes $50,000 or more described their health as fair or poor

- 28.6 percent of males and 43.0 percent of females were trying to lose weight at the time of the survey
- 59.2 percent of women had ever had a mammogram, including 60.7 percent of whites, 55.4 percent of African Americans, and 47.8 percent of Hispanic Americans
- 94.5 percent of women had ever had a Pap smear
- 81.0 percent of white women, 87.5 percent of African-American women, and 86.1 percent of Hispanic-American women had a Pap smear in the past two years
- 71.8 percent of women with incomes less than $15,000; 77.9 percent of women with incomes $15,000–24,999; 83.5 percent of women with incomes $25,000–34,999; 86.9 percent of women with incomes $35,000–49,999; and 89.5 percent of women with incomes $50,000 or more, had a Pap smear in the past 2 years

Source: From *Behavioral Risk Factor Surveillance System Online Prevalence Data, 1995–1998* [On-line], 1999, Division of Adult and Community Health, National Center for Chronic Disease Prevention and Health Promotion, Center for Disease Control and Prevention. Available: http://www2.cdc.gov/nccdphp/brfss/index.asp

Human behavior exists in and is influenced by a complicated set of social, economic, and cultural factors. Smoking is a good example of the result of one such complex web of causation. Most smokers begin the habit as teens or pre-teens. This happens for many reasons, but social influences—such as advertising, desire to demonstrate independence, parental models, and belief that a majority of peers smoke—play a major role in the onset of smoking. Economic status, ethnicity, and gender also appear to be related to beginning the habit. Certain factors such as high cost, effective education programs, and positive role models can reduce likelihood of smoking. Once a person has become a smoker, other factors may contribute to cessation or continuation. Factors encouraging cessation include increased cost, availability of cessation programs, inconvenience caused by people or policies that restrict smoking, family pleas, and health consequences. Addiction, social support, and the pleasure derived from smoking may discourage cessation. Although beginning or continuing to smoke is viewed as an individual choice, this example illustrates that choice is heavily influenced by a number of external and internal factors.

Health promotion—manifested by a variety of strategies—plays a role in reducing risk behaviors. However, behavior change, as noted above, is influenced by a cadre of factors, including variables present in the target group or individual. For example, one behavior that puts teens at great risk of death and injury is driving. Graduated licensing and restricted hours that inexperienced drivers may drive alone are political strategies that are strengthened by parental supervision. These strategies may require additional enforcement and education where cultural norms support underaged driving, such as in rural communities. Improving or expanding education courses is an educational intervention. Peer programs and public service announcements that condemn alcohol use, especially while driving, are social and environmental interventions. Thus, political, cultural, educational, social, and environmental interventions may be implemented to establish or change driving behaviors.

## Official Recognition

*New Perspectives on the Health of Canadians* (Lalonde, 1974)—also called "the Lalonde Report" —identified four factors that influence health: heredity, environment, health care services, and behavior. For several years following that report, health promotion activities emphasized individual behavior. The medical community focused primarily on delivering health care services. However, the Lalonde Report widened the focus from those individuals who appear for illness or injury treatment to the population at risk. Recognition of the role of broad environmental factors in influencing health was another significant contribution. In the United States, *Healthy People* (U.S. Department of Health, Education and Welfare, 1979), although emphasizing individual lifestyle and behavior in the role of development and maintenance of health, followed the lead of the Lalonde Report by addressing the role of environmental factors in individuals' health. Besides the United States and Canada, other countries—notably the Netherlands, Australia, the United Kingdom, and New Zealand—adopted a planning-by-objectives approach to health promotion and disease prevention. Currently, based on the growing evidence of the effect of living conditions and the role of poverty in the health of individuals and communities, health promotion has shifted more of its attention toward correcting environmental causes of health problems, including those associated with income inequity.

The recently expanded nature of health promotion was underscored in the *Ottawa Charter for Health Promotion* (World Health Organization, 1986), which listed the prerequisites for health as peace, shelter, education, food, income, a stable ecosystem, sustainable resources, social justice, and equity. This marked a shift away from proximal **risk factors**—such as poor nutrition, tobacco, and sedentary lifestyle—to what Green and Kreuter (1999) call **risk conditions**—more distant risk factors in time, space, or scope. Risk conditions influence health either through risk factors or by operating directly on human biology over time, but they are much less likely to be under the control of the individuals at risk. Observance of the tenth anniversary of the *Ottawa Charter* placed increased emphasis on social justice, reducing inequalities, and enhancing social cohesion (Rootman & Raeburn, 1997).

The Congressional report *Adolescent Health* (1991) documented the extreme inequalities in health and well-being between poor and nonpoor children. Similar variations have been reported in the United Kingdom (Townsend, Davidson, & Whitehead, 1992) and Canada (Canadian Institute on Children's Health, 1994). The National Research Council (1993) identified such issues as income, employment, quality of families, and quality of neighborhoods as determinants of health.

*The United Kingdom Charter for Health Promotion* (Coronary Prevention Group, 1997) listed justice, inclusion, social capital, enterprise, and "getting local" as priorities and contained the statement,

> Economic and social policies over the preceding decades have contributed to an ever-widening gap between rich and poor. Compelling evidence confirms that exclusion—both societal and material—is inextricably linked to ever-rising health and social problems. . . .

Priority areas identified in *The Action Statement for Health Promotion in Canada* (Canadian Public Health Association, 1996) included reducing inequalities in income and wealth, strengthening communities through local alliances to change unhealthy living conditions, supporting environments that promote healthy lifestyles, and developing a settings approach to practice. *The Jakarta Declaration on Health Promotion into the 21st Century* (World Health Organization, 1997) outlined priorities for promoting social responsibility for health, increasing investments in health development, consolidating and expanding partnerships, increasing community capacity, empowering the individual, and securing an infrastructure for health promotion.

Lifestyle remains a target of health promotion, but the spotlight has shifted to broader determinants of health and a more expansive range of approaches. Robertson and Minkler (1994) referred to the shift in priorities as the "new" health promotion movement and cited some of its prominent features:

- broadening the definition of health and its determinants to include the social and economic context within which health—or, more precisely, non-health—is produced

- going beyond the earlier emphasis on individual lifestyle strategies to apply health to broader social and political strategies

- embracing the concept of empowerment—individual and collective—as a key health promotion strategy

- advocating the community participation in identifying health problems and strategies for addressing those problems

Through these important documents, authorities in most of the world have both validated and initiated the "new" health promotion.

## KEY POINTS

1. Health promotion is a broad field encompassing educational, social, economic, and political efforts to improve the health of a population. It is practiced in a variety of settings by workers of varied backgrounds.

2. Health promotion is composed of three interlocking components: disease and injury prevention, health education, and health protection.

3. Prevention may be primary interventions to avert disease or injury, secondary interventions to identify disease at an early stage and apply treatments to lessen consequences, or tertiary interventions to help sick or disabled people limit the effects of their illnesses or disabilities.

4. The Framework for Health Promotion is a useful way to provide vision and structure to health promotion efforts by delineating three levels of concern and action: health challenges, health promotion mechanisms, and implementation strategies. It offers an opportunity to explore health promotion in light of the biopsychosocial processes that motivate individuals.

5. Empowerment of individuals and communities is a primary theme in health promotion.

6. Viewing health from the social, institutional, and cultural contexts of human–environmental and person–person relations describes the ecological perspective of health promotion. It allows health promoters to view behavior as a complex interplay of social, political, institutional, and interpersonal factors and to develop programs based on reciprocal causation between individuals and their environments.

7. In the process of community organization, community groups produce change and develop their community.

8. Individual behavior and lifestyle are the major contributing factors in reduced health and premature death. A number of factors, internal and external to the individual, contribute to his or her behavior.

9. Many nationally and internationally produced documents have verified the concepts set forth in this chapter. The current approach to health promotion is to influence (more distal) risk conditions instead of (more individual) risk factors.

**risk factors**   human behaviors that put one at risk for disease or injury

**risk conditions**   factors that influence health, either through risk factors or by operating directly on human biology over time, and that are unlikely to be controllable by the individuals at risk

## REFERENCES

*Adolescent Health.* (1991). Washington DC: Congressional Office of Technology Assessment.

The Annie E. Casey Foundation. (1999). *Kids count data book.* Baltimore.

Bracht, N. (Ed.). (1990). *Health promotion at the community level.* Newbury Park, CA: Sage.

Canadian Institute on Children's Health. (1994). *The health of Canada's children: A CICH profile.* Toronto, Canada.

Canadian Public Health Association. (1996). *Action statement on health promotion* [On-line]. Available: http://www.cpha/cpha/docs/ActionStatement.eng.html

Centers for Disease Control and Prevention. (2000) State- and sex-specific prevalence of selected characteristics: Behavioral risk factor surveillance system, 1996 and 1997. *Morbidity and Mortality Weekly Report,* 49(No. SS-6), 1–39.

Cohen, S., & Syme, S.L. (Eds.). (1985). *Social support and health.* Orlando, FL: Academic Press.

Coronary Prevention Group. (1997). *UK charter for health promotion* [On-line]. Available: http://www.healthnet.org.uk/media/press/charter-local.htm

Downie, R.S., Tannahill, C., & Tannahill, A. (1996). *Health promotion: Models and values* (2nd ed.). Oxford, England: Oxford University Press.

Elbaz, G. (1998). Social movements as health-educators. *Journal of Health Education, 29*(5), 295–303.

Eng, E., Briscoe, J., & Cunningham, A. (1990). The effect of participation in state projects on immunization. *Social Science and Medicine, 30*(12), 1349–1358.

Epp, J. (1986). *Achieving health for all: A framework for health promotion. Report of the Minister of National Health and Welfare.* Ottawa, Canada: Department of National Health and Welfare.

Fellin, P. (1995). Understanding American communities. In J. Rothman, J.L. Erlich, & J.E. Tropman (Eds.), *Strategies of community organization* (5th ed.). Itasca, IL: Peacock.

Friere, P. (1970). *Cultural action for freedom.* Cambridge: Harvard Educational Review.

Giroux, H. (1994). Insurgent multiculturalism. In D.T. Goldberg (Ed.), *A critical reader.* Cambridge: Cambridge USA.

Green, L.W., & Kreuter, M.W. (1999). *Health promotion planning: An educational and ecological approach* (3rd ed.). Mountain View, CA: Mayfield.

Green, L.W., & Ottoson, J.M. (1999). *Community and population health* (8th ed.). Boston: WCB McGraw-Hill.

Gutierrez, L. (1990). Working with women of color: An empowerment perspective. *Social Work, 35*(2), 149–154.

Iannantuono, A., & Eyles, J. (1997). Meaning in policy: A textual analysis of Canada's "health for all" document. *Social Science in Medicine, 44*(11), 1611–1621.

Karasek, R., & Thorell, T. (Eds.). (1990). *Healthy work: Stress, productivity, and the reconstruction of working life.* New York: Basic Books.

Labonte, R. (1986). Social inequality and healthy public policy. *Health Promotion, 1*(3), 341–351.

Lalonde, M.A. (1974). *New perspectives on the health of Canadians.* Ottawa, Canada: Information Canada.

Macdonald, G., & Bunton, R. (1992). Health promotion: Discipline or disciplines? In R. Bunton & G. Macdonald (Eds.), *Health promotion: Disciplines and diversity.* London: Routledge.

McLeroy, K.R., Bibeau, D., Steckler, A., & Glanz, K. (1988). An ecological perspective on health promotion programs. *Health Education Quarterly, 15*(4), 351–377.

Minkler, M., & Wallerstein, N. (1997). Improving health through community organization and community building. In K. Glanz, F.M. Lewis, & B.K. Rimer (Eds.), *Health behavior and health education* (2nd ed.). San Francisco: Jossey-Bass.

Monash Health Promotion Unit. (1999). "Health promotion"—What is it? [On-line]. Available: http://www.monash.edu.au/health/course-manual/health.htm

National Research Council. (1993). *Losing generations: Adolescents in high-risk settings. Report of the panel on high risk youth.* Washington, DC: National Academy Press.

O'Donnell, M.P. (1996). Editor's notes. *American Journal of Health Promotion, 10*(4), 244.

Potter, P., & Perry, A. (1993). *Fundamentals of nursing.* St. Louis: Mosby YearBook.

Robertson, A., & Minkler, M. (1994). New health promotion movement: A critical examination. *Health Education Quarterly, 21*(3), 295–312.

Rootman, I., & Raeburn, J. (1997). *People-centered health promotion.* Toronto, Canada: Wiley.

Seffrin, J.R. (1997). Premises, promises, and potential payoffs of responsible health education. *Journal of Health Education, 28*(5), 298–307.

Sharkey, P.W., Graham-Kresge, S., & White, Jr., G.L. (1995). Defining health education: Health, values, and professional responsibility. *Health Values, 19*(6), 23–29.

Sheinfeld Gorin, S., & Arnold, J. (1998). *Health promotion handbook.* St. Louis: Mosby.

Sigerist, H.E. (1946). *The university at the crossroads: Addresses and essays.* New York: Henry Schuman.

Simons-Morton, B.G., & Greene, W.H., & Gottlieb, N.H. (1995). *Introduction to health education and health promotion* (2nd ed.). Prospect Heights, IL: Waveland.

Stokols, D. (1992). Establishing and maintaining healthy environments: Toward a social ecology of health promotion. *American Psychologist, 47*(1), 6–22.

Stokols, D., Allen, J., & Bellingham, R.L. (1996). The social ecology of health promotion: Implications for research and practice. *American Journal of Health Promotion, 10*(4), 247–251.

Tannahill, A. (1985). What is health promotion? *Health Education Journal, 44*, 167–168.

Teague, M.L., & McGhee, V.L. (1992). *Health promotion: Achieving high-level wellness in the later years.* Dubuque, IA: Brown and Benchmark.

Townsend, P., Davidson, N., & Whitehead, M. (Eds.). (1992). *Inequalities in health: The Black report and the health divide.* New York: Penguin.

U.S. Department of Health, Education and Welfare. (1979). *Healthy people: The surgeon general's report on health promotion and disease prevention: Background papers.* Washington, DC: Public Health Service.

U.S. Department of Health and Human Services. (1991). *Healthy people 2000: National health promotion and disease prevention objectives* (Public Health Service Publication No. 91-50212). Washington, DC: U.S. Government Printing Office.

U.S. Department of Health and Human Services. (2000). *Healthy people 2010* (Conference ed.) in two volumes. Washington, DC.

Wallerstein, N. (1992). Powerlessness, empowerment, and health: Implications for health promotion programs. *American Journal of Health Promotion, 6*(3), 197–205.

Working Group on Concepts and Principles of Health Promotion. (1987). Health promotion: Concepts and principles. In T. Abelin, Z.J. Brzezinski, & V.D.L. Corstairs (Eds.), *Measurement in health promotion and protection.* Geneva, Switzerland: World Health Organization.

World Health Organization. (1984). *Report of the working group on concept and principles of health promotion.* Copenhagen, Denmark.

World Health Organization. (1986). The Ottawa charter for health promotion. *Health Promotion, 1*(1), iii–v.

World Health Organization. (1997). *The Jakarta declaration on health promotion into the 21st century* [On-line]. Available: http://rubble.ultralab.anglia.ac.uk/Declare.htm

World Health Organization. (2000). *WHO issues new healthy life expectancy rankings* [On-line]. Available: http//www.who.int/inf-pr-2000/en/pr2000-life.html

Zimmerman, M.A. (1990). Taking aim on empowerment research: On the distinction between individual and psychological conceptions. *American Journal of Community Psychology, 18*(1), 169–177.

# Health Education

During the 1970s and 1980s, health education emphasized altering individuals' behavior. In the 1990s, health education expanded to encompass social action and become more integrated with health promotion. Mayhew Derryberry wrote forty years ago,

> Health education . . . requires careful and thorough consideration of the present knowledge, attitudes, goals, perceptions, social status, power structure, cultural traditions, and other aspects of whatever public is to be addressed. (1960)

Glanz and colleagues (1997) stated that advocacy, policy change, and organizational change have been adopted as central activities of public health education and health promotion. Thus, the merger of health education into the health promotion framework may be blurring the distinction between the two.

It is therefore no wonder that school administrators, parents, community leaders, and employers do not understand what health educators actually do. This misunderstanding often leads to allocating responsibility for health education to people who have little academic background in the field. In schools, people with little health education preparation often get the assignment. In hospitals, and even in health maintenance organizations, administrators are reluctant to trust health education to people who are not clinically trained. Nurses and physicians who often conduct health education—or **patient education**—may lack the aptitude, training, or motivation to do so. Fortunately, most modern nurses take their patient education responsibilities seriously and receive professional preparation in the field. Certainly, health education is best applied by individuals trained to employ its processes.

## WHAT IS HEALTH EDUCATION?

Health education, as does the term "health," has as many definitions as it does practitioners. The term is not easy to define to the satisfaction of all professionals. Health education takes place in a number of settings. Most people believe they can do it well. The actions of every parent, teacher, and role model communicate something about health—but the message may be far from satisfactory. Box 3.1 lists a few definitions of health education.

What do these definitions have in common? Clearly the thread running through them is the notion that health education is a process, not a product. It is a series of planned activities directed toward goals, including an array of deliberate experiences that affect the way people think, feel, and act regarding their own health and the health of their communities.

**patient education**   health education in health care delivery settings to patients and their families

43

**Box 3.1**    Definitions of "Health Education"

The process of providing learning experiences for the purpose of influencing knowledge, attitudes, or conduct relating to individual, community, or world health. (Joint Committee on Health Problems in Education, 1948)

★

The process through which individuals, social groups, and communities attend to and assimilate information about health and disease, and mobilize appropriate behavior for health-promotive ends. (Wilner, Walker, & Goerke, 1973)

★

A process with intellectual, psychological, and social dimensions relating to activities that increase the abilities of people to make informed decisions affecting their personal, family and community well-being. This process, based on scientific principles, facilitates learning and behavioral change in both health personnel and consumers, including children and youth. (Joint Committee on Health Education Terminology, 1973)

★

Planned learning experiences and supportive activities that help people develop their abilities to evaluate behavioral options and their probable consequences and make informed decisions about their responsibilities and actions concerning:

1. Personal practices aimed at promoting vigorous well-being, preventing avoidable disability and premature death, and effectively handling minor diseases and discomforts;

2. Prompt, appropriate use of health services when needed;

3. Selection and carrying out of needed diagnostic, treatment, habilitation, rehabilitation, and maintenance procedures; and

4. Involvement in community efforts (at local, area, state, regional, national and/or international levels) to develop effective, efficient, and appropriate environmental programs, socioeconomic measures, and health services systems that facilitate health improvement. (Bureau of Health Planning and Resources Development, 1973)

★

A process affecting intellectual, psychological, and social dimensions that increases our capacity to make informed health decisions affecting self, family and community well-being. (Bedworth & Bedworth, 1978)

★

Any combination of learning experiences designed to facilitate voluntary adaptations of behavior conducive to health. (Green, Kreuter, Deeds, & Partridge, 1980)

★

Educationally oriented process of planned change which focuses on those behaviors or problems that directly or indirectly affect people's health. (Ross & Mico, 1980)

★

Any activity with clear goals planned for the purpose of improving health-related knowledge, attitudes, or behavior. (Carlyon & Cook, 1981)

★

The process of assisting individuals, acting separately and collectively, to make informed decisions about matters affecting their personal health and that of others. (Henderson & McIntosh, 1981)

★

A deliberately planned, structured learning opportunity about health that occurs in a setting at a given point in time and involves interaction between an educator and a learner. (Bates & Winder, 1984)

★

That continuum of learning which enables people, as individuals and as members of social structures, to voluntarily make decisions, modify behaviors, and change social conditions in ways which are health enhancing. (1990 Joint Committee on Health Education Terminology, 1991)

★

The process of providing the tools to help one approach his or her social, mental, emotional, spiritual, and physical health potentials. (Greenberg & Gold, 1992)

★

Any health-related educational activities, whether in schools, community, clinical, or work settings. (Pollock & Middleton, 1994)

★

The process of developing and providing planned learning experiences in such a way as to supply information, change attitudes, and influence behavior. (Anspaugh & Ezell, 1995)

★

Any combination of learning experiences designed to facilitate voluntary actions conducive to health. (Green & Kreuter, 1999)

Green and Ottoson (1999) brilliantly expressed the moment when health education becomes health promotion:

> The voluntary adoption of behavior conducive to health is the goal of health education. In concert with social and environmental supports for such behavior, health education becomes health promotion.

# THE ESSENCE OF HEALTH EDUCATION

As Oberteuffer, Harrelson, and Pollock (1972) stated:

> The goal of health education is to help each person seek that pattern of behavior which moves him toward an optimal level of health rather than the reverse and to give him the ability to avoid many of the imbalances, diseases, and accidents of life.

Reaching for this worthy goal is the mission of health education and its practitioners. Sharkey and colleagues (1995) pointed out that the purpose of education is to help us understand the relationships among our health **values**, behaviors, and their consequences so that we may make personally responsible choices concerning them. This requires the understanding of relevant, unbiased information as well as the process of applying values. In fact, they claim that health education is unavoidably values education. To seek a "pattern of behavior" and to "make personally responsible choices" implies the voluntary nature of that behavior. Health educators cherish voluntary behavior change.

Whatever definition you choose, one fundamental principle must guide the work of health educators: Individuals, families, and communities can be taught to assume responsibility for their own health and, to some extent, for the health of others. Green and Ottoson (1999) stated that health education is based on the assumption that

> beneficial health behavior in both children and adults will result from a combination of planned, consistent, integrated learning opportunities. This assumption rests on direct evidence from the evaluation of health education programs in schools, at worksites, in medical settings, and through the mass media.

The challenge is to find the most productive ways to influence voluntary individual and community

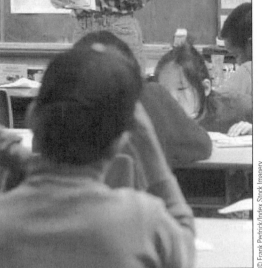

Classroom health instruction is a planned opportunity with goals, objectives, organized activities, and evaluation criteria.

© Frank Pedrick/Index Stock Imagery

behavior without violating individual freedoms guaranteed by the U.S. Constitution.

The process of health education

— is a planned opportunity to learn (intervention) about health with stated goals, objectives, activities, and evaluation criteria

— occurs in a specified setting

— occurs at a specified time

— is part of a sequential program that introduces concepts at appropriate learning levels and that is based upon what was learned previously,

**values**   the underlying constructs of right or wrong that give direction to every decision and result in the action the person takes which forms a basis for what is to be learned in the future

— emphasizes in a comprehensive manner how various aspects of health are interrelated and how all affect the quality of life

— includes interaction between a qualified educator and learner.

Simons-Morton and associates (1995) identified the following interventions of health education:

— teaching

— training: teaching other health educators, other health or education professionals, or volunteers how to accomplish health education objectives or how to employ health education methods

— counseling: the process of helping people learn how to achieve personal growth, improve interpersonal relationships, resolve problems, make decisions, and change behavior

— consulting: the process by which one person's knowledge and experience are used to help another person make better decisions or cope with problems more effectively

Effective health instruction hinges on two interrelated issues: what to teach and how to teach it (Dalis, 1994). One of the main goals of health education is establishing or changing patterns of behavior; therefore, the process of health education must go beyond memorizing information imparted by the educator. Conveying information alone is not sufficient to effect behavior change (Bruhn, 1988; Green & Iverson, 1982; Stone, 1985). Knowledge does not necessarily change attitudes (Kingery, Pruitt, & Hurley, 1993), nor are attitudes always consistent with behavior (Iverson & Portnoy, 1977; Prue et al., 1987). The efficacy of personal and social skills development of students and clients for the purpose of influencing health behavior positively has been supported by research applied to health issues such as AIDS (Botvin & Dusenbury, 1992); teen pregnancy (Schinke, 1984); compliance with sex guidelines (Ahia, 1991); and prevention of tobacco, alcohol, and other drug abuse (Pentz, 1985). Health educators should plan and conduct interventions to reach a number of generic outcomes, including skill development, values awareness,

concept and information acquisition and application, opinion development and discussion, and decision making.

Given the four interventions of health education or the "what to teach and how to teach it" focus, health education obviously carries a message. The source of the message—the educator—is an important determinant of who will attend to the message, how much of the message will be understood, how much will be retained, and whether it will inspire subsequent behavior change (Bettinghaus, 1986). Kelman (1961) identified three characteristics that define an educator's influence: credibility, attractiveness, and power. This would explain how the effectiveness of certain educators and "messengers" (such as actors and athletes appearing in public service announcements) varies according to the audience.

Any modern attempt at education must address the influence of culture. Culture implies shared values, norms, and codes that collectively shape a group's beliefs, attitudes, and behavior during their interactions in and with their environment (Airhihenbuwa, 1995). Individual and group behaviors occur in the context of culture. Any attempt to change or establish behaviors must take culture into account.

# MISCONCEPTIONS ABOUT AND BARRIERS TO HEALTH EDUCATION

The acceptance of health education by decision makers and the public has been stymied by several factors. Many of these are erroneous assumptions and misconceptions; others are impediments erected intentionally or unintentionally by administrators and systems.

## Misconceptions

**Anyone can teach health.**    It is a common belief that, because health is a natural state, anyone can teach it. In fact, in the old style of teaching exclusively by lecture, it may have been true that an individual who was committed to staying current about matters of health could generate the appearance of success by conveying knowledge. However, the modern emphasis on skills development, educational standards, community involvement, cultural sensitivity, and behavior change requires a professionally educated individual.

## Anyone can write an effective health education curriculum.

A corollary to this is "anyone can develop an effective health education program." Structuring learning experiences throughout an academic year or developing a kindergarten-through-high school program requires special expertise. Curricular needs frequently depend upon the needs, resources, values, and principles inherent in a given community. Just as specific expertise is essential to develop a science curriculum, expertise in health education is needed to create curricula in that area. Likewise, the development of a health education program in other settings, such as a health care facility or community agency, requires skills in needs assessment, determining cultural patterns of belief and behavior, designing interventions, and program evaluation.

## Health education is not related to other learning.

A good deal of evidence suggests that children who are healthy are more effective learners. We shall explore the relationship between health and academic achievement in Chapter 7.

## Knowledge is the only result of health education that can be evaluated.

If objectives are clearly written, it is possible to evaluate all outcomes of health education. The use of authentic assessments to evaluate learner behaviors and habits is an accepted practice. Several instruments have been shown to measure changes in attitudes accurately. In addition, such outcomes as changes in disease prevalence, unwanted pregnancies, violent incidents, and other targets of community programs are measured frequently to evaluate the effectiveness of a program.

## Health education is hygiene class.

The old hygiene class dealt mainly with practices such as washing hands and brushing teeth. Though these are necessary activities, today's school health education is much broader and equips students to make decisions affecting their well-being throughout life.

It helps them cope with the challenges of modern life. It imparts the functional knowledge necessary to reach an optimal level of health, influences attitudes so students can appreciate the importance of each decision that affects their health, and provides for the development of skills to carry out those decisions. In patient education, it encourages preventive behavior and compliance with treatment regimens. In work settings, it helps clients develop patterns of behavior that are conducive to health and helps management develop an environment that is supportive of health and safety.

## Health education is sex education.

Although sexuality and family life education are important parts of most school health curricula, they are only one portion of a comprehensive program. Many opponents of health education or family life education overemphasize the role of sexuality education in order to distort the truth about health instruction. Yet, most (80–90 percent) Americans support sexuality education (Donovan, 1998; Hugick & Leonard, 1991), including residents of states considered to be conservative (Lindley et al., 1998; American Social Health Association, 1996; Clark, Houser, & Powell, 1995).

## Barriers

## The accountability movement

This movement seeks to hold schools, teachers, and students responsible for learning. It was spurred by the news of the poor performance by American children on standardized tests and of the loss of U.S. technological supremacy in, and dominance of, world markets. It was initially labeled the "back-to-basics movement," although educators were slow to acknowledge yet another poor performance by American children on measures of the most basic characteristics of successful children: fitness and general wellness.

Nevertheless, during the early stages of the back-to-basics movement, health education was beginning to make gains, despite the lack of general

**accountability** the concept that educators and institutions are answerable for what their clients learn

acceptance that special training was necessary to deliver it effectively. It had not—and in many localities, still has not—reached the status of providing a comprehensive health instruction curriculum within a coordinated health education program.

Current school reform efforts are based on educational standards that are usually established at the state level. Instruction is to be based on the standards, and tests are usually administered to determine if students have reached the standards. Because it is not usually considered a core area, health education is seldom one of the disciplines in which students and teachers are held responsible for meeting standards. Only eight states test students in health education (Bennett, Perko, & Herstine, 2000) This often leads to even less emphasis on health education. However, health educators should look on the reform movement as an ally in reaching their goal of a comprehensive instructional program. The link between healthy children with few risk factors and academic achievement should be emphasized as a rationale for health education. Fortunately, many parents and administrators have recognized that nothing is as basic as the health of their children and that development of mathematical, writing, and reading skills is more likely in healthy children.

## Perceived lack of support  Some school policy makers do not view health education as a high priority, particularly in light of the school accountability reform movement. This low priority may be evidenced by lack of support from citizen boards of education. This leads to a fragmented health curriculum that focuses on mandates for single topics (perhaps AIDS/HIV or drug use prevention). However, most administrators profess to believe in the importance of health education, although many perceive that their community does not. In truth, most parents, students, and school administrators believe that health education is at least as important as other subjects taught in school (Seffrin, 1994).

Leadership has been identified as an important aspect of educational change (Smith, Bibeau, & Altschuld, 1991). Whether in the form of a district person responsible for health education (such as a school health coordinator), backing from a prominent, high-level district administrator, or simply support from principals, visible leadership enhances

curriculum implementation by teachers (Smith et al., 1995).

Some people oppose health education, especially in schools. At times opposition stems from unpleasant experiences in one's own health education, especially if taught by an unqualified individual. The most dangerous opposition comes from organized groups, often instigated from outside the local area. These organizations often distort the nature of health education, accusing the programs of destroying values developed at home, encouraging promiscuity, and undermining religious training.

In many cases, the community approves of health education but is not active in its support. This may give the appearance of apathy or even opposition. However, most parents and students support health education in school, including education related to sexuality. The problem is usually that supporters may not demonstrate their approval vigorously, whereas detractors are much more likely to be vocal, visible, and threatening to elected officials.

## Inadequate professional preparation  Elementary school teachers often are expected to teach health without any college coursework in the discipline. Inservice offerings have the potential for bridging this gap but are often inadequate to acquire the skills and knowledge that a modern approach requires. Quality of teaching in secondary schools often suffers, despite no shortage of professionally prepared health educators, because the class is often assigned to specialists in other subjects—often science or physical education. This is a result of the "anyone can teach health" misconception and the lack of administrative commitment. The professional training, educational background, and access to health resources required for health educators differ from those of science or physical education instructors. This difference exerts a strong influence on the quantity and quality of health instruction (Smith et al., 1995).

When new curricula are adopted, they usually require training. However, teacher preparation for health should not have to depend on the school district's purchase of curriculum materials. The Centers for Disease Control and Prevention (1997) recommended hiring elementary school teachers trained to teach health education and hiring health education specialists to teach in middle and senior high schools.

People who identify themselves as health educators and who practice in other settings are sometimes inadequately prepared. Physicians, social workers, and nurses sometimes engage in patient education without the necessary skills and competencies. Public and community health educators— who may possess degrees in social work, communications, or other disciplines—often learn health education concepts only on the job and at conferences.

## Lack of certification
Although many states mandate health instruction in schools, many do not require that instructors be certified in health education. This has led to a situation in which only 4 percent of lead health education teachers majored in health education and an additional 22 percent majored in health and physical education (Collins et al., 1995), leaving much of health instruction to educators who are unqualified to provide it, typically physical education teachers, coaches, science teachers, and nurses. In 1998, 47 states offered separate certificates in health education, and 18 offered a combined certificate in health and physical education (Bennett, Perko, & Herstine, 2000). However, even when certificates are available, health education is often taught by persons who lack them. If the teacher lacks the training, the students are shortchanged, the taxpayers are cheated, the reputation of health education is tarnished, and students —given the relationship between health and academic performance—may not progress in their other subjects.

The American Association for Health Education holds that health education is a fundamental ingredient in the prevention formula and that primary prevention represents the most rational means to controlling health care costs and improving the health of all Americans. AAHE also notes that health education has become more complex and demanding in recent years. Based on these findings, AAHE (then the Association for the Advancement of Health Education) adopted the following statement in 1991:

Since school health education is a fundamental and indispensable component of basic education, AAHE strongly supports the need for certified teachers in health education. Standards for health education in each state should be the equivalent standards for any other teaching area in terms of adherence to professional standards of preparation. Further, all persons teaching health education at the secondary level or higher, should be required by the State Department of Education to have separate certification in health education. All early childhood and elementary teacher candidates should show evidence of professional preparation in health.

## Encroachment of other disciplines
Other disciplines have made significant inroads into the functions claimed by health educators. This can be beneficial if those involved are willing to share responsibilities, expertise, and diverse approaches so representatives of different professions can collaborate effectively.

The assignment and absorption of health education by a diverse group of practitioners is probably best illustrated in the schools. Perhaps the best example of this is the employment of law enforcement officers, principally in classroom drug prevention. Often these officers have no formal preparation in any type of education other than a few content-related hours of training. School nurses, social workers, and counselors frequently carry out classroom health education services without pedagogical preparation. These individuals would be more effective if working as resources for classes taught by certified health educators. Physical education teachers have historically performed health education. As physical education places more emphasis on wellness, but states require separate certifications for health education and physical education, the potential for the destructive practice of turf-guarding by members of both disciplines may increase.

Other disciplines have intruded into the practice of health education with seldom a thought of cooperation or collaboration. Many sub-specialists within psychology, such as health psychologists and community psychologists, overlap with health education. Home economists have viewed nutrition education and family life education as part of their professional expertise (Livingood et al., 1993). This conviction extends to schools where consumer and family studies (formerly home economics) teachers perform these functions.

The medical establishment has laid claim to anything remotely related to health. Nurses, some physicians, and most chiropractors view health education as a major function of their profession. Fortunately, most nursing programs now contain preservice preparation in patient education. However, what passes for patient education among some providers of alternative remedies is often a sales pitch.

# CONTRIBUTORS TO A UNIQUE DISCIPLINE

Some may argue that health education is not a unique discipline because it is rooted in others, as indicated in Figure 3.1. The behavioral sciences, public health, and education are primary contributors to the discipline of health education. Similar to other fields, health education relies upon and utilizes other disciplines. Health education should therefore be accorded status equal to disciplines such as social studies, language arts, science, physical education, and consumer and family studies in schools.

## The Behavioral Sciences

The behavioral sciences, incorporating psychology, sociology, and cultural anthropology, are concerned with how people behave and why. They define the primary determinants of behavior as

— **psychological predispositions**, including attitudes, knowledge, beliefs, skills, and experiences

— **environmental reinforcement** from family, friends, authority figures, and associates

— **the sociocultural context**, which consists of sustained societal norms about attitudes and behavior

Because behavior change is a desired outcome of health education, these primary determinants become crucial to the practice of health education. Green (1984) suggested that "the dominant contributions to our literature on interventions in health have been, perhaps regrettably, from psychology."

**Figure 3.1**  Contributors to the Discipline of Health Education

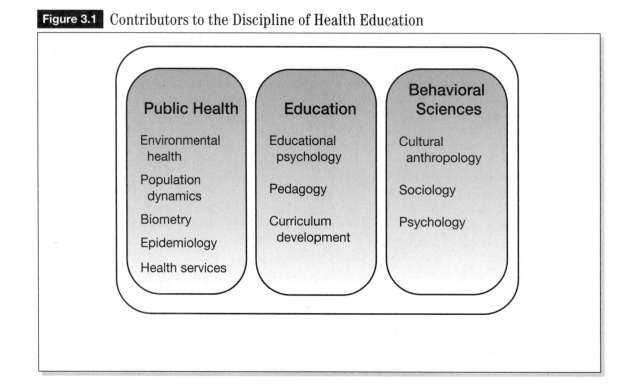

## Public Health

Public health services are provided by government agencies and supported by taxation. Health education relies on public health for, among other things, health statistics for epidemiologic information. Determinants of health problems—environment, medical care, personal lifestyle—often are discovered in the public health realm. Other issues, such as population dynamics, epidemiology, and biomedical science, are deeply rooted in public health. Health promotion is a common function in public health agencies.

## Education

Obviously, education—the study and practice of teaching and learning—plays a role in the development of health education. Learning theory, educational psychology, human development, pedagogy, curriculum development, measurement, and testing are all rooted in the education literature. Health is one of the seven *Cardinal Principles of Secondary Education* (Commission on the Reorganization of Education, 1918/1928).

Nixon (1967) summarized the criteria of a discipline:

1. A discipline has an identifiable domain; it asks vital questions; it deals with immensely significant themes, a specifiable scope of inquiry, a central core of interest; it has a definite beginning point; and it has stated goals.

2. A discipline is characterized by a substantial history and a publicly recognized tradition exemplified by time-tested works.

3. A discipline is rooted in an appropriate structure; it has its unique conceptual structure, and it employs a syntactical structure; the structure organizes a body of basic concepts; and it consists of conceptual relationships as well as appropriate relations between facts.

4. A discipline possesses a unique integrity and an arbitrary quality.

5. A discipline is recognized by the procedures and methods it employs; it utilizes intellectual and conceptual tools as well as technical and mechanical tools; it follows a relevant set of rules; it is recognized by its basic set of procedures, all of which lead to ways of learning and knowing in the domain of the discipline.

6. A discipline is recognized as a process as well as noted for its products (knowledge, principles, generalizations).

7. A discipline relies on accurate language, a participants' language, to provide precise, careful communication both within its ranks and to outsiders.

Based upon these criteria, health education is certainly a unique discipline.

## HEALTH EDUCATION PHILOSOPHY

**Philosophy** shapes the way we look at the world, defines the way we experience our surroundings and events, influences how we act toward others, and helps to form a foundation for reality. Cottrell, Girvan, and McKenzie (1999) stated that a person's philosophy should be synchronous in all aspects of life, maintaining consistency at home, at school, in the workplace, and at play. Piecing together information from (1) experience; (2) education or study; (3) guidance from teachers, religious leaders, and mentors; and (4) lessons from friends and relatives, we synthesize it into a way of thinking, acting, and viewing the world. Our philosophy guides us in solving problems and making decisions. Bensley (1993) related the essence of philosophy when he wrote

> Philosophy can be defined as a state of mind based on your values and beliefs. This in turn is based on a variety of factors which include culture, religion, education, morals, environment, experiences, and family. It is also determined by people who have influenced you, how you feel about yourself and others, your spirit, your optimism or pessimism, your independence and your family. It is a synthesis of all learning that makes you who you are and what you believe. In other words, a philosophy reflects your values and beliefs which determine your mission and purpose for being, or basic theory, or viewpoint based on logical reasoning.

**philosophy** statement summarizing an individual's or group's attitudes, beliefs, values, principles, and state of mind

Even though health education has been defined, the best way to accomplish its mission is less clear. Five philosophies appear to be dominant:

1. **Behavior change**, granted wide acceptance through the work of Green et al.(1980), emphasizes behavioral modification through the use of behavioral contracts, goal setting, and self-monitoring. One reason that educators favor it is that it offers the benefit of allowing easily quantifiable and measurable objectives.

2. **Cognitive-based** is perhaps the most historically established philosophy. This philosophy focuses on content and factual information and on increasing the knowledge base of the student/client. It has the advantage of allowing a large quantity of information to be acquired quickly. It is viewed as a foundation upon which other philosophies can be built (Creswell & Newman, 1993).

3. **Decision making** became a force in health education in the mid-1970s as health educators became disenchanted with the cognitive-based philosophy (Dalis & Strasser, 1977). Its popularity has continued. It is a systematic approach to education that equips students/clients with pragmatic skills, such as problem solving and decision making, and skills necessary to cope with peer pressure that can be utilized in health-related decisions. It also emphasizes lifelong learning and inductive methodologies.

4. **Freeing/functioning** (Greenberg, 1978; Russell, 1976) emphasizes the concepts of freedom, individuality, and lifelong learning. It is grounded in the freedom of the individual to function in a way that is satisfying to him or her and to make the best decisions possible based on his or her best interests, including practices that may not be conducive to health or in the interests of society.

5. **Social change** was developed by Freudenberg and espoused by O'Rourke (1989). By proposing that education is a driving force for social change, this philosophy enlarged the role of health education. As a result, health education became more closely connected to social, political, and economic issues that influence individual health. Social change

philosophy aligned health educators more closely with health promotion.

Welle, Russell, and Kittleson (1995) conducted a study in which the five philosophies described above were presented to a nationwide selection of health education professionals. The first preference of both the academicians and the practitioners was decision-making philosophy. The second choice of both groups was behavior change. The philosophy identified by both groups as the least like their own beliefs was cognitive-based. This startling amount of agreement between health educators in academic settings and those practicing in the field is encouraging to health education as a profession. The next step, choosing how to put decision-making philosophical principles into action, may not be fully realized for many years. The researchers emphasized the significance of this process and of careful consideration of philosophy by writing

> Health educators must remember that every single educational choice reflects a philosophical principle or belief. Educational choices carry important philosophical assumptions about the purpose of health education, the teacher, and also the learner. Thus, health educators should take the time necessary for individual philosophical inquiry, in order to be able to clearly articulate what principles guide them professionally.

In practice, strict separation of philosophies is not always easy. They may overlap. Putting the principles inherent in only one philosophy to work may be difficult at times. It may sometimes appear that an individual educator operates within more than one of the dominant philosophies. This is not necessarily negative, but it may force the individual to fall back on his or her personal values to resolve conflicts.

## WHY HEALTH EDUCATION?

In this age of medical miracles, we may begin to believe health education has little left to teach us. History and statistics prove us wrong. At the turn of the century, the leading causes of death in the United States were contagious diseases. Widespread understanding of the germ theory, development of immunizations, improvements in sanitation and water treatment, and development of treatments such as antibiotics have greatly reduced the risk that humans will succumb to infectious disease. The leading official causes of death in the United States are now heart disease, cancer, stroke, chronic lung disease, and unintentional injury. McGinnis and Foege (1993) demonstrated that the *actual* causes of death (the underlying sources of official causes of death), led by tobacco use (19 percent) and diet/activity patterns (14 percent), are predominantly directly caused by lifestyles and behaviors. Many harmful practices are begun early in life as evidenced by a national survey of high school students, as shown in Box 3.2.

The Youth Risk Behavior Survey (YRBS) data also indicate that deaths among young people are often caused by behavior choices. In fact, 73 percent of all deaths among youth and young adults 10–24 years of age result from only four causes—motor vehicle crashes (30 percent), other unintentional injuries (10 percent), homicide (20 percent), and suicide (13 percent) (Kann et al., 1998). The Behavioral Risk Factor Surveillance System yields some interesting data regarding adult behaviors. Samples of these data are presented in Box 3.3.

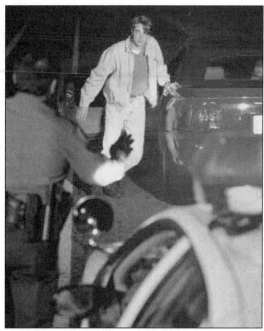

© 2000 PhotoDisc, Inc.

The frequency with which high school students drink alcohol and drive or ride with a driver who has been drinking is alarming. It is an issue for both law enforcement and health education.

## Box 3.2    Youth Risk Behaviors

The 1997 national Youth Risk Behavior Survey of high school students indicated the following:

1. 36 percent of high school students smoked cigarettes in the past month.

2. 25 percent had smoked a whole cigarette before 13 years of age.

3. 9 percent used smokeless tobacco in the past month.

4. 26 percent used marijuana in the past month.

5. 51 percent had at least one drink of alcohol on at least one occasion in the last month.

6. 71 percent ate fewer than 5 servings of fruits and vegetables yesterday.

7. 38 percent ate more than 2 servings of high fat foods yesterday.

8. 36 percent participated in vigorous physical activity on fewer than 3 of the past 7 days.

9. 73 percent did not attend physical education class daily.

10. 40 percent were trying to lose weight during the preceding 30 days.

11. 49 percent had had sexual intercourse during their lifetime.

12. 43 percent of sexually active students did not use a condom during last intercourse.

13. 19 percent of students had rarely or never worn seat belts when riding in a car or truck driven by someone else.

14. 37 percent had ridden one or more times in the preceding 30 days with a driver who had been drinking alcohol.

15. 18 percent had carried a weapon on one or more of the preceding 30 days.

16. 20 percent of students had seriously considered attempting suicide and 8 percent had attempted suicide during the previous 12 months.

Source: From "Youth Risk Behavior Surveillance—United States, 1997," by L. Kann, S.A. Kinchen, B.I. Williams, J.G. Ross, R. Lowry, C.V. Hill, J.A. Grunbaum, P.S. Blumson, J.L. Collins, & L.J. Kolbe, 1998, *Morbidity and Mortality Weekly Report*, 47(SS-3), pp. 1–89.

## Box 3.3    Adult Risk Behaviors

The following information is from the Behavioral Risk Factor Surveillance System, 1995–1998.*

1. 80.8 percent of those ages 18–24, 81.5 percent of those ages 25–34, 77.0 percent of those ages 35–44, 76.5 percent of those ages 45–54, and 71.7 percent of those ages 55–64 have sexual intercourse with only the same partner, leaving large numbers of people having sexual intercourse with multiple partners.

2. Only 78.2 percent of whites, 81.8 percent of African Americans, and 81.2 percent of Hispanic Americans have sexual intercourse with only the same partner.

3. 23.8 percent consume fruit and vegetables at least 5 times a day; 39.6 percent, 3 or 4 times a day; 33.0 percent, 1 or 2 times a day; and 3.5 percent, less than 1 time a day.

4. 52.3 percent of those ages 18–24, 56.6 percent of those ages 25–34, 60.1 percent of those ages 35–44, 64.1 percent of those ages 45–54, 69.0 percent of those ages 55–64, and 79.1 percent of ages 65 and over consumed fruit and vegetables 3 or more times per day.

5. 22.9 percent of adults smoke cigarettes now.

6. 23 percent of whites, 22.8 percent of African Americans, and 23.9 percent of Hispanic Americans smoke cigarettes now.

7. 31.6 percent of those with less than high school education, 27.9 percent of those with high school diploma or GED, 22.6 percent of those with some post–high school, and 12.2 percent of college graduates smoke cigarettes now.

8. In the past 12 months, 9.4 percent of men and 12.1 percent of women had been advised by a doctor, nurse, or other health professional to lose weight.

9. 10 percent had consumed 5 or more alcoholic drinks on 4 or more occasions during the past month.

*Data are presented as the median of the means of the fifty states, District of Columbia, and Puerto Rico.

Source: From *Behavioral Risk Factor Surveillance System Online Prevalence Data, 1995–1998* [On-line], Division of Adult and Community Health, National Center for Chronic Disease Prevention and Health Promotion, Centers for Disease Control and Prevention. Available: http://www2.cdc.gov/nccdphp/brfss/index.asp.

We are killing ourselves with our unhealthy habits and lifestyles—both of which are influenced by environment and economic factors. Demographic, interpersonal, individual, and environmental (including community) factors are associated with physical activity among children and adolescents (CDC, 1997). Age, ethnicity, gender, income, and education are related to some behaviors, as shown in Box 3.3. Health education has a responsibility to help equalize the opportunities for all people to behave in ways which lower risk. We have known for years that health education may improve health knowledge, attitudes, and behaviors (Mullen et al., 1995; Tolsma & Koplan, 1992; Connell, Turner, & Mason, 1985). Perhaps more importantly, well-designed and well-supported health education can help alleviate a number of social ills (Seffrin, 1997).

Poor children are more likely to have problems such as poor nutrition, stunted growth, severe physical or mental disabilities, fatal accidental injuries, iron deficiency, and severe asthma. According to the landmark book *Wasting America's Future: The Children's Defense Fund Report on the Costs of Child Poverty* (CDF, 1994), low-income children are

— 2 times more likely than other children to die from birth defects

— 3 times more likely to die from all causes combined

— 4 times more likely to die from fires

— 5 times more likely to die from infectious diseases and parasites

— 6 times more likely to die from other diseases

Poor children are more likely to experience overcrowding, utility shut-offs, insufficient heating, and pest infestation, all of which contribute to allergies, respiratory problems, infectious diseases, and asthma.

Box 3.4 illustrates some of the negative conditions into which children are born and in which they live and die.

Many of the conditions in Box 3.4 are preventable through health education and other health promotion strategies. Most of these conditions are visited disproportionately on the poor. The human suffering that environmental conditions, poor health decisions, and lifestyles impose on American youth is enough in itself to justify health education in the school, community, clinics, and other settings. The economic effect of health education serves as yet another incentive.

## ECONOMIC BENEFITS OF HEALTH EDUCATION

Health practices may appear to cost money, but in the long run, they save society millions of dollars. Immunization is one of the best defenses we have against diseases and their associated expense. Vaccines are also very cost-effective. For every $1 spent on immunization, as much as $29 can be saved in

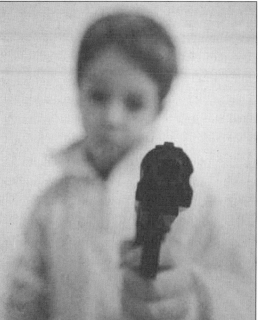

Children carrying guns has become a major issue for American society. This behavior has the potential to result in accidental death, suicide, homicide, and both unintentional and intentional injuries.

© 2000 PhotoDisc, Inc.

---

**Box 3.4    Facts About America's Children**

- Every 25 seconds, a baby is born to an unmarried mother: 1 in 3 babies.

- Every 37 seconds, a baby is born to a mother who is not a high school graduate.

- Every 40 seconds, a baby is born into poverty: 1 in 4 babies.

- Every 56 seconds, a baby is born without health insurance; 1 in 6 children has no health insurance.

- Every 1 minute, a baby is born to a teen mother; 1 in 8 babies.

- Every 2 minutes, a baby is born at low birthweight (less than 5 pounds, 8 ounces); 1 in 13 babies.

- Every 4 minutes, a baby is born to a mother who had late or no prenatal care; 1 in 26 babies.

- Every 4 minutes, a child is arrested for drug abuse.

- Every 10 minutes, a baby is born at very low birthweight (less than 3 pounds, 4 ounces).

- Every 19 minutes, a baby dies.

- Every 41 minutes, a child or youth under 20 dies from an accident.

- Every 2 hours, a child or youth under 20 is killed by a firearm; 1 in 910 children will be killed by guns before age 20.

- Every 4 hours, a child or youth commits suicide.

- Every 19 hours, a young person under age 25 dies from HIV infection.

- One in 138 children will die before his or her first birthday.

- One in 4 children was born poor; 1 in 5 is poor now.

- One in 12 children has a disability.

- One in 24 children lives with neither parent.

Source: Children's Defense Fund. (2000). *The State of America's Children Yearbook 2000*. Washington, DC. Reprinted by permission.

direct and indirect costs (New Jersey Department of Health and Senior Services, 1998). Rotavirus is believed responsible for more than 800,000 deaths annually in developing nations, and about 70 percent of U.S. children ages 1 to 5 years are affected by rotavirus diarrhea. Rotavirus vaccines could yield a net annual savings of $466 million per year in the United States (Jancin, 1997). Despite the fact that vaccine-preventable disease levels have been reduced by over 99 percent since the introduction of vaccines and that all fifty states have legal vaccination requirements, only 76 percent of American infants are fully immunized and more than one million American children remain vulnerable (USDHHS, 1997). Improved health education is one strategy to increase immunization rates and reduce the cost of treating vaccine-preventable diseases.

There is evidence that most of the fifteen leading causes of death, disease, disability, and dysfunction in the United States originate through combinations of diet, smoking, lack of exercise, alcohol, and stress. Any of these can be exacerbated by insufficient or poor health education. Improvement in and provision of quality health education is a good investment in addressing the behaviors that are major factors in death, disease, and disability. Even if health education programs were to result in a modest reduction in risk behaviors, the programs would be cost-effective.

The National Institute on Drug Abuse (1998) estimated the cost of special education to prevent children who were exposed prenatally to cocaine from failing in school to be about $352 million per year nationwide. Every $1 of prevention saves $5 in treatment and other costs. Several inexpensive drug prevention programs are available to schools and community agencies that, if implemented with fidelity, could reduce drug use and its attendant costs.

About one-fourth of pregnant women receive inadequate prenatal care and are three times more likely to deliver low birthweight babies than women who receive adequate care. Almost two-thirds of pre-term and low birthweight births can be prevented or reduced through education, lifestyle change, and early and regular prenatal care. In 1990, U.S. businesses, mostly insurance companies, spent $5.6 billion in costs related to poor birth outcomes.

A basic prenatal education program for 100 pregnancies, including infant car seats and case management, costs about $28,500—the cost of one average pre-term birth, not including long-term costs of the baby (The Willapa Bay Company, 1998).

The cost per student of school health education is relatively low. Even if school health programs produced a modest 10 percent reduction in costs associated with certain risk-taking behaviors, the cost savings would equal billions of dollars.

Medical costs make up a sizable portion of the financial costs of risk-taking behavior. Indirect costs such as lost wages, lower productivity, more absenteeism, high job turnover, and disability payments account for huge expenditures. One has only to look at industry for an economic perspective. Many large American corporations, as well as several of the most successful industrial giants in Japan, provide health promotion programs for employees. These consist of health education, fitness programs, stop-smoking programs, nutrition counseling, and weight-control programs. Companies have found these programs to be cost-effective. If profit-motivated corporations see the benefit of health education, it certainly follows that we should apply this sort of thinking to our schools and other institutions.

# LONG-TERM BENEFITS OF HEALTH EDUCATION

Health education should continue through the life-span and should produce benefits that last a lifetime. Upon developing attitudes conducive to health, acquiring information necessary to make healthy decisions, improving self-efficacy, developing adequate skills, and realizing the other components of health education, people are more likely to

- voluntarily attempt new behaviors and adapt current behaviors to their environment in an effort to improve and maintain a high quality of living
- assume responsibility for their own health, the health of their families, and the health of their communities

- participate in community efforts to improve health

- become role models to others regarding health-related behavior

- support others who attempt to improve or maintain their health

- seek information about health-related matters and use this information to make decisions about their actions and habits

- become more discriminating consumers, including being skeptical about unproven and unsubstantiated treatment regimens and fads

- become active partners with their physicians in their own health care, requiring information from their physicians so that they, as patients, can participate in decisions about their health and treatment

- experience improved self-esteem and self-image

- reduce the effects of stressors

- develop and maintain positive social relationships

- develop a feeling of oneness with nature and the environment

The last benefit in the list above reminds us of the need to use health education as a means of enhancing spirituality. This includes activities that help each individual appreciate his or her unique potential and identify the path that will lead to realization of that potential. It also includes opportunities to develop and strengthen relationships and a sense of connectedness with others, self, or a larger reality.

## KEY POINTS

1. Misunderstanding of the nature of health education has often resulted in allocation of responsibility for it to people with little academic background in the field.

2. Health education is a process, a series of planned activities directed toward goals.

3. There are many misconceptions about health education, including the assumption that it takes no special academic preparation to develop or carry out a health education program.

4. Barriers to health education include competition with other subjects in schools, intensified by the accountability movement; mistaken perception of lack of support from parents and administrators; inadequate professional preparation; and lack of required teacher certification in health education.

5. Health education is a unique discipline with foundations in public health, education, and behavioral sciences.

6. Five philosophies—behavior change, cognitive-based, decision making, freeing/functioning, and social change—dominate the practice of health education.

7. Youth and adults engage in behaviors that put their health and safety at risk. Health education has the responsibility and capacity to reduce these behaviors.

8. Reducing health risks and improving individuals' health has many long-term benefits, some of which are economic.

# REFERENCES

Ahia, R.N. (1991). Compliance with after-sex guidelines among adolescent males: Application of the health belief model and protection motivation theory. *Journal of Health Education, 22*(1), 49–52.

Airhihenbuwa, C.O. (1995). Culture, health education, and critical consciousness. *Journal of Health Education, 26*(5), 317–319.

American Social Health Association. (1996). *N.C. poll: Most voters favor condom education in schools.* News release. May 28.

Anspaugh, D.J., & Ezell, G. (1995). *Teaching today's health* (4th ed.). Boston: Allyn & Bacon.

Association for the Advancement of Health Education. (1991). *Position statement: Teacher certification for health education.* Reston, VA: Author.

Bates, I.J., & Winder, A.E. (1984). *Introduction to health education.* Palo Alto, CA: Mayfield.

Bedworth, D.A., & Bedworth, A.E. (1978). *Health education: A process for human effectiveness.* New York: Harper & Row.

Bennett, J.P., Perko, M.A., & Herstine, J.H. (2000). 1988–1998 national practices in K–12 health education and physical education teacher certification. *Journal of Health Education, 31*(3), 143–148.

Bensley, L.B. (1993). This I believe: A philosophy of health education. *The Eta Sigma Gamma Monograph Series, 11*(2), 1–7.

Bettinghaus, E.P. (1986). Health promotion and the knowledge-attitude-behavior continuum. *Preventive Medicine, 15*(5), 475–491.

Botvin, G.J., & Dusenbury, L. (1992). Substance abuse prevention: Implications for reducing risk of HIV infection. *Psychology of Addictive Behaviors, 6*(6), 70–80.

Bruhn, J. (1988). Life-style and health behavior. In D. Gochman (Ed.), *Health behavior.* New York: Plenum Press.

Bureau of Health Planning and Resources Development. (1973). *Educating the public about health: A planning guide* (DHEW Pub. No. 78-14004). Washington, DC: Dept. of Health, Education and Welfare.

Carlyon, W., & Cook, D. (1981). *Science education and health instruction.* Colorado Springs, CO: Biological Sciences Curriculum Study, 4.

Centers for Disease Control and Prevention. (1997). Guidelines for school and community programs to promote lifelong physical activity among young people. *Morbidity and Mortality Weekly Report, 46*(RR–6).

Children's Defense Fund. (1994). *Wasting America's future: The children's defense fund report on the costs of child poverty.* Washington, DC: Author.

Children's Defense Fund. (2000). *The state of America's children yearbook: 2000.* Washington, DC: Author.

Clark, J.E., Houser, C.M., & Powell, K.D. (1995). *We the people.* Charlotte, NC: Pregnancy Prevention Coalition of North Carolina.

Collins, J.L., Small, M.L., Kann, L., Pateman, B.C., Gold, R.S., & Kolbe, L.J. (1995). School health education. *Journal of School Health, 65*(8), 302–311.

Commission on the Reorganization of Education. (1928). *Cardinal principles of secondary education.* Washington DC: Government Printing Office. (Originally published 1918, Department of Interior, Bureau of Education, Bulletin no. 35.)

Connell, D.B., Turner, R.R., & Mason, E.F. (1985). Summary of findings of the school health education evaluation: Health promotion effectiveness, implementation, and costs. *Journal of School Health, 55*(8), 316–321.

Cottrell, R.R., Girvan, J.T., & McKenzie, J.F. (1999). *Principles and foundations of health promotion and education.* Boston: Allyn & Bacon.

Creswell, W.H., & Newman, I.M. (1993). *School health practice* (10th ed.). St. Louis: Times Mirror/Mosby College Publishing.

Dalis, G.T. (1994) Effective health instruction: Both a science and an art. *Journal of Health Education, 25*(5), 289–294.

Dalis, G.T., & Strasser, B.B. (1977). *Teaching strategies for values awareness and decision making in health education.* Thorofare, NJ: Charles B. Slack.

Derryberry, M. (1960). Health education: Its objectives and methods. *Health Education Monographs, 8*(1), 5–11.

Division of Adult and Community Health, National Center for Chronic Disease Prevention and Health Promotion, Centers for Disease Control and Prevention. *Behavioral Risk Factor Surveillance System Online Prevalence Data, 1995–1998* [On-line]. Available: http://www2.cdc.gov/nccdphp/brfss/index.asp

Donovan, P. (1998). School-based sexuality education: The issues and challenges. *Family Planning Perspectives, 30*(4), 188–193.

Glanz, K., Lewis, F.M., & Rimer, B.K. (1997). The scope of health promotion and health education. In K. Glanz, F.M. Lewis, & B.K. Rimer (Eds.), *Health behavior and health education* (2nd ed.). San Francisco: Jossey-Bass.

Green, L.W. (1984). Modifying and developing health behavior. In L. Breslow, J. Fielding, & L. Lave (Eds.), *Annual Review of Public Health, 5.* Palo Alto, CA: Annual Reviews.

Green, L.W., & Iverson, D.C. (1982). School health education. *Annual Reviews in Public Health, 3*, 321–338.

Green, L.W., & Kreuter, M.W. (1999). *Health promotion planning: An educational and ecological approach.* (3rd ed.) Mountain View, CA: Mayfield.

Green, L.W., Kreuter, M.W., Deeds, S.G., & Partridge, K.B. (1980). *Health education planning: A diagnostic approach.* Palo Alto, CA: Mayfield.

Green, L.W., & Ottoson, J.M. (1999). *Community and population health* (8th ed.). Boston: WCB McGraw-Hill.

Greenberg, J. (1978). Health education as freeing. *Health Education, 9*(2), 20–21.

Greenberg, J., & Gold, R. (1992). *The health education ethics book.* Dubuque, IA: Wm. C. Brown.

Henderson, A.C., & McIntosh, D.V. (1981). *Role refinement and verification for entry-level health educators: Final report.* San Francisco: National Center for Health Education.

Hugick, L. & Leonard, J. (1991). Sex in America. *Gallup Poll Monthly, 313*, 1–9+.

Iverson, D.C., & Portnoy, B. (1977). Reassessment of the knowledge/attitude/behavior triad. *Health Education, 8*(6), 31–34.

Jancin, B. (1997). Rotavirus vaccine could save $466 million per year. *Pediatric News, 31*(11), 8.

Joint Committee on Health Education Terminology. (1973). *Health Education Monographs, 33*, 63–70.

Joint Committee on Health Problems in Education of the National Education Association and the American Medical Association. (1948). *Health education.* Washington, DC: National Education Association.

Kann, L., Kinchen, S.A., Williams, B.I., Ross, J.G., Lowry, R., Hill, C.V., Grunbaum, J.A., Blumson, P.S., Collins, J.L., & Kolbe, L.J. (1998). Youth risk behavior surveillance—United States,

1997. *Morbidity and Mortality Weekly Report, 47*(SS-3), 1–89.

Kelman, H.C. (1961). Processes of opinion change. *Public Opinion Quarterly, 25*(1), 57–78.

Kingery, P.M., Pruitt, B.E., & Hurley, R.S. (1993). Adolescent exposure to school health education: Factors and consequences. *Journal of School Health, 24*(6-Supplement), S42–S46.

Lindley, L.L., Reininger, B.M., Vincent, M.L., Richter, D.L., Saunders, R.P., & Shi, L. (1998). Support for school-based sexuality education among South Carolina voters. *Journal of School Health, 68*(5), 205–212.

Livingood, W.C., Woodhouse, L.D., Godin, S., Eickneier, J., Cosgrove, W., & Howard, M. (1993). Credentialing and competition for social jurisdiction. *Journal of Health Education, 24*(5), 282–284.

McGinnis, J.M., & Foege, W.H. (1993) Actual causes of death in the United States. *JAMA, 270*(18), 2207–2212.

Mullen, P.D., Evans, D., Forster, J., Gottlieb, N.H., Kreuter, M., Moon, R., O'Rourke, T., & Strecher, V.J. (1995). Settings as an important dimension in health education/promotion policy, programs, and research. *Health Education Quarterly, 22*(3), 329–345.

National Institute on Drug Abuse. (1998). *Prevention could save $352 million annually* [On-line]. Available: http://oasas.state.ny.us/pio/ma-1022.htm

New Jersey Department of Health and Human Services. (1998). *Childhood immunization facts* [Online]. Available: http://state.nj.us/health/cd/immfacts.htm

1990 Joint Committee on Health Education Terminology. (1991). Report of the 1990 Joint Committee on Health Education Terminology. *Journal of School Health, 61*(6), 251–254.

Nixon, J.E. (1967). The criteria of a discipline. *Quest, 9*(Winter), 42–48.

Oberteuffer, D., Harrelson, O.A., & Pollock, M.B. (1972). *School health education* (5th ed.). New York: Harper & Row.

O'Rourke, T. (1989). Reflections on directions in health education: Implications for policy and practice. *Health Education, 28*(6), 4–14.

Pentz, M.A. (1985). Social competence skills and self-efficacy as determinants of substance use in adolescence. In S. Shiffman & T.A. Wills (Eds.), *Coping and substance abuse.* New York: Academic Press.

Pollock, M.B., & Middleton, K. (1994). *School health instruction: The elementary and middle school years* (3d ed.). St. Louis: Mosby-Year Book.

Prue, D.M., Wynder, E.L., Scharf, L.S., & Resnicow, K.A. (1987). Health education and behavioral analysis. *Education and Treatment of Children, 10*(1), 19–32.

Ross, H.S., & Mico, P.R. (1980). *Theory and practice in health education.* Palo Alto, CA: Mayfield.

Russell, R.D. (1976). *There is no philosophy of health education! Rather . . . our strength and our weakness is in the many.* Paper presented at AAHE session on philosophy in health education, Milwaukee, WI.

Schinke, S.P. (1984). Preventing teenage pregnancy. In M. Hersen, R.M. Eisler, & P.M. Miller (Eds.), *Progress in Behavioral Modification, 16.* New York: Academic Press.

Seffrin, J.R. (1994). America's interest in comprehensive school health education. *Journal of School Health, 64*(10), 397–399

Seffrin, J.R. (1997). Premises, promises and potential payoffs of responsible health education. *Journal of Health Education, 28*(5), 298–307.

Sharkey, P.W., Graham-Kresge, S., White, Jr., G.L. (1995). Define health education: Health, values, and professional responsibility. *Health Values, 19*(6), 23–29.

Simons-Morton, B.G., Green, W.H., & Gottlieb, N.H. (1995). *Introduction to health education and health promotion* (2nd ed.). Prospect Heights, IL: Waveland.

Smith, D.W., Bibeau, D.L., & Altschuld, J.W. (1991). An analysis of health instruction in selected schools and the personal health characteristics of principals. *Health Values, 15*(1), 21–30.

Smith, D.W., Steckler, A.B., McCormick, L.K., & McLeroy, K.R. (1995). Lessons learned about disseminating health curricula to schools. *Journal of Health Education, 26*(1), 37–43.

Stone, E.J. (1985). School-based health research funded by the National Heart, Lung, and Blood Institute. *Journal of School Health, 55*(5), 168–174.

Tolsma, D.D., & Koplan, J.P. (1992). Health behaviors and health promotion. In J.M. Last & R.B. Wallace (Eds.), *Public health and preventive medicine* (13th ed.). Norwalk, CT; Appleton & Lange.

U.S. Department of Health and Human Services. (1997). *U.S. celebrates national infant immunization week* [On-line]. Available: http://news.medscape.com/govmt/DHHS/1997/apr/InfantImmunizationWeek.html

Welle, H.M., Russell, R.D., & Kittleson, M.J. (1995). Philosophical trends in health education: Implications for the 21st century. *Journal of Health Education, 26*(6), 326–332.

The Willapa Bay Company, Inc. (1998). *Health education information* [Online]. Available: http://twbc.com/healthed.html

Wilner, D.M., Walker, R.P., & Goerke. L.S. (1973). *Introduction to public health* (6th ed.). New York: Macmillan.

# History of Health Education and Health Promotion

Health promotion has been with us for a long time: Religious texts contain stories, parables, and directives concerning health, health behavior, methods to prevent illness, and cleanliness. Learning behaviors that protect health has been a major factor in the development of civilization.

Other steps in our advancement were to require services that improved health status and to insist that others practice health behaviors.

Efforts to educate people regarding health have taken many avenues over the years. When efforts to educate failed to produce the desired result, authorities—backed either by law or by superior numbers—compelled compliance. This might include restrictions such as quarantine. The evolution of health education and health promotion in the United States is inextricably linked to the history of general education and of society at large and must be considered in relation to those events.

Many individuals, including educational theorists who conceived of the mind and body as dependent and inseparable entities, have contributed to health education. Europeans have had particular influence on American education. Jacques Rousseau's ideas about health and physical activity were outlawed in eighteenth-century France but later

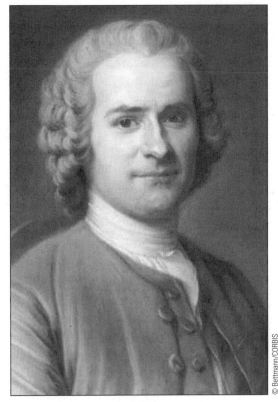

© Bettmann/CORBIS

Jacques Rousseau's ideas led to major reform in educational thought and practice.

contributed to practical reform in educational thought and practice. Strongly influenced by Rousseau, Johann Bernard Basedow was an education reformer who established the *Philanthropinum*—a school that strove to improve the quality of education by relating schoolwork to the world outside the classroom. Basedow is considered the originator of physical education. Johann Heinrich Pestalozzi, also influenced by Rousseau, is considered the father of elementary education. In 1799, he opened a school in Burgdorf, Switzerland, which served as a testing ground for the Pestalozzian system, in which the child is guided to learn through practice and observation and through the natural employment of the senses. Friedrich Froebel worked with Pestalozzi in Switzerland and, in 1816, founded the Universal German Educational Institute, where he developed ideas for the education of preschool children. He is known as the originator of the kindergarten.

Varying from region to region and school to school, American education was often simply the passage of information; at others, it was immersed in religion. Health instruction was often haphazard and steeped in traditions and superstition. We shall begin our discussion of American health instruction with conditions as they were found by European explorers.

## THE PRE-MODERN ERA

Among Native Americans, health information was communicated orally from generation to generation. Group concern for health was evidenced in the selection and preparation of food, recognition of the need for pure water, and procedures for burial. Most tribes had regulations relating to family responsibilities. Nonetheless, Europeans considered Native American medical practices primitive because they were frequently based upon religion and what the explorers considered superstition. Nonetheless, European explorers found a generally healthy population in North America.

With the Europeans came disease and epidemics. Native Americans possessed none of the immunity that comes from generations of exposure to microorganisms, and they were unprepared to take protective measures. Neither culture knew anything about germs; neither had formal health promotion technology as we know it today although both had practitioners of crude medicine. To compound the problem, the settlers had little interest in the health of the native peoples. By the time the Pilgrims landed at Plymouth, the Native Americans of the surrounding countryside had been all but eliminated, apparently by smallpox introduced by the Cabot and Gosnold expeditions. European arrivals had similar effects in Central America and the Caribbean.

The early colonists in North America found life fraught with hardships. They faced the necessity of clearing land and building homes, securing food and transportation, as well as problems brought by the weather and the indigenous peoples. Many starved, died violent deaths, or expired from infectious diseases, which often were of epidemic proportions. Many of the early settlements were eliminated completely by diseases, most notably smallpox.

Smallpox was a deadly enemy, producing several pandemics, most conspicuously in the Massachusetts Bay colonies in 1633, New Netherlands

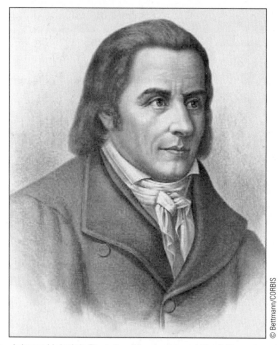

© Bettmann/CORBIS

Johann Heinrich Pestalozzi is considered the father of elementary education.

(New York) in 1663, and Boston in 1752. During the Boston attack, only 174 of the city's 15,000 residents completely escaped smallpox. During the life of George Washington, 90 percent of the people age 21 and older had contracted smallpox at some time in their lives. Boston suffered five epidemics of measles between 1657 and 1740. Epidemics brought by the colonists came close to eliminating Native Americans—and any threat they posed to colonial expansion—as disease spread through the tribes.

Community health action in the colonies was taken only during epidemics and consisted of isolation and quarantine. Otherwise, measures to protect community health were feeble and mostly ineffective.

## Early Records and Boards of Health

As a way of keeping track of the population, causes of death, and maintaining property rights, the Massachusetts colony passed an act in 1639 requiring that each birth and death be recorded. The Plymouth colony followed suit.

In 1701, Massachusetts passed legislation providing for the isolation of smallpox victims and for ship quarantine. In 1746, the Massachusetts Bay colonies passed regulations to prevent the pollution of Boston Harbor.

Local boards of health were established in several cities in the late 1790s. Some of these, most notably those in New York and Massachusetts in 1797, were a result of the spread of yellow fever. It had become a worse pestilence than smallpox during the eighteenth century (and would continue as such during the nineteenth century.) In 1793, for instance, Philadelphia, the capital of the nation, was virtually abandoned as yellow fever killed 10 percent of the population. The disease returned for several years as warm weather supported the mosquito population.

## Education

Harvard College was founded in 1636 and remained the only college in the country for fifty years. It holds special importance to health educators, because it was home to the first required course in hygiene in American higher education. The course consisted of five lectures.

It is noteworthy that an institution of higher education was founded in the United States before compulsory schooling for children was installed. In 1642, Massachusetts was the first of the colonies to establish a law requiring all children to read and write—meant mainly to force the population to understand religion and law. In 1647, the "Old Deluder" law was passed in Massachusetts, requiring towns with at least 50 families to have an elementary school and those with at least 100 households to have a Latin grammar secondary school. The name for the law was a euphemism for Satan, whose efforts to prevent people from reading the scriptures would be hampered if they were taught to read as children.

In 1751, one of Benjamin Franklin's lifelong dreams came to pass with the founding of the Academy. Located in Philadelphia, the Academy was the first institution of secondary education in America. Like Franklin himself, the Academy advocated "healthful situation" and physical exercise. In 1821, the American high school was founded.

In the early days of American education, only boys went to school. Days and terms were short. Individual needs received little attention. Literacy and religion were the major subjects taught. Oral recitation was the primary means of instruction, because few printed materials were available. The schools frequently had no sanitary facilities, used wood stoves, and were poorly built, ventilated, and lighted. Health and hygiene were not emphasized in the colonial or early American school.

## THE PRE-INDUSTRIAL ERA: 1800–1850

The United States underwent significant changes during this period: Land acquisitions—the Louisiana Purchase and others—expanded the size of the country. Inventions and the growth of industry changed American life. However, physicians still practiced the medicine of the ancient Greeks by starving, bleeding, and purging their patients. Surgery was conducted without anesthesia. Often physicians went from one surgery to another without washing their hands. Only a few effective drugs were available, among them digitalis for heart failure and quinine for malaria. Nevertheless, the nineteenth century brought some major advances in medicine and health.

The United States was swept by epidemics of smallpox, typhus, yellow fever, cholera, and typhoid during the first half of the nineteenth century. Tuberculosis also took thousands of lives. Shattuck (1850/1948) reported that the average age at death in Boston decreased from 27.85 years in 1820–1825 to 21.43 in 1840–1845. In New York, the average age at death decreased from 26.15 to 19.69 during the same period. Medical problems were met by physicians with poor training and sometimes questionable motives. Superstition, misconception, and reliance on the supernatural ruled much of the treatment of disease.

Political and social changes led to changes in education, which varied a great deal among the states. States moved toward greater financial support for schools, particularly in the elementary grades. In 1840, Rhode Island passed a law making education mandatory. Other states soon followed suit, although conditions, facilities, and methods remained shoddy. At the same time, teaching as a profession gained attention as new ideas, including those from abroad, influenced the schools. The principles and policies upon which health education would be built were starting to form.

In 1823, the first professional preparation book for health education was published. William A. Alcott, the "father of school health education" in the United States, wrote a widely acclaimed book in 1820 on the healthful construction of schoolhouses, and he was the first to write a health book suitable for children.

Horace Mann, the first secretary of the first state board of education in the United States and probably the most influential educator of his day, discussed the problem of school hygiene in his *First Annual Report of the Secretary of the Board of Education* (Massachusetts) in 1837. In all six of his annual reports between 1837 and 1843, he made powerful recommendations that physiology and hygiene be added to the curriculum of the common (elementary) school. Subsequently, in 1850, Massachusetts became the first state to require mandatory physiology and hygiene by law in all public schools

(Pollock, 1987). Mann also wrote, in several ensuing works, about the value of physical strength, health, and education for health.

Legislation relating to community sanitation was passed in England in 1837. With that legislation, public health was recognized officially for the first time. Soon thereafter, partly because of a devastating cholera epidemic, Parliament appointed the Factory Commission to study the health conditions of the laboring population of England. Child employment conditions were of particular interest to the commission. Edwin Chadwick, author of Britain's draconian Poor Law of 1834, was made secretary of the Factory Commission. In 1842, the commission published *Report on the Sanitary Condition of the Labouring Population of Great Britain*, a milestone in public health history that pointed out that half of the children of the working classes died before age 5. Chadwick's distinctive descriptions of the wretched conditions of the working class, both at home and at work, kindled a resolve in compassionate people to address these problems. This may not have been Chadwick's motivation, given that he held fiercely to the view that the filth and immorality of the poor—not economic policies—were principal causes of disease (Chadwick, 1842/1965). However, William Farr and other new public health professionals and advocates vigorously disputed Chadwick's view, arguing that poverty was not only the direct cause of disease (for example, via starvation) but also a critical determinant of family discord and alcohol abuse (Hamlin, 1995, 1998). Chadwick was the author of the 1848 Public Health Act, which authorized the newly created General Board of Health to establish local boards to deal with water supply, sewerage, and control of offensive trades, as well as to institute surveys and investigations of sanitary conditions in particular districts (Rosen, 1993; Calman, 1998). The impetus for the act lay not only in the growing filth of rapidly industrializing and more densely populated cities, but also in response to a labor movement that demanded improved working conditions, better pay, and decent housing.

## THE MODERN ERA: 1850–1910

Community health promotion in the United States was first widely publicized with publication of the

*Report of the Sanitary Commission of Massachusetts* (Shattuck, 1850/1948), which served as a guide in the health field for a century. Although technically a layperson, Lemuel Shattuck was intelligent, talented, and highly interested in sanitation. According to Pickett and Hanlon (1990):

> Among the many recommendations made by Shattuck were those for the establishment of state and local boards of health; a system of sanitary police or inspectors; the collection and analysis of vital statistics; a routine system for exchanging data and information; sanitation programs for towns and buildings; studies of the health of school children; studies of tuberculosis; the control of alcoholism; the supervision of mental disease; the sanitary supervision and study of problems of immigrants; the erection of model tenements, public bathhouses, and washhouses; the control of smoke nuisances; the control of food adulteration; the exposure of nostrums; the preaching of health from pulpits; the establishment of nurses' training schools; the teaching of sanitary science in medical schools; and the inclusion of preventive medicine in clinical practice, with routine physical examinations and family records of illness.

Well over half of Shattuck's fifty recommendations have become established parts of public health practice. The endorsement of an ambitious program of health education in schools is particularly noteworthy.

Shattuck's report signaled the beginning of the modern era of health. Society began to attack health problems in a disciplined way, even though this attack at first was based upon untrue assumptions. The modern era of health can be divided into five phases:

1. **Miasma phase** (1850–1880), when disease was thought to be caused by noxious vapors

2. **Bacteriology phase** (1880–1910), when it was discovered that specific microorganisms cause specific diseases, enabling the use of more specific means to prevent disease

3. **Health resources phase** (1910–1960), during which enormous financial investments were made in hospitals, health staffing, and biomedical research

4. **Social engineering phase** (1960–1975), when equal access to health services was given priority in legislation and policy so economically, socially,

and educationally disadvantaged people were less likely to lose out on health care

5. **Health promotion phase** (late 1970s until present), when focus has been directed to innovative programming to change behavior that poses risks to health and encourage behaviors that are beneficial to health.

This section juxtaposes these five phases with developments in health education and health promotion. Events are presented mostly in chronological order.

## The Miasma Phase

Epidemics historically were dealt with by quarantine and isolation, partly because of the notion persisting during the miasma phase that diseases were caused by unhealthy vapors. So extreme was this belief that people often used herbs and incense to perfume the air and body in the hope that the smells would fill the nose and crowd out the miasma. Local and state powers were marshaled to fight infectious diseases. In an effort to reduce the outbreaks of yellow fever introduced through the port of New Orleans, the state of Louisiana established a commission to deal with quarantine issues. Though this often is referred to as the first state board of health, it did not function as such because of its narrow focus on quarantine. The first true state health department or board of health was established in 1869 in Massachusetts, with Dr. Henry I. Bowdich as the first head. The board concerned itself with public and professional education in hygiene, various aspects of housing investigation and prevention of various diseases, methods of slaughtering animals for food, sale of poisons, and conditions of the poor.

Florence Nightingale, a true pioneer in health care and health promotion, defined the laws of nursing and the concept of nursing as a profession. She was well known for her hospital reform during the Crimean War (1854–1856) and for advocacy

> **miasma phase** the period of time from 1850 to 1880, when disease was thought to be caused by noxious vapors

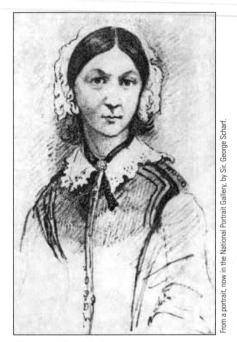

From a portrait, now in the National Portrait Gallery, by Sir. George Scharf.

Florence Nightingale

The American Public Health Association was founded in 1872. The association, still a leader today in the arena of public health, proposed to go far beyond the current quarantine mentality. It projected the interests of hospital hygiene, sanitation, prevention of disease transmission, and other concerns of the public. Today, the APHA is a pacesetter in program development, information sharing, health education, and legislative action and advocacy.

### Scientific Temperance Movement

This movement began with the founding of the Women's Crusade in 1874 by Dr. Dio Lewis. The Women's Christian Temperance Union, as it later was called, became one of the most important pressure organizations in history. It preached the evils of alcohol, tobacco, and narcotics using every medium, including the schools. As a result of the work of the WCTU, led by Mary Hanchett Hunt, 38 states and territories passed laws between 1880 and 1890 requiring the teaching of hygiene and physiology, and in 16 states these subjects were required in all grades of all pupils (Rogers, 1933). Every state passed legislation requiring instruction on the effects of alcohol and narcotics, and Congress established a comparable law for the territories (Rogers, 1930). Many of these laws remained in effect, even after the temperance movement became less influential. The curricula on alcohol often contained myths and fallacious information (Payne & Schroeder, 1925), but it focused attention on health and hygiene education. Not coincidentally, by 1880, more than 35 textbooks had been written specifically for the study of health.

In 1874, a Kalamazoo, Michigan, court case established the right of the community to tax its citizens to support public schools. The present system of class credits was initiated in 1892, based on the recommendation of the Committee of Ten appointed by the National Education Association. The compulsory tax-supported education system that exists today was coalescing.

## The Bacteriology Phase

Beginning in the 1850s, bacteriologists Louis Pasteur and Robert Koch ushered in the bacteriology phase by demonstrating that microorganisms cause

regarding nursing education for hospital nurses. She established the Nightingale Training School for nurses at St. Thomas Hospital in London, which had quite high standards for the time. Nightingale also is known as a social reformer and as an initiator of public health nursing (Monteiro, 1985). In her book *Notes on Nursing*, Nightingale (1859/1946) established the concept that nursing the healthy was even more important than nursing the sick and that preventive hygiene superceded curative care. This notion forms the backbone of much of health promotion and patient education today.

By 1860, most large U.S. cities divided schoolchildren into grades and, by 1870, the concept had spread almost everywhere there were enough students to classify. By the Civil War, state governments in the North generally had created common (public) school systems by enacting laws for tax-supported elementary schools and appointing state school officers. Such support for public schooling came later to the South. Although sixteen states had compulsory attendance laws (for white people) by 1885, most of those laws were sporadically enforced (Olson, 1999).

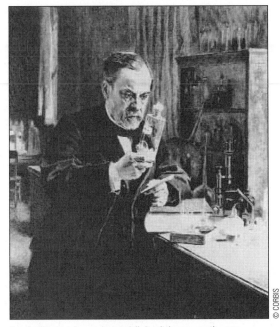

© CORBIS

Louis Pasteur's work established the germ theory of disease.

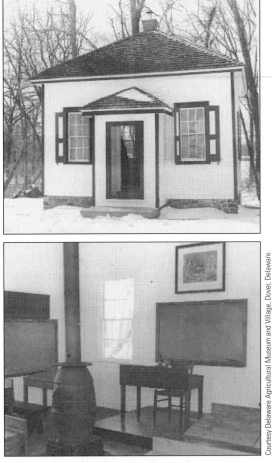

Courtesy Delaware Agricultural Museum and Village, Dover, Delaware.

The tiny one-room school with its pot-bellied stove survived well into the twentieth century.

infectious diseases. Even given these momentous discoveries, old methodologies, such as isolation, quarantine, and placarding, were still the rule of disease prevention, and health education as we know it was virtually nonexistent in this country. Numerous epidemics toward the end of the nineteenth century took a terrible toll among U.S. children. Even survivors were handicapped in their capacity to learn.

## Physical Education Movement
The physical education movement had tremendous impact on health education. The roots of the physical education movement can be traced to the 1866 founding of the American Association for the Advancement of Physical Education (which became the American Physical Education Association in 1903). In 1892 in Ohio and 1899 in North Dakota, those states passed laws making physical education a mandatory part of public school curricula. During the next thirty years, virtually all states passed legislation similar to that of Ohio and North Dakota. Even before 1900, the practice of physical education included health instruction.

One of the early crusaders for health and a leader of the physical education movement was Catherine Esther Beecher, often referred to as the "originator of the first American system of gymnastics and as the first woman physical education leader in America" (Rice, Hutchinson, & Lee, 1958). At age 22, she opened the Hartford (Connecticut) Female Seminary and developed a system of physical education that incorporated calisthenics and

**bacteriology phase**   the period of time between 1880 and 1910, when means to counteract specific diseases were made possible by the discovery that specific microorganisms cause specific diseases

physiology. Her textbook, *Physiology and Calisthenics for Schools and Families* (Beecher, 1856), included 26 lessons on physiology for schools, families, and health establishments. Among Beecher's recommendations were the daily teaching of physical education and physiology, appointment of a coordinator or head of the school health program, and instruction methods beyond the simple dissemination of information.

Another pioneer in the physical education movement was Thomas Denison Wood, a medical doctor. In 1891, at age 26, Wood developed the Department of Physical Training at Stanford University. At the 1883 International Congress on Education at the Chicago World's Fair, where the National Education Association gathered physical educators from all over the country, Wood presented a vision for a "new" physical education (188X):

> Physical education must have an aim as broad as education itself and as noble and inspiring as human life. The great thought in physical education is not the education of physical nature, but the relation of physical training to complete education, and then the effort to make the physical contribute its full share to the life of the individual, in environment, training, and culture.

This conference marked the end of the era in which gymnastics dominated the physical education curriculum and the beginning of a modern era, symbolized by Wood's view of physical education having broad goals to contribute to a student's complete education. From 1911 to 1938, he chaired the Joint Committee (of the National Education Association and the American Medical Association) on Health Problems in Education. Under his leadership, the joint committee moved toward a focus on health instruction, health services, and healthful environment and defined the roles schools were to play in the nation's drive to promote health. In 1927, Wood published *The New Physical Education* with Rosiland Cassidy. The work described a new, progressive philosophy of physical education that participation in fitness, sport, and physical education was important because it contributed to the child's intellectual, social, physical, and moral development and prepared the individual for efficient living in present-day civilization. Wood was also

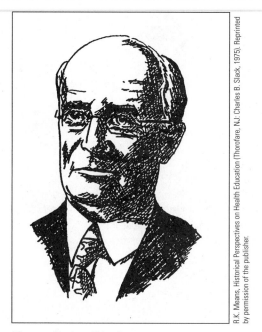

R.K. Means, Historical Perspectives on Health Education (Thorofare, NJ: Charles B. Slack, 1975). Reprinted by permission of the publisher.

Thomas Denison Wood

head of the physical education department at Teachers College, Columbia University, where he initiated undergraduate and graduate programs that were recognized as the training ground for leadership in physical education. According to LaSalle (1960), Wood was renowned for

> his crusade to have school administrators accept their responsibility for the promotion of child health; his labors to help physicians and educators identify and interpret problems of school health; his concept of the school health program as embracing health services, healthful environment (including hygiene instruction), and health instruction, all of which must be coordinated; his concept of improved behavior, rather than mere knowledge, as the ultimate goal in health instruction; his definition of health as "an abundance of life rather than freedom from disease"; his viewpoint that health is a means which enables humans to move toward their goals, and that it is never an end in itself; his realization that the school, the home, and the community must work together if the health of the child is to improve.

In 1894 a Department of Child Study was founded within the National Education Association. A year later, a Department of Physical Education was founded within the NEA (Means, 1975). Both new departments focused on health.

## Era of Medical Inspection

The era of medical inspection actually had its genesis before 1900 because of the prevalence of communicable diseases in children and the recognition that the (now-compulsory) schools could be useful in reducing the transmission of disease. The unsanitary conditions of nineteenth-century schools undoubtedly contributed to epidemics of childhood illnesses. Physicians and nurses worked to identify and exclude from school those pupils who were unequivocally dangerous to others. School physicians and teachers became involved with the health of their students, but in a manner oriented much more toward crisis intervention than toward prevention. These were the beginnings of what we now know as school health services.

During this period, some cities appointed physicians and public health workers to examine children and teachers in the schools. In many locations, teachers were instructed to make daily health inspections of their pupils and report suspected cases of serious disease (Haag, 1972). For instance, in 1899, Connecticut required vision examinations of school children. In 1902, New York City required routine inspections of pupils to detect contagious eye and skin diseases. Connecticut and Vermont began similar programs. In 1902, Lillian Wald demonstrated in New York City that nurses working in schools could reduce absenteeism due to contagious diseases by 50 percent in a matter of weeks (Lynch, 1977). By 1911, more than 100 cities had school nurses. In 1906, Massachusetts made medical inspections compulsory in public schools. Although the medical inspection movement made some progress, it was hampered by a number of problems, not the least of which was inadequate funding.

## Modern Health Crusade

By the beginning of the twentieth century, awareness of children's health problems led to greater acceptance of the need for health education. The Modern Health Crusade of the National Tuberculosis Association was a massive organized effort at improving the health behavior of school children. Simple health rules were printed and distributed to children. Prizes, buttons, and toothbrushes were awarded as incentives. In 1914, these crusaders organized in southern Illinois and were encouraged to practice four rules (Means, 1975):

1. Sleep with your window open.

2. Have fresh air where you work or play.

3. Breathe through your nose with your mouth closed.

4. Get the rest of your family to do the same.

The movement soon was taken up by other states and spread nationally.

The Christmas Seal Campaign to raise funds to fight tuberculosis was initiated in Wilmington, Delaware, in 1907 and was adopted nationally the following year. Beginning in 1915, each child buying or selling 10 cents worth of seals was enrolled as a Modern Health Crusader and was given a certificate with the following health rules (Strachan, 1932):

1. Always breathe fresh air. Never sleep, study, work, or play in a room without a window open.

2. Eat nourishing food and drink plenty of pure water. Avoid food that is hard to digest, like heavy pastries. Never eat or drink anything that weakens the body, like alcoholic drinks.

3. Make sure that everything you put in your mouth is clean. Wash your hands always before eating and bathe your whole body often. Clean your teeth every day. Do not smoke before you grow up.

4. Exercise every day in the open air. Keep your shoulders straight. Take 10 deep breaths every day.

The Record for Health Chores became the basis for the Modern Health Crusaders. Children were encouraged to perform several health chores each day, and various levels of achievement were recognized. The program soon became international in membership. In 1924, the Joint Committee on Health Problems in Education published *Health Education—A Program for Public Schools and Teacher Training Institutions*, which outlined responsibilities and facets of a comprehensive school health program. The crusade owns a particular place in history, however, because through it the National Tuberculosis Association brought health education based upon behavioral aspects of learning into the school—an approach for the future.

Open-Air Classrooms   As a result of the high rates of airborne infections such as tuberculosis, the nation became infatuated with outdoor *open-air classrooms* and schools shortly after the end of the nineteenth century. The practice originally was intended to promote the care and instruction of children whose state of health was below normal. The first open-air classroom in the United States was in the Sea Breeze Hospital on Coney Island in 1904 (Brannon, 1931), which specialized in treating children with tuberculosis. Open-air classrooms later were found in other types of hospitals.

Many cities began providing open-air classrooms in regular schools, including some mandated by local law. As late as 1930, over 1,100 open-air schools existed in the United States, caring for more than 31,000 pupils with health needs. Early in the history of open-air schools and classrooms, health education was integrated into their overall educational plan, including emphasis on the development of positive attitudes toward health.

# THE MODERN ERA: 1910–PRESENT

## Health Resources Phase

### The New Field of Health Education   Anderson (1972) suggested that health education and physical education were considered synonymous until 1910. Then the American Physical Education Association recognized a distinction between the two fields by making "School Hygiene and Physical Education" the theme for its seventeenth annual meeting. Further evidence of the separation between physical education and health education was the awarding of college degrees in health education. Health education still was not fully established in American schools, though. According to the Report of the Committee on the Status of Physical Education in Public Normal Schools and Public High

Schools (1910), 16 percent of high schools gave regular instruction in hygiene, 11 percent prescribed such instruction, and 8 percent granted credit for these courses.

According to the Report of the Committee on the Status of Physical Education in American Colleges (1916), 80 percent of institutions of higher education offered hygiene instruction and 80 of them gave credit toward the bachelor's degree for those courses. In 1917, under the direction of Kathleen Wooten, the Health Department of the Georgia Normal and Industrial College offered courses in "Personal Hygiene and Mothercraft," later titled "Health of the Family." In 1918, the course "Health Education for Teachers" was added to the curriculum. The college was the first institution to grant an undergraduate degree in health education in 1921. Soon thereafter, Teachers College of Columbia University and the Harvard University–Massachusetts Institute of Technology combined program began to award degrees in health education.

## Social Reforms   The period 1900–1920 demonstrated much social reform in the United States. Upton Sinclair's *The Jungle* exposed the unsafe and unhealthy plight of immigrants in the meat packing industry as well as the contamination of food. This led to the passage of the Pure Food and Drug Act of 1906, which provided greater regulation of the food industry. States passed workman's compensation laws.

World War I provided the first large-scale measure of the health status of Americans. The induction examinations of candidates for the armed forces produced dismal results. Approximately 34 percent were rejected because of physical or mental disabilities. This finding led to a change of course in public health in the United States and contributed to the health resources phase. Results of the preinduction physical exams demonstrated clearly that health problems were often the result of chronic conditions such as heart disease, cancer, and cirrhosis of the liver rather than infectious diseases, as had been the case until this time. Many of these health problems could have been prevented, and many of the disabilities could have been corrected.

The shock of finding that a significant number of its supposed fittest and strongest were unfit for military service led to enactment of laws concerning health and physical education in the schools and sparked widespread acceptance of school health education. It also helped make medical examinations a conspicuous part of school programs.

Preventing and controlling communicable diseases clearly were not enough. In addition to chronic conditions, the war helped expose problems of poverty such as malnutrition and the abysmal health condition of children. Providing the highest level of the health resources the nation could muster became the new direction. Health departments began to direct programs toward personal health services such as those for mothers, infants, and children. Most important, the ideas of individual behavior and responsibility were planted in the American consciousness.

One of the most important education documents ever published was the *Cardinal Principles of Secondary Education* (National Education Association, 1918). It marked a significant turning point in secondary education in the United States. The seven principal objectives, as identified by the Commission on the Reorganization of Secondary Education of the National Education Association, were

1. Health
2. Command of fundamental processes
3. Worthy home membership
4. Vocation
5. Citizenship
6. Worthy use of leisure time
7. Ethical character

The cardinal principles provided direction for secondary education and further legitimized and influenced the course of health education.

## Health Education Movement

Early in the century, health administrators recognized that one of the most effective sites for disseminating information and for changing health status was the school (see "Era of Medical Inspection," p. 69). The Child Health Organization of America was formed in 1918 as the Modern Health Crusade was waning. Founding of the CHO often is considered the beginning of the health education movement. The CHO was founded on the recommendation of the Committee on War Time Problems of Childhood of the Pediatrics Section of the New York Academy of Medicine. The committee itself, chaired by L. Emmett Holt, was created as a result of concern over childhood malnutrition. The CHO was founded to proliferate the ideal that knowledge is not always enough to result in practice, and that teachers are the logical source to provide the kind of health instruction that will be effective in establishing acceptable practices.

In 1919, the CHO conducted a national campaign to better the health of American children. The program emphasized the positive rather than the negative. The Rules of the Game (Reaney, 1922) became the basis for further development of health education programs:

1. A full bath more than once a week
2. Brushing the teeth at least once every day
3. Sleeping long hours with windows open
4. Drinking as much milk as possible, but no coffee or tea
5. Eating some vegetables or fruit every day
6. Drinking at least four glasses of water a day
7. Playing part of every day out of doors
8. A bowel movement every day

Publications containing cheerful, health-proclaiming messages were disseminated, and children were encouraged to voice them and adopt their messages. The campaign's approach was summed up by Van Ingen (1935):

> Health education was considered an essential part of the school curriculum and recognition was given both to the possibility and to the necessity of coordinating physical education, home economics, school lunches and other subjects and activities to this important end. Instead of supplying a definite program for teachers to follow, the aim was to develop interest, initiative, and originality on the part of the teacher. . . . In its 5 years, the popular

**health resources phase**   the period of time between 1910 and 1960, characterized by enormous financial investments in hospitals, health personnel, and biomedical research

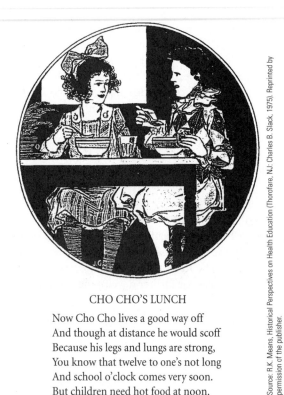

Source: R.K. Means, Historical Perspectives on Health Education (Thorofare, NJ: Charles B. Slack, 1975). Reprinted by permission of the publisher.

### CHO CHO'S LUNCH

Now Cho Cho lives a good way off
And though at distance he would scoff
Because his legs and lungs are strong,
You know that twelve to one's not long
And school o'clock comes very soon.
But children need hot food at noon.

Rhyme of Cho Cho's lunch, a Child Health Organization activity from *Rhymes of Cho Cho's Grandma* by Mrs. Frederick Peterson, 1922.

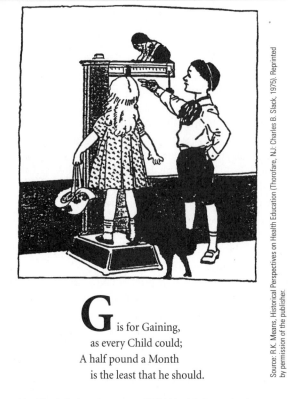

Source: R.K. Means, Historical Perspectives on Health Education (Thorofare, NJ: Charles B. Slack, 1975). Reprinted by permission of the publisher.

**G** is for Gaining,
   as every Child could;
A half pound a Month
   is the least that he should.

Health alphabet rhyme—a Child Health Organization activity from *Child Health Alphabet* by Mrs. Frederick Peterson, New York: Child Health Organization, 1921.

campaign had extraordinary influence on the transformation of information into impact, the promotion of health in schools, and teacher education.

This era marked a turning point in school health programming. The term "health education," which replaced "hygiene," was first proposed at a New York conference of the Child Health Organization in 1919. The word "hygiene" had become unpopular in schools, and it was believed that a new, more definitive term would be helpful in popularizing health practices (Jean, 1946). Between 1918 and 1921, almost every state enacted laws related to health education and physical education for school children. In addition, a new approach to health education was taking root, based on motivational psychology and the understanding of behavior. This approach was to form a philosophical foundation that reaches to the present.

In 1920, the National Education Association's Committee on Standards for Use in the Reorganization of Secondary School Curricula selected health as the first of four objectives—an indication of the priority the most powerful education organization in the United States placed on health. Still, recognition of the professional preparation for health educators was slow in coming; in 1924, only four states had certification requirements for health education teachers in the secondary school (Haag, 1972).

The temperance movement, which provided the impetus for so much early health education, was still evident in health education curricula throughout the 1920s. Its influence was lessening, though, as other topics gained attention.

Curriculum and research in health education was undergoing significant changes in the 1920s. The report issued by the Joint Committee on

Health Problems in Education of the NEA and the AMA (1924), in *Health Education—A Program for Public Schools and Teacher Training Institutions*, clearly demonstrated a change in emphasis with its statement of purpose for health education. According to the committee, the broad aims of health education were

— to instruct children and youth so that they may conserve and improve their health

— to establish in them habits and principles of living which throughout life, and in later years, will assure that abundant vigor and vitality which provide the basis for the greatest possible happiness and service in personal, family, and community life

— to influence parents and other adults, through the health education program for children, to better habits and attitudes, so that the school may become an effective agency for the promotion of the social aspects of health education in the family and community as well as the school itself

— to improve the individual and community life of the future; to insure a better second generation and a still better third generation; a healthier and fitter nation and race

*A Health Survey of 86 Cities*, begun in 1923 (American Child Health Association, 1925), was done to determine what organized activities were being conducted by private and public agencies, including schools, to improve the health of school children. Health education was judged to be mostly a hit-or-miss proposition, consisting mostly of propaganda, pamphlets, and publicity, with little systematic planning of programs. The study led communities to analyze the efficiency of their own work, though. In 1925, the researchers launched a follow-up study involving 70 cities to provide data for administrators to use in evaluating local school health activities.

As *A Health Survey of 86 Cities* showed, public health education in the early 1920s was not consistent. In 1922, however, the American Public Health Association formed a section on Health Education. Believing that the schools were much more systematic in their approach to health education, public

health workers eventually began to adopt the schools' more successful organized approaches and gradually eliminated the propagandizing.

During the 1920s, several commercial companies became interested in health education. They naturally looked upon education largely as a means to augment their sales, and commercial companies often have benefited from the health education of children. Many industries, such as dairy groups, food manufacturers, and insurance companies, began producing health education materials. A number of high-quality curricula and audiovisual materials were funded or designed and disseminated by private companies and by institutes and councils representing industry. They have provided exhibits at the Smithsonian Institution, EPCOT Center in Walt Disney World, and other prominent sites.

The American School Health Association (ASHA) was founded in 1927. From an initial membership of 325 physicians, ASHA has grown to over 3,000 members in 56 countries. A multidisciplinary organization, ASHA counts among its membership administrators, counselors, dentists, health educators, school nurses and physicians, physical educators, and advocates for high-quality school health programs. The mission of the association is to protect and improve the well-being of children and youth by supporting coordinated school health education programs.

By 1929, health and physical education had grown in stature in the schools. Thirty-six states had laws dealing with health and physical education in schools; and 33 states made health and physical education mandatory. Regarding health and physical education, 27 states had standards for time to be allotted for instruction, 30 had published courses of study, 27 had standards for teacher training, 18 had standards for teacher certification, and 20 had general standards for school programs (Meredith, 1933).

In 1937, the National Education Association gave official recognition to school health education. The American Association for Health and Physical Education was formed by the merger of the NEA and the American Physical Education Association. A year later, recreation was added to the title, making it the American Association for HPER. Now the

American Alliance for Health, Physical Education, Recreation and Dance, it is a leading professional organization.

**Research Studies**    The Locust Point Demonstration, beginning in 1914 in a low-income section of Baltimore and continuing for three years, was one of the earliest school health demonstrations. The objective of the project was to increase the level of health in the community. The local Department of Health assigned one part-time physician and one full-time nurse to work with a principal in a school of 900 pupils. Teachers disseminated information to students about various aspects of health, such as balanced diet, importance of sufficient sleep, and the benefits of outdoor exercise. Its team approach proved successful at improving children's and teachers' health. The demonstration attracted national and international attention and visitors from near and far to learn about the project's innovative methods and approaches. Three facts emerged from the demonstration. In Jean's (1946) words, it showed that

> [t]he interest of the teacher in promoting health can be secured; that the interest of the child himself is an essential in influencing his health behavior; and that the child does influence the health behavior of the family.

Other researchers include Clair Turner, a profuse contributor to nearly all areas of public health. His most noteworthy research in health education was the Malden studies, which grew from a health education project in the schools of Somerville, Massachusetts, from 1921 to 1931 (Turner, 1925; Means 1975). The Malden studies are recognized as the first significant research that attempted to demonstrate whether the health of school children could be improved by health education (Hahn, 1982). They contributed in a major way to the philosophy that formal health education in early school years can affect health and health behavior and were instrumental in developing programs still used in school health education today. The study led to the first school health textbook series, re-evaluation and refinement of height/weight tables as growth measures, and the use of audio-visual aids in school health education (Hahn, 1982).

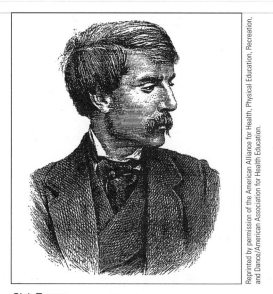

Reprinted by permission of the American Alliance for Health, Physical Education, Recreation, and Dance/American Association for Health Education.

Clair Turner

Delbert Oberteuffer, a true giant in health education, added to the momentum by producing one of the most significant early investigations in health education in the United States. The Ohio Research Study (Oberteuffer, 1932) represented the first attempt to discover students' health needs and interests and use them as a basis for curriculum development. Begun in 1929 and completed three years later, the study's purpose was to determine what to teach in health in secondary schools and where to teach it, and to supply Ohio secondary schools with a practical course of study based on the findings.

Using 24 junior and senior high schools, Oberteuffer gathered student health questions and questions from several health texts and popular books on health. He also analyzed data from health examinations, vital statistics, and judgments from an expert panel to provide information for curricular decisions. The study provided a graded health education curriculum for grades 7–12 free of charge to teachers and schools in Ohio and eventually all over the United States. The Ohio Research Study served as a model for other research into curriculum for many years.

The Cattaraugus County (New York) Studies, sponsored by the Milbank Memorial Fund, was another important research project. The five-year study began in 1931 under the direction of Ruth Grout. The first phase demonstrated the superiority of health instruction in improving health practices and knowledge of health. It also showed that older pupils exposed to health education for a longer time had greater changes in health habits than younger pupils (Grout & Pickup, 1938). The second phase of the project demonstrated the positive influence of a well-planned and -organized health education program on physical conditions in the school environment. This was true especially of sanitary and hygienic conditions in the year that the teaching program directed special emphasis to problems of the environment (Greenleaf & Grout, 1938). The third phase of the Cattaraugus County project showed the value of inservice education for teachers (Strang, Grout, & Wiehl, 1937). Taken together, the Cattaraugus County Studies, through the techniques they utilized and their results, added immensely to knowledge about school health education.

Under the direction of Dorothy Nyswander, the Astoria Study ran from 1936 through 1940. It dealt primarily with school health services in the Astoria Health District of New York City. The study led to significant advancements in cooperation and interaction among school screening methods; health instruction and curriculum; school health personnel ratios; staff training; and cooperation of health counselors.

## Economic Collapse and Medical Advances
The Great Depression wreaked havoc on all parts of the economy, including education. Schools made drastic cuts in education personnel and in program offerings. Many schools, especially in rural areas, were closed. Salaries were cut, and curricula were revised to fit scaled-down budgets. Conditions forced a kind of reconstruction in education, trying new ideas, plans, and fads. All states had established compulsory education. The Depression forced society and schools to focus on children's health needs, with concern shifting to the individual child and his or her needs. Junior high schools and junior colleges developed rapidly, and the vocational rehabilitation school movement also began to unfold.

Medically, tremendous advances took place during the health resources phase. Many were supported by or took place at the National Institutes of Health, which was created in 1887. New treatments were developed, such as insulin treatment of diabetes mellitus by Dr. F. G. Bunting's team in 1921. Dr. Alexander Fleming discovered penicillin in 1929. Means of early detection, such as the Pap smear for cervical cancer, were made available in the 1940s. New drugs, improved medical technology, and prosthetic devices emerged from World War II. The Salk vaccine against poliomyelitis was developed in 1954 and was followed in 1962 by the Sabin oral polio vaccine. Improved surgical techniques and medical discoveries were frequent.

The largest federal health investment during this phase was in hospitals, health personnel, and biomedical research. With the passage of the 1946 Hill-Burton Act, Congress provided huge appropriations to construct medical facilities—although lack of planning, allowed some of these hospitals to be built too close together and thus provide overlapping and unnecessary services (McKenzie & Pinger, 1997). Voluntary health agencies became more involved in health promotion, particularly through health education.

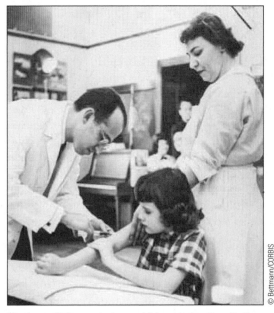

Dr. Jonas Salk vaccinates a child against polio with the vaccine he developed.

**National Conferences and Projects**    A series of important conferences was held between about 1930 and 1960. Among a series of White House Conferences on Child Health and Protection, one stands out as most significant. Its purpose was to study the status of the health and well-being of children, to report what was being done, and to recommend what ought to be done and how to do it (Means, 1975). This 1930 conference produced the most comprehensive list of statements regarding children's needs ever derived from a single conference. It pointed to the teacher's responsibility to guide the child toward healthy living and to select materials for health teaching and health education curriculum; it recommended school health services, including health examinations, immunizations, dental care, school lunch, and adequate guidance; and it called for healthful school living, including fire safety, clean drinking water, ventilation, heating, shower facilities, and gymnasiums.

After an eight-year study, the Progressive Education Association concluded in 1938 that health should be the first of eleven educational goals. In the same year, the Educational Policies Commission of the NEA included personal and community health as objectives under one of the four purposes of education in American democracy (Johnson et al., 1969). These recognitions of the importance of health education were important to the reputation of the fledgling profession.

The School Community Health Project, sponsored by the W.K. Kellogg Foundation, began in 1942. A teacher in a Battle Creek, Michigan, suburb organized a class to teach girls to be nurses' aides. Through the cooperation of community agencies, including hospitals, the class became highly successful. As word of the idea spread, the Michigan Department of Public Instruction solicited the Kellogg Foundation for support. By the 1943–44 school year, 150 Michigan high schools taught the program. Later, 24 additional states received grants from the foundation to start similar projects. The project demonstrated that effective health education is accomplished best through cooperative services of professional personnel of schools and agencies and that this cooperation can be achieved through a health council. It also demonstrated the importance of community understanding and support of health education to its effectiveness (W.K. Kellogg Foundation, 1950).

World War II reinforced, through military pre-induction examinations, the need to improve health and fitness of the population. During World War II, high school and college enrollments dropped dramatically, accompanied by decreased financial support for education. The war, however, did stimulate interest in the health of high school students (Strachan & Jordan, 1947).

A number of significant events combined to align health education with other fields of education in the 1940s and 1950s. The Office of Education initiated the Physical Fitness program in 1941, with the aid of the army, navy, Public Health Service, and the U.S. Children's Bureau. The Victory Corps, launched in 1942, emphasized fitness and vocational studies in high schools. The Committee on Wartime Health Education for High School Students was appointed, and a program titled High School Victory Corps was developed. Materials and resources were developed for health education. Health programs in schools and colleges enlarged, providing a wider variety of content, new activities and services, and an emphasis on healthful school living. General education recognized and supported health education as an essential part of the curriculum during these troubled times.

Throughout the 1940s, Oberteuffer and others vigorously proposed stronger teacher preparation in health education. He also acted to dispel the idea (still held by many) that only physicians should give health information.

By 1945, most schools offered expanded class time for health education. Compulsory education in health, first aid, social hygiene, and occupational health problems was becoming the norm. By 1950, health education generally was becoming an integral part of elementary, secondary, and collegiate curricula (Means, 1975).

The United Nations Conference of 1945 in San Francisco led to the founding of the World Health Organization in 1948, a milestone in the history of international health. At the urging of Clair Turner, a Health Education section was established. Most of the early health education work of that organization was in the area of public health education. The WHO has been a world leader in providing health services to disadvantaged people throughout the world and in stimulating and conducting medical research. The WHO also did some work in school health in cooperation with the United Nations Educational, Scientific, and Cultural Organization, which was created at the same time as the WHO to promote the three areas identified in its title.

During the 1950s, a number of studies were conducted to evaluate the role of school health services and health service personnel, particularly the school nurse. The Committee on School Nurse Policies and Practices of the American School Health Association (1956) published a paper entitled "Recommended Policies and Practices for School Nursing," which has been a useful guide over the years.

The President's Conference on the Fitness of American Youth in 1956 was the first of several President's Conferences on Fitness. The initial conference, held in Annapolis, Maryland, explored fitness issues, including the role of schools and health education. One of the outcomes of this conference was establishment of the President's Council on Youth Fitness. The council promotes fitness programs in schools, initiates new programs, and coordinates the efforts of individuals and groups interested in fitness.

## Social Engineering Phase

**Equal Access**   Health advances brought about by technology and resources obviously were not distributed evenly throughout the population. Therefore, provision of equal access to health services was given priority in legislation and policy during the social engineering phase. Economically, educationally, and socially disadvantaged people frequently had missed the benefits of community health programs. Outreach programs—designed to deliver services to the doorstep of those in need—became the mainstay of local health departments.

By this time, the insurance industry was an integral part of the health care delivery system. Those who could afford insurance usually received medical care. As part of the New Frontier legislation of the Kennedy administration and the War on Poverty of the Johnson administration, Congress enacted numerous laws to funnel federal monies through state and county agencies to provide

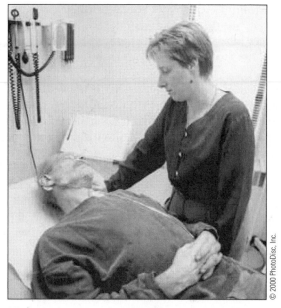

Medicare ensures a level of health care for the elderly.

medical and social services to people previously deprived of these services.

Perhaps the most significant legislation in the history of providing medical care was the creation of Medicare and Medicaid in 1965. The two groups most likely to be without health insurance, the elderly and the poor, were to be covered by these two programs. But although much of the gap in the utilization of medical services between high- and low-income people had closed by the end of the 1960s, the differences in death and disease rates between rich and poor, white and non-white, urban and rural populations lingered.

The decade of the 1960s presented unique challenges to health education. An eruption of social and health problems provided tremendous need for health instruction. The use of illicit drugs raged, characterized by widespread use of both new and familiar drugs, increased availability, epidemic addiction, and increasing defiance of authority and social order. Spurred by the newly marketed birth

**social engineering phase**   the period of time between 1960 and 1975, when legislation and policy prioritized equal access to health services

control pill, patterns of sexual behavior changed. Even with the pill so accessible, the teenage pregnancy rate increased dramatically.

The social engineering phase was characterized by large expenditures of state and federal monies for health care and the design of a "system" of health care built around federal and state financing (Medicare and Medicaid), regional planning, sophisticated delivery of services, and improved quality control. Virtually ignored in the legislative scheme was prevention. Health education and preventive behaviors were far down the list of federal priorities. Partially as a result of this line of thinking, health-care costs have continued to exceed the rate of inflation for years and have become an ever-larger percentage of the gross national product.

In 1960, just prior to the massive increase in drug use and adolescent pregnancy, the White House Conference on Education specified health as one of the fourteen areas about which American youth should be educated (Johnson et al., 1969). In the same year, the Golden Anniversary of the White House Conference on Children and Youth announced as its purpose "to promote opportunities for children and youth to realize their full potential for creative life in freedom and dignity" (Brown, 1959). Among the 1,400 recommendations emerging from this conference, a good deal of attention was given to all aspects of school health education programs, especially school health services and healthful school living.

The health consumer was beginning to want more of a voice in decisions affecting his or her health. The combination of an inflationary spiral of the economy, the need to reduce health care costs, and the growing evidence that health education could reduce costs and that preventing disease was cheaper than treating it led to more interest in health education. Health education became a mandated service in some organizations and states and a recommended, rapidly growing service in others (Breckon et al., 1998). Both the demand for and the supply of health educators grew, particularly in community health settings. Many of those appointed to positions designated as health education were not qualified, although functional definitions and standards of preparation and practice were virtually absent. Professionally trained health educators

began to clamor for improvements in professional preparation. The emphasis on accountability sustained interest in advancing preparation. This situation presented an opportunity for colleges and universities to develop health education undergraduate and graduate programs at a rapid pace.

**The Concept Approach: SHES**    One of the major developments in health education was the introduction in the mid-1960s of the concept approach, which stemmed from the School Health Education Study (SHES). The project—inspired by Deputy Commissioner of the State Health Department of New York Granville Larimore, MD; Herman Hilliboe, MD, head of public health practice, Columbia University; and three educators working in school and college health education—was funded by the Samuel Bronfman Foundation and Minnesota Mining and Manufacturing (3M) and directed by Elena Sliepcevich. The SHES was the first attempt to determine what children and youth in the United States know about health and scientifically develop a health education curriculum following the basic principles used for all other educational curricula. Taking part in the study were 135 school systems, 1,460 schools, and more than 840,000 students from 38 states (Sliepcevich, 1967).

The first phase of the study involved a survey of health education in the nation's schools, evaluation of instructional practices, and testing of student health behavior. The findings revealed dreadful conditions. Health education had been viewed as a benign hygiene and physiology course. Practices more applicable to physical education were applied to the organization of health education, grouping of students, number of periods allotted for health education, preparation of those assigned to teach, and titles given to courses (Means, 1975). In some cases, state requirements for certification of elementary school teachers did not require any preparation in health education. The SHES demonstrated obvious inadequacies in instructional materials, as well as lack of time in the curriculum and unqualified staff. Some health topics were omitted, and others were repeated grade after grade with no increase in level of sophistication. The findings indicated problems and weaknesses so huge that immediate action was crucial.

In the second phase, the SHES dealt with development of curriculum materials. The result was a concept approach that became a model for health education curriculum development for grades K–12. The conceptual approach was predicated on three key concepts: growing and developing, decision making, and interaction. Part of the beauty of the SHES format is that the conceptual statements (presented in Box 4.1) represent major ideas under which health subject matter could "fit"; the framework need not be revised for each new health problem or crisis (Cortese, 1993). It also produced a cycle plan delineating the scope and sequence of health education for K–12 curriculum development. Many teaching materials and publications flowed from the SHES.

In 1967, the Connecticut State Board of Education initiated a study to determine the health interests and concerns of school children in all grades.

---

**Box 4.1**  **Ten Conceptual Statements from the School Health Education Study**

1. Growth and development influences and is influenced by the structure and functioning of the individual.
2. Growing and developing follows a predictable sequence, yet is unique for each individual.
3. Protection and promotion of health is an individual, community, and international responsibility.
4. The potential for hazards and accidents exists, whatever the environment.
5. There are reciprocal relationships involving people, disease, and environment.
6. The family serves to perpetuate humans and to fulfill certain health needs.
7. Personal health practices are affected by a complexity of forces, often conflicting.
8. Utilization of health information, products, and services is guided by values and perceptions.
9. Use of substances that modify mood and behavior arises from a variety of motivations.
10. Food selection and eating patterns are determined by physical, social, mental, economic, and cultural forces.

---

The report, called *Teach Us What We Want to Know* (Byler, 1969), quantified in detail the health areas of interest or concern to students of various ages. The study continues to influence curriculum development in health education. Student input in curriculum development has become accepted as a positive and useful principle.

During the decade of the 1970s, the nation continued to mature educationally and try new ideas. The open classroom experiment met with some success, but little popularity. The decade saw tremendous growth in community colleges. Higher education became less a refuge for the elite and more of a training ground for the general population. Educational and medical research continued to flourish. In 1977, smallpox became the first infectious disease to be eradicated by public health efforts.

The nation had not yet approached the real potential of health education. After more than a year of study, the President's Committee on Health Education identified serious shortcomings in health education. The committee reported the following (U.S. Department of Health, Education, and Welfare, 1973):

> Although the major causes of illness and death can be affected by individual behavior, health education is a neglected, under-financed, fragmented activity with no agency inside or outside of government responsible for establishing short- or long-term goals.

> Virtually no component of society makes full use of health education. That includes the health care delivery system, the educational system, voluntary health agencies . . .

> School health education in most primary and secondary schools either is not provided at all, or loses its proper emphasis because of the way it is tacked onto another subject such as physical education or biology, assigned to teachers whose interests and qualifications lie elsewhere.

> There has been little effort to bring together the fields of health education, parent education and early childhood education for planning and evaluation.

Sadly, nearly three decades later these words still apply in many parts of the country. However, the committee recommended that model state laws for school health education be developed and adopted, the feasibility of matching state funds for health education with federal funds be explored, and that the federal government initiate research and evaluation in school health education.

A major shift occurred in health education during the decade of the 1970s. Health education began to move away from the emphasis on acquisition of facts toward a curriculum model based on the affective domain, which consists of emotions, feelings, and attitudes. This shift paralleled a general trend in education that sprang from humanistic psychology.

Further clarification of health instruction goals continued in the late 1970s and into the 1980s. Health instruction became viewed as a two-phase process that first motivated students to make a choice relative to health behavior and then helped them to practice and adopt the chosen behavior. The behavior evaluated was students' ability to use the process rather than the overt personal health behavior exhibited when they were away from school (Lohrmann, Gold, & Jubb, 1987).

## Medical Cost Containment
During the early 1970s, the search for ways to contain costs of medical care became a major federal priority. The late 1960s and early 1970s produced health planning acts, peer-review requirements for quality control, and new forms of medical care delivery. The health maintenance organization, pushed by the Health Maintenance Organization Assistance Act of 1973, was the most noticeable new form of medical care delivery, one that was supposed to emphasize health education. As attention turned to fine-tuning the medical care system, state and local health departments lost much of their financial and political base. However, it became evident that, as medical costs escalated, attention had not yet been focused on health promotion. Interest in a positive, nationwide strategy to help Americans gain control of their own health led to the formation of the President's Committee on Health Education.

The first vision of health promotion emerged in 1974 in response to several factors, including growing disillusionment with the limits of medicine, pressures to contain medical care costs, and a social and political climate emphasizing self-help and individual control over health. Almost simultaneously with the passage of legislation regarding health

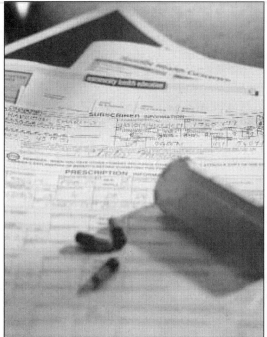

© 2000 PhotoDisc, Inc.

As insurers try to hold down costs, patients suffer increased out-of-pocket expense for prescription drugs and other health care.

planning and health care delivery, renewed interest in disease prevention and health promotion arose in Great Britain, Canada, and the United States.

Control of medical care costs will continue to be a policy issue well into the twenty-first century. Few people doubt that health promotion and disease prevention can reduce costs, but they receive very little of the health care dollar in the United States. Given that health care finances are finite, the public and government must make choices. For instance, do we want to spend large amounts of money to treat a chronic disease at the end of life or do we want to fund programs for those who are healthy, such as immunization for children in need or worksite wellness programs? Such questions are not easy to answer when we realize that it is people with genuine pain and loving family members who are at stake. Further, the attempt at health care reform in the early 1990s demonstrated the political extremes of citizens with no health insurance versus the interests of an industry straining under the weight of increasing costs.

**Comprehensive Education**   The 1970s produced a number of significant events in health education. Although the SHES study produced a marvelous plan for comprehensive school health instruction, most school districts were unwilling to provide time in the curriculum, faculty trained professionally in health education, and supporting services (Cortese, 1993). The 1970s saw much promotion of legislation on the state and local levels to mandate delivery of health education and implementation of a comprehensive approach. Several states were successful. A national task force developed a handbook for state policymakers on planning and implementing "comprehensive school health education." That phrase, along with "comprehensive school health program," became important parts of the language of school health in the 1980s.

The National Center for Health Education (NCHE) was created in 1975 at the recommendation of a President's Committee on Health Education as an independent nonprofit organization. NCHE's mandate was to encompass advocacy for health education, convening health educators, technical assistance for health educators, research and evaluation of health information, and information exchange. One of NCHE's primary contributions was national leadership of the School Health Curriculum Project, which produced the *Growing Healthy* curriculum. The President's Committee also recommended that health education be explored for preschool children, that model state laws for school health education be developed and adopted, and that the feasibility of matching state funds with federal funds to support school health education be explored.

The Coalition of National Health Education Organizations was formally established in 1972. The coalition of eight organizations provides consultation regarding health education program planning and implementation. Each organization sends a representative to the coalition to act when all organizations agree to speak together for the profession.

## Health Promotion Phase

In 1976, the Society for Public Health Education approved and published the first genuine code of ethics for health educators. Although the code did not gain acceptance by other professional organizations, it marked the beginning of a new era in the evolution of health education as a full-fledged profession.

**The Groundwork for Health Promotion**   Although the origins of health promotion practice occurred in the 1940s, it was not given institutional expression or a name until publication of *A New Perspective on the Health of Canadians*, usually referred to as the Lalonde Report (1974) after its author. This publication ushered in both a new concept and a new era in public policy, the health promotion phase. It also popularized the concept that the "health field" consisted of four equally weighted elements to which death and disease could be attributed: human biology (heredity), environment, lifestyle (behavior), and inadequacies in current health care provision. (The health field concept was summarized in Chapter 1.)

The Lalonde Report laid the groundwork for broader reconceptualizations of health that were to follow by elevating biology, environment, and lifestyle to the same level as medical care. Arising from the old public health movement, which was sparked by the reports of Chadwick and Shattuck and nurtured by health education, health promotion became a matter of public policy only with Lalonde's document. The report was hailed as "the first official government statement of policy that recognized the beginning of a new era in public health" (Terris, 1984). As a result of this report, the Canadian government shifted its emphasis away from treatment to prevention of illness and, ultimately, to health promotion.

The U.S. government officially entered the health promotion arena with publication of *Healthy People: The Surgeon General's Report on Health Promotion and Disease Prevention* by the U.S. Department of Health, Education and Welfare (1979).

**health promotion phase**   the period of time beginning in 1975 and continuing into the present, when educational, political, social, and economic interventions are employed to promote adaptations that will improve or protect individuals' health

This report argued that "we are killing ourselves," not only by "our own careless habits," but also by polluting the environment and permitting harmful social conditions to exist. Like the Lalonde Report, the Surgeon General's Report called attention to the substantial role individuals can play in modifying their personal behaviors, and it articulated governmental support for health education and health promotion to influence change in those behaviors.

A year after publication of *Healthy People,* the U.S. Department of Health and Human Services issued *Promoting Health/Preventing Disease: Objectives for the Nation.* The year 1990 was targeted for meeting the objectives. These two publications indicated that some members of federal government recognized the importance of preventive behavior.

International Conferences    Prompted by the Lalonde Report, the World Health Organization was the principal mover in the field of health promotion, especially on the international level, for the next fifteen years. Meeting in Alma Ata in the Soviet Union in 1978, representatives of 134 nations forming the World Health Assembly committed all member countries to the principles of the *Declaration of Alma Ata* to strive for health for all by 2000. The declaration stated that primary health care was the key to attaining health for all, and it also incorporated a commitment to community participation and intersectoral action—currently recognized elements of any earnest health promotion program. Lifestyle and structuralist approaches were combined in HFA (World Health Organization and United Nations Children's Fund, 1978). More equitable access, health education, and maternal and child care were also listed as essential elements of primary health care. Unfortunately, the member states' commitment to the HFA has been irregular, with only moderate success at meeting regional targets. Volatile international political and economic circumstances, limited resources, and lack of political will has attributed to poor progress (Rathwell, 1992).

Ottawa, Canada, was the host for the first international conference on health promotion in November 1986. The Ottawa conference produced a charter outlining five principal areas for health promotion action that provide a useful framework for delivering health promotion programs:

— building healthy public policy
— creating supportive environments
— strengthening community action
— developing personal skills
— reorienting health service

The Ottawa Charter included three processes through which people could start to take control of their own health: mediation, enablement, and advocacy.

The second international conference on health promotion was held in Adelaide, Australia, in April 1988. The main thrust of this conference was healthy public policy as an arm of health promotion. It delineated certain policy priorities, including support of health for women, nutrition policies, policies on alcohol and tobacco, and policies concerning the environment. Health equity and policy accountability were designated as underpinnings of these priority areas. Also, an implicit assumption—one that has been shown to be faulty—is that only central government policymaking had any real effect on measures for health promotion.

The third international conference on health promotion was convened in Sandsvall, Sweden, in June 1991. With the theme "Supportive Environments for Health," it produced a handbook on action to improve public health and the environment. The conference and the handbook explored practical ways to create physical, social, and economic environments compatible with sustainable development.

The fourth international health promotion conference was assembled in Jakarta, Indonesia, in July 1997. Its focus was directions and strategies required to address the challenges of promoting health in the twenty-first century. The priority areas identified were (WHO, 1997)

• promote social responsibility for health (including restriction of production and trade in tobacco and armaments)

• increase investment for health development (especially in housing and education and for women, children, older adults, and poor and marginalized populations)

- consolidate and expand partnerships for health
- increase community capacity and empower the individual (including more practical education, leadership training, and access to resources)
- secure an infrastructure for health promotion (including new mechanisms for health promotion funding and incentives for action)

Participants in the Jakarta Conference endorsed the formation of a global health alliance, the goal of which is to advance the priorities for action in health promotion. Priorities of the alliance include:

- raising awareness of the changing determinants of health
- supporting the development of collaboration and networks for health development
- mobilizing resources for health promotion
- accumulating knowledge on best practice
- enabling shared learning
- promoting solidarity in action
- fostering public accountability in health promotion

## Foundations for Health Education   The "back to basics" movement in the early 1980s questioned the roles of health education and physical education in schools. Nevertheless, during the 1980s, health education had its share of bright moments. The health education establishment was moved to action by publication of health objectives for the nation (U.S. Department of Health and Human Services, 1980). (See Chapter 8 for a discussion of this publication.) The PRECEDE model (Green et al., 1980) set the standard for health planning frameworks. The office of the Surgeon General, U.S. Department of Health and Human Services (1981) expressed strong support for school health education.

In 1982, the Centers for Disease Control (CDC) reorganized and included a School Health Section, demonstrating further federal interest. In the same year, the National School Health Education Coalition (NaSHEC) was formed to enhance networking and cooperation among health agencies for the improvement of health education. The Office of Disease Prevention and Health Promotion (ODPHP)

entered into an agreement in 1985 with the American School Health Association (ASHA) to develop model strategies to relate the 1990 health education objectives for the nation to the school population. ODPHP, ASHA, the Association for the Advancement of Health Education (AAHE), and the Society for Public Health Education (SOPHE) entered into a cooperative agreement for an ongoing national survey of knowledge, attitudes, and practices in school health.

Although the epidemic of acquired immune deficiency syndrome (AIDS), which struck in the late 1970s, was a worldwide tragedy, it provided the opportunity for health educators to demonstrate their skill and expertise. Once researchers identified human immunodeficiency virus (HIV) as the cause of the disease and recognized its risk factors, the most exhaustive education efforts against any single health entity were mustered. Mass media campaigns and federal publications directed to the home and schools carried the message that HIV is usually contracted as a result of chosen behaviors, such as sexual activity and injectable drug use and, therefore, is mostly preventable. However, the power of certain groups that have fought against any form of sex education in schools, and particularly have battled HIV/AIDS education, has driven home a remarkable point: The health and lives of children may be at risk because of reluctance to educate them about the realities of life. At present, rates of HIV infection continue to rise. In 1987, the CDC established cooperative agreements with fifteen organizations for AIDS education.

In 1991, the landmark *Healthy People 2000* (U.S. Department of Health and Human Services, 1991) was released, containing several objectives related directly to health education. (This publication is discussed in Chapter 8.) The Drug Free Schools and Communities Act of 1986 provided more than $200 million to fight drug abuse. The U.S. Department of Education was designated to offer the funding to schools and communities. The initiative was later expanded and renamed the Safe and Drug Free Schools and Communities Act with escalating funding.

During the 1980s, particularly the latter part of the decade, a number of curricula were developed by foundations, corporations, and voluntary health organizations. Many of these complete and packaged curricula were donated to school districts or were made available at low cost. This trend continued in the 1990s. Three examples are the National Dairy Council nutrition curriculum and the *Project ALERT* and *Project Northland* substance use prevention curricula.

In the 1980s, the practice of health instruction moved toward incorporation of affective education and personal skills development in concert with other theoretical modes from psychology, including social learning theory, inoculation theory, and problem behavior theory (Parcel & Baranowski, 1981; Botvin & Wills, 1985). The various shifts in planning that began in the 1960s illustrate a progressive process whereby previously held ideas are refined, retained, and subsumed as new research and theory emerge. During the 1980s, this resulted in the development of research-based curriculum models founded solidly in various aspects of educational and behavioral psychology (Lohrmann, Gold, & Jubb, 1987).

The evaluation of *Teenage Health Teaching Modules*, conducted from 1986 to 1989, provided evidence of positive effects on knowledge, attitudes, practices, and some self-reported behaviors in selected sub-groups of students (Nelson, Cross, & Kolbe, 1991). Although this is not a comprehensive K–12 grade evaluation, it provides powerful evidence of what can be expected from school-based education.

It had become necessary for health educators to "speak with one voice," to possess a common language. In this spirit, five professional organizations and one representative from the American Academy of Pediatrics produced a widely disseminated document, *Report of the 1990 Joint Committee on Health Education Terminology* (1990 Joint Committee, 1991), which defined numerous terms associated with the discipline.

The Goals 2000: Educate America Act, a result of a 1989 education summit of state governors and President George Bush, was passed in 1991. The act provides funding to schools or school districts for standards-based school improvement efforts. Although it has been stymied somewhat by political events, content standards for various subject areas have been developed. Through the sponsorship of the American Cancer Society and the cooperation of four professional organizations, *National Health Education Standards: Achieving Health Literacy* was published in 1995. (This outstanding document is discussed in Chapter 7, and the standards are contained in Appendix C.) Certainly, by implementing a coordinated school health program with emphasis on national standards, schools can address directly or indirectly all of the Education Goals.

**Education Reform**   Since the early 1980s, education reform has focused on producing an educated and productive workforce to ensure the nation's competitiveness in the world economy (Greene & McCoy, 1998). This movement has been spurred by American students' disappointing performance on standardized tests in comparison with those of other industrialized nations and with those of students of the past. Best-selling books (e.g., Bloom [1987] and Hirsch [1987]) bemoaned how today's youth are intellectually, morally, and academically inferior compared with earlier generations. This led in the 1990s to a movement to reform the education system in the United States and to demand accountability from those responsible for student performance. The Goals 2000: Educate America Act spurred the movement and supported state efforts to develop clear and rigorous standards for what every child should know and be able to do. These goals are listed in Box 4.2. A number of models of school reform have been proposed and implemented across the U.S. Forty-seven states plus the District of Columbia and Puerto Rico have comprehensive Goals 2000 plans for education reform (U.S. Department of Education, 1998).

More recently, school reform focus has shifted somewhat to structural change. This would allow more flexibility in implementing programs, shared decision making within each school, links between curriculum standards and assessment and accountability, family involvement, and options for which schools students attend (Greene & McCoy, 1998).

The connection of health and education is gaining advocates and momentum in discussions of education reform. Business leaders, who helped initiate the school reform process, recognize that one of the essential components of a successful education system is "health and other social services sufficient to reduce significant barriers to learning." Schools should address students' health and well-being in partnership with families and other persons in the community. Schools cannot and should not be

---

**Box 4.2** Education Goals 2000

By the year 2000,

1. All American children will start school ready to learn.

2. The high school graduation rate will increase to 90 percent.

3. All students will leave grades 4, 8, and 12 having demonstrated competency over challenging subject matter including English, mathematics, science, foreign languages, civics and government, economics, arts, history, and geography, and every school in American will ensure that all students learn to use their minds well, so they may be prepared for responsible citizenship, further learning, and productive employment in our nation's modern economy.

4. The nation's teaching force will have access to programs for the continued improvement of their professional skills and the opportunity to acquire the knowledge and skills needed to instruct and prepare all American students for the next century.

5. United States students will be first in the world in mathematics and science achievement.

6. Every adult American will be literate and will possess the knowledge and skills necessary to compete in a global economy and exercise the rights and responsibilities of citizenship.

7. Every school in the United States will be free of drugs, violence, and the unauthorized presence of firearms and alcohol and will offer a disciplined environment conducive to learning.

8. Every school will promote partnerships that will increase parental involvement and participation in promoting the social, emotional, and academic growth of children.

Source: From *The National Education Goals Report: Building a Nation of Learners*, National Education Goals Panel, 1994. Washington, DC: U.S. Government Printing Office.

---

expected to do the job alone (Business Roundtable, 1992).

It has been argued very convincingly (McKenzie & Richmond, 1998) that each of the education goals has a direct or indirect link to the objectives of a coordinated school health program. The most obvious examples are Goals 1 and 7. Coordinated school health programs also contribute to Goal 2 by providing quality prevention programs that keep more young people in school. They also contribute to Goals 3 and 6 by preparing students to be critical thinkers and problem solvers; responsible, productive citizens; self-directed learners; and effective communicators (Boyett & Conn, 1991; Secretary's Commission on Achieving Necessary Skills, 1991).

Despite their relationship to national education goals, health education issues—reducing student health risk behavior, changing student attitudes, and increasing knowledge and health-related skills—are not typically a part of the standards used to measure student and teacher achievement. They are not a part of the accountability process. When health education is not integrated into overall goals, we risk school health education being relegated to a lesser position than it held before the accountability movement began. By January 1998, 38 states had drafted academic standards in core subjects (English, mathematics, science, and social studies), and 34 states used standards-based assessments of math and English (The Center for Education Reform, 1999). Many states require that students pass tests constructed to conform to the standards before they can progress to the next grade or graduate. Unfortunately, in some schools, any subject, content, or skill not found on the achievement test, may not merit time in the school schedule. Few states and districts require that health-related information, let alone behavior, be measured on achievement tests used to evaluate student, teacher, and administrative performance. This, of course, produces a troubling and contradictory picture when (as will be discussed further in Chapter 7) strong evidence supports the idea that healthy students perform better academically.

Barriers to school reform include loss of demonstration project funding, teacher opposition, parental apathy, leadership turnover, and the feeling that one model fits all communities. Added to these is resistance from people, including educators, who observe that, when standardized tests become the primary measurement of student and teacher performance, teachers concentrate on teaching to the tests to the exclusion of other important issues.

The long-term effects of school reform are unknown, although it is certain that education reform and pursuit of the Education Goals 2000 will continue well into the twenty-first century. School districts and states must find ways to incorporate the coordinated school health program (the phrase that replaced "comprehensive school health program"). In the long run, it may be the key to successful reform.

*Healthy People 2010* (2000), which contains the national health objectives for the year 2010, has the potential to further the implementation of school reform and strengthen school health programs during the reform process. The objectives include numerous references to school health education, school nurses, school health environment, nutritious school meals and snacks, and physical education, as well as to increasing high school completion rates.

People of the future may look back at the 1990s and beyond as a period of **social ecology** (Cottrell, Girvan, & McKenzie, 1999). The ecological perspective takes into account social, political, and economic surroundings. Given that the focus on altering individuals' behavior has produced mixed results, some educators suggest that a more complex approach—that recognizes important supports to behaviors and requires health educators to address them—is in order. This approach was broached in the 1990s, principally in the public health arena. If the ecological perspective continues to be featured in health promotion, we may be seen as initiating the sixth phase of the modern era.

# A BRIEF HISTORY OF SEXUALITY EDUCATION

No discussion of health and health education would be complete without including issues relating to the family and sexuality. Throughout this century, either through legislative mandate or social evolution, women have gained more social freedom.

Traditional mores have been questioned, probably first as a result of large numbers of people coming in contact with other societies during World War I. As a result, family roles were brought into question and sometimes altered. The view of sexual behavior as being sinful declined, and arguments were advanced supporting sexual expression as natural and meaningful. The family structure started to shift from a patriarchal form to a somewhat more democratic style. Dating influenced the selection of a mate and afforded opportunities for people to know each other better before forming permanent relationships.

The story of sexuality education in the United States has been one of controversy and hard-fought battles. Because sexuality has been entangled with other social forces historically addressed by education, it could be argued that sexuality education has existed for centuries. In an expansive sense, perhaps this is true. Sexuality education in a formal organized sense, however, can be traced back about a century. As early as the 1880s, several groups, including the YMCA, YWCA, American Purity Alliance, and the Child Study Association sponsored lectures and panels on topics related to human sexuality. The National Congress of Parents and Teachers and the National Education Association conducted discussions on school-based sexuality education in the early 1890s (Carrera, 1971).

Early in the twentieth century, the topic of sexuality education began to appear somewhat regularly in educational literature. References often were made to sexuality education in school and to the importance of instruction in sexual hygiene and preparation for marriage and parenthood—so-called sex hygiene. Boys and girls were usually separated for this instruction. The 1919 White House Conference on Child Welfare, at which it was stated that "the problem of [sex] instruction becomes more properly a task of the school" (Means, 1962), provided impetus for instruction in human sexuality in the schools. Two publications, titled *The Problem of Sex Education in Schools* and *A High School Course in Physiology in Which the Facts of Sex Are Taught*, were published in 1919 by the U.S. government.

Margaret Sanger gave energy to the contraceptive movement in the 1920s and 1930s. She opened clinics designed to make birth control information and services available. Her writing, emphasizing the right of women to control their own bodies and the positive effects that fertility control could have on marriage, influenced thinking on many family-related issues. Sanger's work inevitably led to contraception education in many venues.

Despite the heightened interest in sexuality education, the majority of school systems in the United States did not provide sexuality education by the mid-1920s. Even in the late 1920s, courses in physiology and hygiene frequently omitted any mention of sex. During the 1930s, a number of significant statements were made supporting sexuality education in the schools, including that from the 1930 White House Conference that the school should provide instruction in "social hygiene, including sex; and in the preparation for potential parenthood" (Means, 1962). These statements were

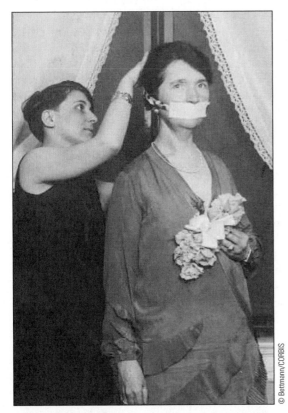

Margaret Sanger was a pioneer in the provision of contraception for women. Here she dramatizes the silencing of women about issues regarding their reproductive health.

not transformed into action in most instances. In 1940, a pamphlet titled *High Schools and Sex Education* was published by the U.S. Public Health Service. It broadly covered methods, materials, planning, organization, and integration of sexuality education within many fields, along with a suggested outline of a course for teachers of sexuality education in secondary schools (Bruess & Greenberg, 1994).

Some important action finally occurred in 1950, when the Mid-Century White House Conference on Children and Youth accentuated the importance of family life education, indicating that well-prepared teachers should emphasize sexuality in a humanistic and psychologically oriented fashion. The American School Health Association launched a nationwide program in family life education in 1953 with the support of several other organizations. A number of important pamphlets on sexuality education were published by prestigious organizations such as the American Medical Association and the Joint Committee on Health Problems in Education of the National Education Association.

The decade of the 1960s brought widespread availability of the birth control pill and, with it, more permissive attitudes about sex. "Free love" was one of the slogans of the youth of that decade. The need for education regarding sexuality was even more important and, though inroads were made into school curricula, vocal opposition to sexuality education persisted. Organizations such as the John Birch Society, the Christian Crusade, and Mothers Organized for Moral Stability were active in their opposition to sex education, sometimes referring to such programs as "smut," "immoral," and "a filthy communist plot" (Haffner & de Mauro, 1991; People for the American Way, 1994). Their goal was to eliminate all sex education in schools, and they achieved some success.

The birth of two significant organizations provided momentum for the movement for comprehensive sexuality instruction through their publications and educational programs: The Sex Information and Education Council of the United

**social ecology**   the health perspective that takes into account the social, political, and economic milieu in which people exist

States (SIECUS) and the American Association of Sex Educators, Counselors, and Therapists. Although gains were being made, a survey of teacher preparation institutions indicated that less than 10 percent of them offered coursework specifically designed to prepare instructors to teach sexuality education, despite the U.S. Department of Education's encouragement and support of family life and sex education programs and teacher training programs (Bruess & Greenberg, 1994).

Despite the many advances in sexuality education, the opposition groups clearly had an impact. By the early 1970s, legislatures in twenty states had voted to restrict or abolish sexuality education programs (Haffner & de Mauro, 1991) and only three states and the District of Columbia required schools to provide sex education (Kenny & Alexander, 1980).

Widespread fear of HIV/AIDS sparked interest and support for school sexuality education in the 1980s. It became politically untenable to argue that sexuality education should not be taught in schools in light of the fact that the deadly disease is transmitted through sexual intercourse. A 1993 assessment of state sex education programs by the SIECUS revealed that 48 states either mandated or recommended sexuality education programs in schools through state law or policy (Gambrell & Haffner, 1993). By December 1997, 19 states and the District of Columbia had laws or policies that *required* schools to provide sexuality education, and 34 states and the District of Columbia mandated instruction about HIV, AIDS, and other sexually transmissible diseases (NARAL, 1998) The SIECUS assessment found that 38 states had developed state sexuality curricula, although many exclude such topics as abortion, homosexuality, and masturbation. Virtually all teens now receive some sexuality education in high school. Box 4.3 provides a summary of historical events relating to sexuality education.

Although significant progress has been made in the area of educating children and adults about their sexuality, and though a large majority of parents and students support sexuality education (Adolescent Pregnancy Prevention Coalition of North Carolina, 1993; Hugick & Leonard, 1991; Public Agenda, 1994), a vocal minority of opposition remains. This opposition takes the form of

criticism of textbooks, curricula, teachers, and even board of education members. In some cases, it is orchestrated by groups who are not even residents of the community. Some conservative groups have published their own family life curricula, which are often laden with misinformation and material designed more to promote guilt than to inform and educate.

Research into the effects of sexuality education programs suggests that one of the most important requirements for success of the program is the quality of the teacher (Carrera, 1971). The likely effects of well-planned and implemented programs now can be predicted with a great deal of accuracy. As a result of this research and of supporting statements from influential organizations such as the Alan Guttmacher Institute and the Planned Parenthood Federation of America, sexuality education programs have become more prominent and are being instituted into comprehensive health instruction programs across the continent. One of the consistent and historical arguments against sexuality education is its alleged contribution to or encouragement of early sexual activity. Several studies show that sexual intercourse did not increase after presentation of pregnancy prevention programs that included discussions of abstinence, contraception, and disease prevention and that taught teens decision-making and communication skills (Kirby, 1997; Frost & Forrest, 1995). In fact, such programs can help teens delay the onset of intercourse, can reduce the frequency of sex, and can increase the likelihood that they will use condoms and other contraceptives when they do become sexually active (Jemmott, Jemmott, & Fong, 1998; Kirby, 1997; Main et al., 1994). A report by the World Health Organization found no evidence that sexuality education in schools leads to earlier or increased sexual activity among young people. This review of 35 studies indicated that sexuality education is most effective when given before a young person becomes sexually active, and programs promoting postponement of sexual intercourse and protected sexual intercourse were more effective than those promoting abstinence alone (Howard & McCabe, 1990). Recent research has indicated that "safe sex training" courses administered at clinics can significantly increase the number of adults who avoid unprotected sex (MSNBC, 1999). Moreover, researchers have found no methodologically sound studies that show abstinence-only programs delay initiation of sexual intercourse (Kirby, 1997; Wilcox, 1996). Nevertheless, in 1996 Congress appropriated $250 million to promote abstinence-only education programs over a five-year period, an amount which was increased the next year.

Despite government funding for abstinence-only programming, recent data indicate that the main message emphasized in both school district policy and curricula today is most likely to be a comprehensive one—that is, to include both abstinence and contraception versus presenting abstinence as the only option. However, fewer than half of the junior and senior high schools provided

---

**Box 4.3   Sexuality Education: Important Historical Events**

| | |
|---|---|
| 1892 | National Education Association promoted sexuality education as a needed part of a national curriculum and passed a resolution favoring "moral education in the schools." |
| 1899 | PTA promoted sexuality education before puberty. |
| 1906 | YWCA promoted sexuality education as part of a total health program. |
| 1910 | American Federation of Sex Hygiene founded; renamed American Social Hygiene Association in 1913. |
| 1913 | YWCA created a Commission on Sex Education. |
| | Fourth International Congress on School Hygiene promoted publicly funded sexuality instruction for parents to get support for sexuality education. |
| 1919 | U.S. government supported sexuality education as part of White House Conference on Child Welfare Standards. |
| 1920 | U.S. Public Health Service conducted fifty regional conferences on sexuality education in high schools and colleges. |
| 1922 | U.S. Public Health Service published the *Manual on Sex Education in High Schools*. |
| | American Birth Control League founded. |
| 1930 | U.S. government supported sexuality education as part of White House Conference on Child Health and Protection. |
| 1940 | U.S. Public Health Service labeled school sexuality education as "urgent need." |
| 1942 | American Birth Control League renamed Planned Parenthood Federation of America, Inc. |
| 1952 | International Planned Parenthood Federation founded. |
| 1953 | American School Health Association launched a national family life education program. |

| | |
|---|---|
| 1960s | A concerted effort to stop sexuality education was launched by John Birch Society, Christian Crusade, Parents Opposed to Sex and Sensitivity Education, Sanity on Sex, and Mothers Organized for Moral Stability. |
| 1964 | Sex(uality) Information and Education Council of the United States incorporated. |
| 1967 | American Association of Sex Educators, Counselors and Therapists founded. |
| 1968 | Center for Family Planning Program Development founded. |
| 1970 | U.S. Congress enacted Title X of the Public Health Service Act, providing support and funding for family planning services and educational programs. |
| 1977 | Center for Family Planning Program Development renamed the Alan Guttmacher Institute. |
| 1980s | Interest in sexuality education increased because of the relationship between sexual activity and HIV/AIDS. |
| 1985 | Alan Guttmacher Institute published *Teen Pregnancy in Industrialized Countries*, which showed that the U.S. teen pregnancy rate is the highest in the industrialized world. |
| 1986 | U.S. Surgeon General declared a need for school sexuality education. |
| 1990 | National Coalition to Support Sexuality Education established by SIECUS. |
| 1996 | U. S. Congress appropriated $250 million to promote abstinence-only sexuality education programs as a part of welfare reform (the next year the amount was raised to $500,000 for the next five years). |

information about where to get and how to use contraception and condoms, and as many as half of schools do not address issues such as abortion and sexual orientation (The Henry J. Kaiser Family Foundation, 1999). An Alan Guttmacher Institute study (Landry, Kaeser, & Richards, 1999) indicated that, among the 69 percent of public school districts that have a district-wide policy to teach sexuality education, 14 percent have a comprehensive policy that treats abstinence as one option for adolescents in a broader sexuality education program; 51 percent teach abstinence as the preferred option for adolescents, but also permit discussion about contraception as an effective means of protecting against unintended pregnancy and disease; and 35 percent (23 percent of all U.S. school districts) teach abstinence as the only option outside of marriage, with discussion of contraception either prohibited entirely or permitted only to emphasize its shortcomings.

# PROFESSIONAL CREDENTIALING

The qualifications necessary to become a health educator have long been debated. As programs developed in institutions of higher education to prepare professions, many came to appreciate the need to establish some degree of uniformity. Perhaps this need also reflected a desire for means of comparing one program to another. Issuing formal credentials became the favored method of evaluating professionals. This led to the later establishment of certain criteria for professional preparation programs.

The actual process of formal credentialing of health educators was initiated in 1948 (Cleary, 1986) with the National Conference on Undergraduate Professional Preparation in Health Education, Physical Education, and Recreation, held in Jackson's Mill in Reston, Virginia. The conference was co-sponsored by nine educational organizations (Patterson, 1992). The Jackson's Mill Conference focused on improving professional preparation programs and recognizing professional competencies needed by teachers and leaders in health education, physical education, and recreation (Athletic Institute, 1948). This conference was followed by several others,

including the Conference of the Undergraduate Professional Preparation of Students Majoring in Health Education, in December 1949, and the National Conference on Graduate Study in Health Education, Physical Education, and Recreation, in January 1950 —all of which focused on professional preparation with emphasis on identifying competencies.

The American Public Health Association's Committee on Professional Education, chaired by Clair Turner, released a report in 1957 that recommended adding standards for educational evaluation, adding at least one year of graduate education in public health for qualification as a public health educator, and recognizing that the need for health educators was six to seven times greater than the supply. Furthermore, the report recommended that health educators' preparation emphasize social, biological, and health sciences as well as education and educational psychology (Creswell, 1986).

In 1962, the American Association for Health, Physical Education, and Recreation (AAHPER) sponsored a national conference titled "Professional Preparation in Health Education, Physical Education and Recreation Education." Professional competencies were defined for each of seven areas (Patterson, 1992):

1. Philosophy and objectives of professional preparation

2. Organization and administration

3. Student personnel

4. Faculty

5. Curricula

6. Professional laboratory experiences

7. Facilities and instructional materials

During the 1960s, a number of significant reports were issued on the subject of professional preparation of health educators. These reports came principally from the Society for Public Health Education and AAHPER. In 1967, professional standards were being developed for community health educators. Community health leaders were considering having their programs accredited, a step that would be helpful in placing graduates in the workforce and would allow accredited programs to be eligible for public health traineeship funds. To provide a mechanism for accrediting programs, the Public Health Service subcontracted with the National Commission on Accrediting to develop accreditation criteria and guidelines. Based on the result of this action, the American Public Health Association in 1969 issued its criteria and guidelines for accrediting graduate programs in community health education (Creswell, 1986).

In 1971, President Richard Nixon, responding to the failure of the nation to keep pace with other Western nations in vital areas such as infant mortality, childhood immunization, and life expectancy, created the President's Committee on Health Education. The resulting committee report recommended the creation of public and private organizations to stimulate, coordinate, and evaluate health education programs. The upshot was the formation of the Federal Bureau of Health Education at the Centers for Disease Control and the National Center for Health Education, which was formed as an independent organization from the research arm of the SOPHE (which was known as the Health Education Research Council). The administration believed it could preserve the health of Americans, control escalating health care costs, and present a less costly alternative than national health insurance, which was being proposed at the time (Guinta & Allegrante, 1992). A presidential report (Nixon, 1971) at that time stated

> It is in the interest of our entire country . . . to educate and encourage each of our citizens to develop sensible health practices. Yet we have given remarkably little attention to the health education of our people.

In 1973, AAHPER sponsored a conference to improve professional preparation by identifying guidelines for undergraduate teacher preparation programs. The conference also produced recommended competencies and personal qualifications of health teachers (AAHPER, 1974).

Based on a 1977 SOPHE report titled "Guidelines for the Preparation and Practice of Professional Health Educators" and visits to several SOPHE chapters, society President-Elect Helen Cleary (1995) wrote,

> The field was in desperate need of implementation of the concepts delineated in the report. What I found . . . was a profession in disarray. Many health educators could not define themselves nor their role. It was clear that the preparation of most was so varied that there was no common core.

Clearly, the time had arrived to upgrade professional practice and preparation. Box 4.4 presents significant events in this process.

The upgrade took a significant turn in February 1978, establishing a direction that led more directly to the birth of a true credentialing process. The federal government sponsored a workshop that has come to be known as the First Bethesda Conference, at which a representative group of health educators met to discuss the "commonalities and differences in preparation and practice of community, patient, and school health educator" (Hoover, 1980). The result of this workshop was a major recommendation that the roles and competencies of entry-level health educators be defined as the initial step in a credentialing process. The Division of Associated Health Professions of the Health Resources Administration and the National Center for Health Education entered into a contract in September 1978 that resulted in the Role Delineation Project. The National Task Force on the Preparation and Practice of Health Educators was an outgrowth of the First Bethesda Conference. The task force, consisting of representatives of eight professional organizations, was given the responsibility of developing a credentialing system for health educators (Patterson, 1992).

Developing a credentialing system required delineation of the roles of health educator and verifying those roles. This was accomplished as the Role Delineation Project, which established the concept of training a generic health educator. The concept held that all health educators, regardless of audience or setting, should have common roles, competencies, and skills. At a 1981 meeting, information on curriculum content utilized in institutions that prepare health educators formed the basis for a resource document titled *A Guide for the Development of Competency-Based Curricula for Entry Level Health Educators*. The guide, subsequently revised and retitled *A Competency Based Curriculum Framework for the Professional Preparation of Entry-Level Health Educators*, defined the competencies and

| Box 4.4 | Development of Certification for Health Education Specialists |
|---------|---------------------------------------------------------------|

| | |
|------|-----|
| 1978 | First Bethesda (MD) Conference: Workshop on Commonalities and Differences in the Preparation and Practice of Health Educators |
| | National Task Force on the Preparation and Practice of Health Educators, Inc., established to develop a credentialing system for health educators |
| 1980 | Role delineation and refinement by the National Task Force on the Preparation and Practice of Health Educators, Inc. |
| 1981 | National Conference for Institutions Preparing Health Educators, Birmingham (AL), to discuss the delineated role and its potential impact on the field |
| 1983 | Dissemination of "A Guide for the Development of Competency-Based Curricula for Entry-level Health Educator" |
| 1985 | Dissemination of revised document "A Framework for the Development of Competency-Based Curricula for Entry-level Health Educators" |
| 1986 | Second Bethesda (MD) Conference: Workshop on Quality Assurance in the Delivery of Health Education Services: Credentialing Health Education Specialists |
| 1988 | National Commission for Health Education Credentialing, Inc., (NCHEC) was established. |
| 1989 | Charter Certification Phase; certification through examination of credentials |
| 1990 | First certification examination for Health Education Specialists |
| 1991 | National Council for the Accreditation of Teacher Education adopted NCHEC responsibilities and competencies for accreditation of programs preparing school health educators |
| 1992 | Joint Committee for Graduate Standards established |
| 1998 | Competency Update Project commenced to review and evaluate the responsibilities and competencies and establish entry-level and advanced competencies |

skills the Role Delineation Project deemed essential to entry-level health educators.

The Second Bethesda Conference met to decide future directions and goals of the Task Force (National Task Force on the Preparation and Practice of Health Educators, 1986). It was decided that the Task Force should develop a plan of action for establishing a credentialing process for health educators, including raising money, developing self-assessment instruments, identifying the most appropriate structure to carry out credentialing in health education, and bringing together the organizations involved in credentialing for health education.

In June 1988, the National Commission on Health Education Credentialing (NCHEC) was established. NCHEC grants the credential titled Certified Health Education Specialist (CHES). The Role Delineation Project is the basis for the examination that leads to the CHES designation. (Chapter 13 discusses this and other issues relating to credentialing.) The first examination for CHES was given in 1990. The Responsibilities and Competencies for Entry-Level Health Educators formed the basis for accreditation for undergraduate professional preparation programs in health education.

The process is underway to revise the responsibilities and competencies. This effort will produce both entry-level and advanced competencies.

In 1997, the Standard Occupational Classification Policy Review Committee approved the creation of a new, distinct classification for the occupation of health educator (Auld, 1997/1998). This means that all federal agencies that collect occupational data, including the Bureau of Labor Statistics and the Bureau of the Census, will now collect data on health educators. Many state and local governments will follow suit. It is unlikely that this recognition would have occurred had the profession not developed and published a set of unique competencies.

## KEY POINTS

1. The evolution of health education and health promotion is tied to historical events of general education and society at large.

2. The modern era of health is divided into five phases: miasma, bacteriology, health resources, social engineering, and health promotion.

3. Pioneers such as Catherine Esther Beecher, Thomas Denison Wood, Kathleen Wooten, and L. Emmett Holt helped develop a foundation for health instruction and school health services.

4. Health education was recognized as distinct from physical education during the early part of the twentieth century, the seminal event being the recognition of "school hygiene and physical education" by the American Physical Education Association in 1910.

5. Rejection of large numbers of inductees for military service in World War I led to a change in public health direction, enactment of laws covering health and physical education in schools, acceptance of school health education, and inclusion of medical exams as part of school health programs. The publication of the *Cardinal Principles of Secondary Education* in 1918 marked a turning point in U.S. secondary education and further legitimized school health education.

6. Between 1918 and 1921, almost every state enacted laws related to health education and physical education for school children. By 1929, 33 states made health and physical education mandatory in school.

7. Several studies and demonstration projects extended the body of knowledge about health education. Turner's Malden studies were instrumental in development of modern school health education. Oberteuffer's Ohio Research Study determined what should be taught in secondary school health programs and provided a health education curriculum for grades 7–12. The Cattaraugus County Studies contributed mightily to the body of knowledge about school health education. The Astoria Study led to significant advances in school screening methods, health instruction, and staff training.

8. Inequities in health care services among Americans spurred the development of many programs in the 1960s, including Medicare and Medicaid. Although vast expenditures were devoted to the redesign of the health care system, prevention and health education remained lower priorities.

9. The School Health Education Study demonstrated enormous problems and weaknesses in school health education and provided a conceptual model for health education.

10. The 1970s saw governments and professional organizations pushing for "comprehensive school health education."

11. The Lalonde Report ushered in a new concept in health promotion and a new era in public policy. The report prompted a series of international conferences that brought international commitments to health promotion.

12. Inclusion and utilization of health education to further education reform and the pursuit of Education Goals 2000 has not been fully accomplished.

13. The ecological perspective of health promotion may result in the 1990s and beyond being recognized as the social ecology phase of the modern health era.

14. Sexuality education, though opposed by many groups, is favored by most parents and students. Comprehensive sexuality education programs have been shown to delay onset of intercourse, reduce the frequency of intercourse, and increase the likelihood of using condoms and other contraceptives among those who are sexually active.

15. A decades-long process culminated in the adoption of a profession-wide set of responsibilities and competencies for health educators and the Certified Health Education Specialist credential.

# REFERENCES

Adolescent Pregnancy Prevention Coalition of North Carolina. (1993). *We the people.* Charlotte, NC.

American Association for Health, Physical Education, and Recreation. (1974). *Report of the national conference on undergraduate professional preparation in dance, physical education, recreation education, safety education and school health education.* Washington, DC: National Education Association.

American Cancer Society. (1995). *National health education standards: Achieving health literacy.* Atlanta: Author.

American Child Health Association. (1925). *A health survey of 86 cities.* New York.

American School Health Association. (1956). Recommended policies and practices for school nursing, ASHA committee on school nurse policies and practices. *Journal of School Health, 26*(1), 13–26.

Anderson, C.L. (1972). *School health policies.* St. Louis: C. V. Mosby.

Athletic Institute. (1948). *Report on the national conference on undergraduate professional preparation in physical education, health education and recreation.* Chicago.

Auld, E. (1997/1998). Executive edge. *SOPHE News & Views, 24*(4), 4.

Beecher, C.E. (1856). *Physiology and calisthenics for schools and families.* New York: Harper and Brothers.

Bloom, A. (1987). *The closing of the American mind.* New York: Simon and Schuster.

Botvin, G.J., & Wills, T.A. (1985). Personal and social skills training: Cognitive-behavioral approaches to substance abuse prevention. In C.S. Bell, & R. Battjes (Eds.), *Deterring drug abuse among children and adolescents.* Washington, DC: U.S. Government Printing Office.

Boyett, J.H., & Conn, H.P. (1991). *Workplace 2000: The revolution reshaping American business.* New York: Dutton.

Brannon, J.W. (1931). Open-air schools in the United States. *Proceedings of the Fifth Congress of the American School Health Association.* Springfield, MA: American School Health Association.

Breckon, D.J., Harvey, J.R., & Lancaster, R.B. (1998). *Community health education: Settings, roles, and skills for the 21st century.* Gaithersburg, MD: Aspen.

Breuss, C.E., & Greenberg, J.S. (1994). *Sexuality education: Theory and practice* (3rd ed.). Dubuque, IA: Brown and Benchmark.

Brown, E.G. (1959). The 1960 White House Conference on Children and Youth. *National Parent-Teacher, 54*(2), 16–19.

The Business Roundtable. (1992). *The essential components of a successful education system: Putting policy into practice.* Washington, DC.

Byler, R.V. (1969). *Teach us what we want to know.* New York: Mental Health Materials Center.

Calman, K. (1998, August 29). The 1848 public health act and its relevance to improving public health in England now. *British Medical Journal, 317,* 596–598.

Carrera, M. (1971). Preparation of a sex educator: A historical overview. *Family Coordinator, 20*(2), 99–108.

The Center for Education Reform. (1999). *Answers to frequently asked questions about state and local reform issues* [On-line]. Available: http://edreform. com/faq/reform.htm

Chadwick, E. (1842/1965). *Report on the sanitary condition of the labouring population of Great Britain.* Edinburgh, Scotland: Edinburgh University Press.

Cleary, H. (1986). Issues in the credentialing of health education specialists: A review of the state of the art. In W.B. Ward, *Advances in health education and promotion: A research manual 1,* Part A (pp. 129–154). Greenwich, CT: Jai Press.

Cleary, H. (1995). *The credentialing of health educators: An historical account 1970–1990.* New York: The National Commission for Health Education Credentialing.

Cortese, P.A. (1993). Accomplishments in comprehensive school health education. *Journal of School Health, 63*(1), 21–23.

Cottrell, R.R., Girvan, J.T., & McKenzie, J.F. (1999). *Principles and foundations of health promotion and education.* Boston: Allyn & Bacon.

Creswell, W. (1986). Professional preparation: A historical perspective. *National Conference for Institutions Preparing Health Educators.* Washington, DC: U.S. Department of Health and Human Services.

Frost, J.J., & Forrest, J.D. (1995). Understanding the impact of effective teenage pregnancy prevention programs. *Family Planning Perspectives, 27*(5), 188–195.

Gambrell, A., & Haffner, D. (1993). *Unfinished business: A SIECUS assessment of state sexuality education programs.* New York: SIECUS.

Green, L.W., Kreuter, M.W., Deeds, S.G., & Partridge, K.B. (1980). *Health planning: A diagnostic approach.* Palo Alto, CA: Mayfield.

Greene, B.Z., & McCoy, K.I. (1998). The national role in coordinated school health programs. In E. Marx, S.F. Wooley, & D. Northrop (Eds.), *Health is academic: A guide to coordinated school health programs.* New York: Teachers College Press.

Greenleaf, C.A., & Grout, R.E. (1938). Evaluation of a rural school health education project: II. A study of the effectiveness of a rural school health program in improving the school environment. *Milbank Memorial Fund Quarterly, 16*(2), 156–172.

Grout, R.E., & Pickup, E.G. (1938). Evaluation of a rural school health education project: III. A study of pupil health practices. *Milbank Memorial Fund Quarterly, 16*(4), 382–402.

Guinta, M.A., & Allegrante, J.P. (1992). The President's Committee on Health Education: A 20-year retrospective on its politics and policy impact. *American Journal of Public Health, 82*(7), 1033–1041.

Haag, J.H. (1972). *School health program* (3rd ed.). Philadelphia: Lea and Febiger.

Haffner, D.W., & de Mauro, D. (1991). *Winning the battle: Developing support for sexuality and HIV/AIDS education.* New York: SIECUS.

Hahn, D.B. (1982). The Malden studies: The first experimental research project in school health education. *Health Education, 13*(4), 8–9.

Hamlin, C. (1995). Could you starve to death in England in 1839? The Chadwick-Farr controversy and the loss of the "social" in public health. *American Journal of Public Health, 85*(6), 856–866.

Hamlin, C., (1998). *Public health and social justice in the age of Chadwick: Britain 1800–1854.* Cambridge, England: Cambridge University Press.

The Henry J. Kaiser Family Foundation. (1999) *Policy and politics: Sex education in public secondary schools* [On-line]. Available: http://www.kff.org/ content/1999/1560

Hirsch, Jr., E. (1987). *Cultural illiteracy.* Boston: Houghton Mifflin.

Hoover, D.B. (1980). *The initial role delineation of health education: Final report.* Bethesda, MD: U.S. Department of Health and Human Services.

Howard, M., & McCabe, J.B. (1990). Helping teenagers postpone sexual involvement. *Family Planning Perspectives, 22*(1), 21–26.

Hugick, L., & Leonard, J. (1991). Sex in America. *Gallup poll monthly 313,* 1–9+.

Jean, S.L. (1946). Health education—some factors in its development. *News Letter, 5,* School of Public Health, University of Michigan, 1–4.

Jemmott, J.B., Jemmott, L.S., & Fong, G.T. (1998). Abstinence and safer sex: A randomized trial of HIV sexual risk-reduction interventions for young African-American adolescents. *Journal of the American Medical Association, 279*(19), 1529–1536.

Johnson, J.A., Collins, H.W., Dupuis, V.L., & Johansen, J.H. (1969). *Introduction to the foundations of American education.* Boston: Allyn & Bacon.

Joint Committee on Health Problems in Education of the National Education Association and the American Medical Association. (1924). *Report of joint committee on health problems in education of the national education association and the American medical association: Health education—a program for public schools and teacher training institutions.* New York: NEA.

Kenny, A.M., & Alexander, S.J. (1980). Sex/family life education in the schools: An analysis of state policies. *Family Planning/Population Reporter, 9*(3), 44.

Kirby, D. (1997). *No easy answers: Research findings on programs to reduce teen pregnancy.* Washington, DC: National Campaign to Prevent Teen Pregnancy.

Lalonde, M. (1974). *A new perspective on the health of Canadians.* Ottawa, Canada: Government of Canada.

Landry, D.J., Kaeser, L., & Richards, C.L. (1999). Abstinence promotion and the provision of information about contraception in public school district sexuality education policies. *Family Planning Perspectives, 31*(6) 280–286.

LaSalle, D. (1960). Thomas D. Wood. *Journal of Health, Physical Education, and Recreation, 31*(4), 61+.

Lohrmann, D.K., Gold, R.S., & Jubb, W.H. (1987). School health education: A foundation for school health programs. *Journal of School Health, 57*(10), 420–425.

Lynch, A. (1977). Evaluating school health programs. In A. Levin (Ed.), *Health services: The local perspective.* New York: Academy of Political Science.

Main, D.S., Iverson, D.C., McGloin, J., Banspach, S.W., Collins, J.L., Rugg, D.L., & Kolbe, L.J. (1994). Preventing HIV infection among adolescents: Evaluation of a school-based education program. *Preventive Medicine, 23*(4), 409–417.

McKenzie, F.D., & Richmond, J.B. (1998). Linking health and learning: An overview of coordinated school health programs. In E. Marx, S.F. Wooley, & D. Northrop. *Health is academic: A guide to coordinated school health programs.* New York: Columbia College Press.

McKenzie, J.F., & Pinger, R.R. (1997). *An introduction to community health.* Boston: Jones and Bartlett.

Means, R.K. (1962). *A history of health education in the United States.* Philadelphia: Lea and Febiger.

Means, R.K. (1975). *Historical perspectives on school health.* Thorofare, NJ: Charles B. Slack.

Meredith, W.F. (1933). Some trends in acceptance of credits in health and physical education for college entrance. *Research Quarterly, 4*(1), 68–77.

Monteiro, L.A. ( 1985). Florence Nightingale on public health nursing. *American Journal of Public Health, 75*(2), 181–186.

MSNBC. (1999). *Safe sex education prevents AIDS* [On-line]. Available: http://www.msnbc.com/news/174141.asp

National Abortion and Reproductive Rights Action League. (1998). *A state by state review of abortion and reproductive rights.* Washington, DC.

National Education Association, Committee on Reorganization of Secondary Education. (1918). *Cardinal principles of secondary education* (U.S. Department of Interior, Bureau of Education, Bulletin No. 35). Washington, DC: Government Printing Office.

National Task Force on the Preparation and Practice of Health Educators. (1986). *Proceedings of the second Bethesda conference: Quality assurance in health education.* New York.

Nelson, G., Cross, F., & Kolbe, L. (1991). Teenage health teaching modules evaluation. *Journal of School Health, 61*(1), 3–4.

Nightingale, F. (1946). *Notes on nursing: What it is, what it is not.* Philadelphia: J. B. Lippincott. (Original work published 1859).

1990 Joint Committee on Health Education Terminology. (1991). Report of the 1990 joint committee on health education terminology. *Journal of School Health, 61*(6), 251–254.

Nixon, R.M. (1971). National health insurance: Message from the President of the United States. *Congressional Record, 117*(Part 3), 3119–3125.

Oberteuffer, D. (1932). *A program for Ohio secondary schools.* Columbus, OH: F.J. Heer Printing.

Olson, L. The foundation of universal education. *Education Week 18*(20), 29.

Parcel, G.S., & Baranowski, T. (1981). Social learning theory and health education. *Health Education, 12*(3), 14–18.

Patterson, S.M. (1992). An historical perspective of selected professional preparation conferences that have influenced credentialing for health education specialists. *Journal of Health Education, 23*(2), 101–108.

Payne, E.G., & Schroeder, L.C. (1925). *Health and safety in the new curriculum.* New York: American Viewpoint Society.

People for the American Way. (1994). *Teaching fear: The religious right's campaign against sexuality education.* Washington, DC.

Pickett, G., & Hanlon, J.J. (1990). *Public health administration and practice* (9th ed.). St. Louis, MO: Times Mirror/Mosby.

Pollock, M. (1987). *Planning and implementing health education in schools.* Palo Alto, CA: Mayfield.

Public Agenda. (1994). *What Americans expect from public schools.* New York.

Rathwell, T. (1992). Realities of health for all by the year 2000 (review). *Social Science and Medicine, 35*(4), 541–547.

Reaney, B.C. (1922) *Milk and our school* (*Health Education* No.11). Washington, DC: U.S. Department of the Interior, Bureau of Education, Health Education.

Report of the committee on the status of physical education in American colleges. (1916). *American Physical Education Review, 21,* 155–157.

Report of the committee on the status of physical education in public normal schools and public high schools. (1910). *American Physical Education Review, 15,* 453–454.

Rice, E.A., Hutchinson, J.J., & Lee, M. (1958). *A brief history of physical education* (4th ed.). New York: Ronald Press.

Rogers, J.F. (1930). *State-wide trends in school hygiene and physical education* (U.S. Department of the Interior, Office of Education, Pamphlet #5 rev.). Washington, DC: Government Printing Office.

Rogers, J.F. (1933). *Health instruction in hygiene in grades IX–XIII* (U.S. Department of the Interior, Office of Education, Pamphlet #43). Washington, DC: Government Printing Office.

Rosen, G. (1993). *A history of public health.* Baltimore, MD: Johns Hopkins University Press.

Secretary's Commission on Achieving Necessary Skills. (1991). *What work requires of schools: A SCANS report for America 2000.* Washington DC: U. S. Department of Labor.

Shattuck, L. (1948). *Report of the sanitary commission of Massachusetts, 1850.* New York: Cambridge University Press. (Original published in 1850.)

Sliepcevich, E.M. (1967). Health education: A conceptual approach to curriculum design. In E.M. Sliepcevich, *School health education study.* St. Paul: 3M Education Press.

Strachan, M.L. (1932). *Fifteen years of child health education.* New York: National Tuberculosis Association.

Strachan, M.L., & Jordan, E.F. (1947). *From pioneer to partner.* New York: National Tuberculosis Association.

Strang, R.M., Grout, R.E., & Wiehl, D.G. (1937). Evaluation of a rural school health education project. III. Evaluation of teachers' work in health education. *Milbank Memorial Fund Quarterly, 15*(4), 355–370.

Terris, M. (1984). New perspectives on the health of Canadians: Beyond the Lalonde report. *Journal of Public Health Policy, 5*(3), 327–337.

Turner, C.E. (1925). Malden studies in health education: A preliminary report. *American Journal of Public Health, 15*(5), 405–414.

U.S. Department of Education. (1998). *Goals 2000: Reforming education to improve student achievement: Executive summary* [On-line]. Available: http://www.ed.gov/pubs/ GwKReforming/g2exec.html

U.S. Department of Health, Education, and Welfare. (1973). *The report of the President's committee on health education.* Washington, DC: Government Printing Office.

U.S. Department of Health, Education, and Welfare. (1979). *Healthy people: The surgeon general's report on health promotion and disease prevention* (PHS Publication No. 79-55071). Washington, DC: Public Health Service.

U.S. Department of Health and Human Services. (1980). *Promoting health/ preventing disease: Objectives for the nation.* Washington, DC: Public Health Service.

U.S. Department of Health and Human Services. (1981). *Better health for our children: A national strategy: Vol. 1, Major findings and recommendations.* Washington, DC: Superintendent of Documents.

U.S. Department of Health and Human Services. (1991). *Healthy people 2000: National health promotion and disease prevention objectives* (PHS Publication No. 91-50212). Washington, DC: Public Health Service.

U.S. Department of Health and Human Services. (2000). *Healthy people 2010* (Conference ed.). Washington, DC: Author.

Van Ingen, P. (1935). *The story of the American child health association.* New York: American Child Health Association.

Wilcox, B.L. (1996, March 10). *Federally funded adolescent abstinence promotion programs: An evaluation of evaluations.* Paper presented at biennial meeting of Society for Research on Adolescents, Boston, MA.

W.K. Kellogg Foundation. (1950). *An experience in health education.* Battle Creek, MI.

World Health Organization. (1997). *The Jakarta declaration on leading health promotion into the 21st century* [On-line]. Available: http://who.int/ hpr/documents/jakarta/english.html

World Health Organization and United Nation's Children's Fund. (1978). *Primary health care. Report of the International Conference on Primary Health Care, Alma Ata, USSR, September 6–12.*

# Health Education and Promotion as a Profession

Every working person likes to regard himself or herself as professional. The word "professional" could be used to describe anyone who does work for money, such as a professional baseball player; it may also describe someone who carries on his or her work in a manner that is distinguished from the ordinary. Usually, however, it means that the practitioner is held to certain standards by others in the same line of work, or **profession**. Greene and Simons-Morton (1984) listed the characteristics of professionals:

- They believe in what they are doing.
- They want to see the job done properly.
- They do their best.
- They feel a sense of responsibility for the quality of work done by others in the field.

Two definitions stand out among the many available. Livingood (1996) defined a **profession** as "the sociological construct for an occupation that has special status." Wilensky's (1964) definition is

one which requires an abstract body of knowledge, a base of systematic theory, work which is challenging, for which long training is necessary, and which has a code of ethics and an orientation toward service.

Simons-Morton and colleagues (1995) listed three essential characteristics followed by six related characteristics of a profession:

**Essential**

- A service mission

- A unique body of knowledge
- A prolonged period of training

**Related**

- Continuing education
- Code of ethics
- Standards of education
- Shaping of legislation
- Freedom from lay control
- Strength of identity

The remainder of this chapter will examine the development of health promotion/education as a profession. We will attempt to apply each of the nine characteristics listed above to health promotion/education and discuss the progress made in achieving each to evaluate the discipline's standing as a profession.

## A SERVICE MISSION

Health education and health promotion provide a unique and essential service. The mission statement of the Society for Public Health Education reads, " . . . to promote the health of all people . . . " (SOPHE, 1997). Other associations have similar

---

**profession**  the sociological construct for an occupation that has special status

97

aims. Indeed, the essential outcome of health education/promotion is the improvement of the status of clients, students, and the community. In this context, the term "community" can be applied to small groups with a common characteristic or location or to large populations, including the world at large.

The uniqueness of health education/promotion stems from the combination of its efforts and variety of practice settings. Health educators work diligently to help individuals establish health-enhancing behaviors. They also work on a larger scale to affect the social conditions of people and to reduce the effects of economic deprivation on health. They carry out these efforts in schools, community organizations, clinics and other medical care facilities, places of worship, worksites, public health facilities, and elsewhere.

Many health educators work for little pay, or even volunteer, in international and national programs. Many work with boards of education to develop school health programs and request nothing in return for these services. Patient educators, including nurses, often spend long hours developing and implementing programs for patients and community groups with the goal of lifting the quality of life for those clients.

Health educators/promoters are engaged daily in providing services to clients. Many lay people claim to provide these services, but those who are academically prepared and who continually upgrade their skills and knowledge form an uncommon group of practitioners who work with great expertise and commitment.

## A UNIQUE BODY OF KNOWLEDGE

The body of knowledge associated with health education/promotion is based upon the combination of its content (e.g., nutrition and physical fitness), an underlying theoretical base, and contributions from other disciplines.

Deeds, Cleary, and Neiger (1996) wrote that health education's body of knowledge "represents a synthesis of facts, principles, and concepts drawn from biological, behavioral, sociological, and health sciences, but interpreted in terms of human needs, human values and human potential." They also stated that health education borrows from other disciplines, principally the behavioral sciences, education, public health, and health sciences. The combination of knowledge gleaned from these contributing disciplines may make health education/promotion unique, and the body of knowledge is still developing.

Wilensky's definition proposes that a fundamental characteristic of a profession is that it has a theoretical base underlying its practice within whose parameters the profession operates. Although no single theory forms the underpinning of health education/promotion, a number of theories that are applicable to altering human behavior to reduce health risks are discussed in Chapter 10, and several models applied to health planning are presented in Chapter 11.

## A PROLONGED PERIOD OF TRAINING

The length of training for entry into health promotion/education is not agreed upon at this time. This factor leads some practitioners to describe health education/promotion as an "emerging profession" (Cottrell, Girvan, & McKenzie, 1999; Simons-Morton, Greene, & Gottlieb, 1995). Some believe that completion of a bachelor's degree is sufficient to entry; others claim that a master's degree is the minimum requirement. Although there is no clear or authoritative position, requirements for entry do appear to vary somewhat by practice setting. For instance, school teachers usually gain state certification and practice with a bachelor's degree. Those in public health settings are often required to possess a graduate degree.

During the development of competencies used for awarding the Certified Health Education Specialist credential, there was a good deal of discussion of the different criteria for entry-level and advanced level practitioners. There was no clear consensus on the issue of training and educational requirements for the two levels.

More than 140 different institutions in the United States offer degrees in community health or public health, such as the Master of Public Health

(M.P.H.), Doctor of Public Health (Dr.P.H.), and Doctor of Philosophy (Ph.D.) in Public Health. The approach of these degrees usually is directed toward preparing professionals to achieve group change and collective goals rather than focusing on individuals and frequently places less emphasis on education and more emphasis on service delivery and ecological change. Of the 300 or more institutions that grant degrees in Health Education or Health Promotion, many are located in departments titled Health Education, Health Science, or Health and Human Performance. They frequently are linked to a College of Education or School of Public Health. These institutions grant a variety of degrees, including Bachelor of Science (B.S.), Master of Education (M.Ed.), Doctor of Education (Ed.D.), and Doctor of Philosophy (Ph.D.) in Health Education. These degrees usually are rooted in the process of education (teaching) and frequently are preparatory for school health education.

Some "health educators," unfortunately, emerge from other programs with little or no health education preparation *per se*. Some of these individuals are assigned health education duties by virtue of their backgrounds in nursing, medicine, home economics, biology, or psychology. In order to become effective, the most dedicated of these people acquire skills through on-the-job training, workshops, conferences, and college courses. The least effective situation is when lack of funding forces someone with no interest in health education to teach it.

Fortunately, those who enter the field of health education/promotion are increasingly doing so after completing a concentrated and extended preparation program. In order for the field to mature as a profession, such preparation must become a minimum criterion for practicing.

## CONTINUING EDUCATION

Members of a profession are expected to keep current with changing knowledge and practice in their areas of expertise. In many professions, such as medicine or nursing, continuing education is a requirement to retain one's license.

Certified Health Education Specialists are required to pursue continuing education in order to maintain their certification. Opportunities are available at conventions and conferences, universities, and professional publications. However, it should be noted that the certification is not a requirement to practice, although recently a few states have entertained legislation requiring a person identifying himself or herself as a health educator to be CHES.

Health promoters/educators can continue their professional development in more formal settings as well. Many colleges and universities offer courses that allow the individual to maintain currentness in the field. Some of these courses are offered through distance learning via computers and satellites. Often, governmental agencies hold teleconferences that offer opportunities for practitioners to increase their knowledge of current practice.

Professional organizations publish journals that contain research, practice, and perspective articles. Some of these articles are appropriate for continuing education credits for CHES. Regardless of acceptance for credit, the professional health promoter/educator is obligated to read the contemporary literature in the field.

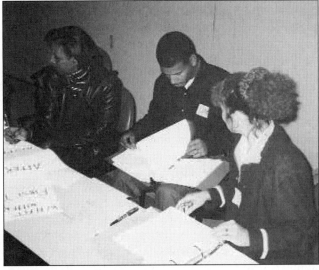

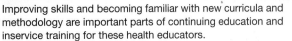
Improving skills and becoming familiar with new curricula and methodology are important parts of continuing education and inservice training for these health educators.

# CODE OF ETHICS

It is often held that a **code of ethics** is one of the final steps in the establishment of a profession. It is doubtless necessary and valuable. However we should keep in mind that the presence of a code of ethics is hardly sufficient for optimal practice. According to Newman and Brown (1996),

> [c]odes, unfortunately, are too often designed to protect professionals from outside regulation and are often conservative. They are more likely to focus on what should not be done and on the minimal behavior rather than on what should be done and on ideal behavior. . . . Another reason why ethical codes and rules for professionals may lack comprehensiveness is that they usually represent a consensus of opinions. . . . Despite these limitations, statements of ethical codes and rules are a hallmark of maturity for a profession, serving as useful guidelines for both experienced and new professionals.

## Why Study Ethics?

Greenberg and Gold (1992) asserted that, "For any profession to be worthy of the name, it must have a code of ethics as a standard by which it is judged." Indeed, any occupation that wishes to claim the respect bestowed by the title "profession" must have a code of ethics that is studied adequately by its membership and applied consistently in its practice. A code of ethics ensures minimum standards of practice for the practitioner, provides consumers with an understanding of what they should expect from the provider, and helps the professional know what is generally considered to be acceptable in the profession (Thomasma, 1979).

**Ethics** becomes an important criterion for the profession of health education/promotion because of the relationships between the practitioner and the client/student, employee, and the profession. Students and clients depend upon educators to practice in an ethical manner. Ethics are tied to values; values are unavoidably a part of teaching (Fain, 1992).

Historically, codes of ethics have been used for a number of important purposes. They have been used

— to state the ideals of a profession,

— to legitimize the profession in the face of skepticism or uncertainty,

— to regulate the practices of its practitioners toward each other,

— to delineate the relationship that should exist between a practitioner and client,

— to define the nature of the profession, and

— to establish some internal rules for regulating the practice of that profession (Callahan, 1982).

The study of ethics should be a requirement of professional preparation programs in health education/promotion for several reasons. First, society is asking for greater accountability from all professions, particularly education. Second, the nature of health education/promotion involves content areas and issues that are debatable and controversial and provide opportunities for discussing ethical issues and reasoning. Third, as Pigg (1994) stated, " . . . we belong to a profession with a mission to serve the individual." There should be guidelines and standards to govern that service. Fourth, ethical issues do not always provide a single correct resolution.

Part of the dilemma health educators face is the necessity of dealing with sensitive issues in ways that satisfy community standards. Professional responsibility in the face of community resistance requires difficult decisions. Many health-related issues, such as death, violence, and sex, demand attention but generate controversy. We might miss the opportunity to develop values, morals, and aesthetic standards in clients/students if we fail to address these issues and experiences. The role of the health educator in utilizing this opportunity begs for a code of ethics for guidance.

Health educators/promoters face an imposing set of ethical questions. Some examples are

- Because health educators have as their primary goal the change of behavior or establishment of healthy behavior, should grading be based upon student behavior outside the classroom?

- How do we confront topics that may have no definite answers, such as dealing with death, options relating to sexual behavior, and use of legal or illegal chemical substances?

- How much detail is appropriate in discussing certain topics, such as domestic violence, sexual assault, and drug use, when working with students/clients and their families?

- How do we handle situations that may represent conflicts of interest?

- What is our responsibility in evaluating the work of colleagues and pointing out when they are less than competent or less than ethical?

- Should our students/clients have the right of informed consent before participating in health education/promotion activities? What about research subjects?

- What are our ethical responsibilities in reporting and taking credit for results of evaluative studies and research?

- Do we have an obligation to balance the rights of smokers against the rights of nonsmokers?

- Is it proper for those not formally trained in health education to take on the duties of and claim to be health educators? Is there an ethical way to deal with this situation?

Ethics involves making right choices. Health educators seem to be more involved in ethical decisions than other contemporary educators—partly because of our increasing involvement in behavior-change strategies, the expanding knowledge of behavior change and control, and society's pragmatic willingness to use these methods with little concern for the consequences. Given our stated mission to change behavior and society's increasing willingness to have individuals' behavior changed, health educators have to possess principles to guide us in this mission. Therefore, we need a code of ethics to guide our practice, and we need to study the code so we can understand its application.

Bayles (1981) made useful distinctions among standards, principles, and rules.

- **Standards** are prescribed by codes of ethics and guide human and professional codes by stating desirable traits to be exhibited and undesirable ones to be avoided.

- **Principles** prescribe responsibilities but do not specify what the required conduct should be.

- **Rules** are defined by codes of ethics to express duties of the professional.

Whereas professionals must judge what conduct is desirable based upon principles laid out in their codes of ethics, rules designate the specific conduct that is not presented by principles. Rules do not allow latitude for professional judgment.

Bayles' definitions could be applicable to a useful code of ethics for health educators/promoters. Relative to standards, a code of ethics for health educators would help describe traits desired in health educators, such as honesty, respect for others, and conscientiousness and cite undesirable traits, such as dishonesty, deceitfulness, and exaggerated self-interest (Greenberg & Gold, 1992). The code would communicate the principles that should govern health education activities, including the professional's responsibility to clients, to employers, to colleagues, and to the profession. The code of ethics for health education should explicate rules required for ethical behavior in the profession.

In short, a code of ethics for health educators/promoters should clearly inform the public and members of the profession as to the rules, principles, and standards that govern their activities. This could set up a mechanism to discipline and screen out unethical practitioners. Any useful code of ethics allows consumers (clients/students) and employers to know what to expect from practitioners. All involved in the process—students, clients, employers, and health educators/promoters—benefit from a clear, concise code of ethics.

Codes of ethics have value only if actively used, applied, and interpreted. O'Connell and Price (1983) described four ethical theories of behavior change, which are summarized in Box 5.1. These theories can be applied to the practice of health education/promotion.

## Ethical Principles

Greenberg and Gold (1992) deviated from Bayles by defining ethical principles as guidelines that can

**code of ethics**  a statement of principles prescribing the responsibilities of a profession in general terms

**ethics**  a branch of philosophy that deals with systematic approaches to understanding morality

be applied to situations to decide whether they are moral or immoral. Simply put, we utilize ethical principles in practicing ethics. Four examples of ethical principles discussed prominently in the health education and biomedical literature (e.g., Beauchamp & Childress, 1989; Greenberg & Gold, 1992) are nonmalificence, beneficence, autonomy, and justice.

Nonmalificence    The principle of **nonmalificence** instructs us to do no harm or take no intentional risk of harm. Nonmalificence has been applied to several major issues in biomedical ethics, including the distinction between withholding and withdrawing life-sustaining treatments, the role of judgments of quality of life, the treatment of seriously ill newborns, and the duties of proxy decision makers for incompetent patients (Beauchamp & Childress, 1989). The principle could be applied to health education/promotion settings in deciding when counseling is appropriate for clients, in deciding matters of sequence and age-appropriate content in curricula, and selection or elimination of learning strategies that have the potential for causing friction in the home. Nonmalificence consists of three components:

1. Not inflicting harm, such as not lowering a person's self-esteem when emphasizing the importance of attaining suitable weight.

---

**Box 5.1    Ethical Theories for Promoting Health**

**Natural law**    Based on the principle of self-determination or autonomy, this theory holds that individuals have the right to select their personal health behavior or lifestyle. Natural law presumes that, even when we disagree strenuously with a decision, health educators must ensure clients' rights to choose how they want to live and die and their right to act on their personal decisions at any given time. External restraints on an individual's behavior are justified and necessary when the behavior is no longer a question of harm only to self but also harm to others. Society at large and health educators in particular are justified in intervening when a person's actions threaten the well-being of others.

**Utilitarianism**    This theory places the overall benefit to society as the standard for curtailing certain self-destructive behaviors. Utilitarianism provides society with an opportunity to enjoy significant economic gains and to avoid losses rather than to rely on claims that less-healthy people are at fault or violating the rights of others. For instance, prohibiting three-wheeled all-terrain vehicles is a utilitarian choice that seeks to avoid medical treatment, increased insurance premiums, and lost workdays. Wikler (1978) encapsulated the health promoter's role within this theory by stating, "We will not err if we give priority to utility over liberty where the benefit is high, the loss of liberty is small, and the practice affected is relatively unimportant."

**Paternalism**    This theory maintains that the government may intervene into personal lives and liberties by invoking the *parens patriae* power of the state. For example, schools routinely govern children's behavior much as a parent would. Some health educators/promoters claim a similar paternalistic duty to intervene in the life choices of their clients/students. Advocates of paternalism claim that many choices are not voluntary. Examples are decisions to smoke based on advertisements aimed at children and teenagers or consumption of a high-fat diet because of environmental factors such as peer pressure and family examples. Proponents claim that lack of information also renders some unhealthy behavior choices not fully voluntary.

**Distributive justice**    This theory advances the ideal of just distribution of goods, needs, punishment, and reward to all. This theory is illustrated by the fact that, in today's world, it would be unrealistic to expect most individuals to pay the entire cost of treating a serious medical condition. Others, in the form of insurance companies and their customers who pay premiums, must help. To avoid an unfair burden on citizens who remain healthy and take active steps to do so, insurance companies assess surcharges, special taxes, and increased premiums on individuals who engage in high-risk behaviors. Advocates of distributive justice would institute coercive behavior change interventions by health educators for people who did not pay the taxes, premiums, and charges.

2. Preventing harm, such as conducting educational activities to encourage the use of bicycle helmets for safety. A dangerous area of health educators' responsibility is teaching about environmental tobacco smoke without risking a child's security in a home where smoking is routine.

3. Removing harm when it is present. This final component may be the most difficult to implement. Suppose a teacher in a different but related discipline is teaching inaccurate information. The health educator's task is to eliminate the harm done by this colleague and still maintain a professional relationship.

## Beneficence

The principle of **beneficence** requires that we do more than simply doing no harm; we must contribute to the health and welfare of people. Beauchamp and Childress (1989) identified two components of this principle: providing benefits and balancing benefits and harms. Differentiating the benefits and the risks is critical, because benefits of an endeavor often are accompanied by potential risks. Many of the things we love—food, sex, sports—carry risks. Health educators/promoters should help students/clients recognize the risks and benefits of a behavior option so they can make well-informed decisions. The discipline struggles to help people determine whether the benefits of behaviors outweigh the risks. In addition, health professionals, including health educators, must strive to ensure that the benefits of a learning activity are worth the risks involved.

## Autonomy

**Autonomy** is the principle that people should be free to decide their own course of action as long as they do no harm to others. Absolute autonomy means the person is fully free to function. Relative autonomy means the person is free to function to a limited extent. To be absolutely autonomous means that every morally relevant act stems from the person's own character, totally determined by his or her own freedom, and that his or her pure conscience or pure reason is the sole guide. Of course, none of us in a modern world is absolutely autonomous. Social constraints bind our autonomy. Educators must find the proper set of

social constraints that will maximize the relative autonomy of our clients/students. One social constraint is the requirement of some sort of state-approved education for children. Relative autonomy, however, is practiced in the notion of "informed consent," which not only recognizes the individual's capacity to comprehend risks but also his or her need for adequate and complete understanding before deciding on a course of action, whether it is a medical or an educational procedure.

If children are involved, the principle of informed consent resides with the parents. In schools, we exercise informed consent policies, such as obtaining parental consent for field trips, utilizing school-based clinics, and counseling. Many school districts require parental consent for children to be instructed in matters of health, particularly matters relating to family living and sexuality.

If complete information necessary to make a decision is not available or the individual cannot read or understand the information provided, he or she has not acted autonomously. If a person is coerced, such as with the anticipation of a high grade or the threat of having some benefit withheld, his

**nonmalificence**  the ethical principle that a professional should do no harm or impose unreasonable intentional risk of harm

**natural law**  the theory that individuals have the right to select their personal health behavior or lifestyle

**utilitarianism**  the theory that uses overall benefit to society as the criterion for curtailing self-destructive behaviors

**paternalism**  the theory that the government may intervene into personal lives and liberties by invoking *parens patriae* power of the state

**distributive justice**  the theory advancing the ideal of just distribution of goods, needs, punishment, and reward to all

**beneficence**  the ethical principle that people, especially professionals, should contribute to the health and welfare of others; not doing harm is not enough

**autonomy**  the ethical principle that people should be free to decide their own course of action as long as they do no harm to others

or her decision is not autonomous. The more coercion, the less autonomy.

## Justice

To adhere to the principle of **justice**—that every person should be treated fairly and similarly—norms and rules must be applied to every member of a group consistently and continuously. When application of norms and rules is inconsistent or discontinuous, injustice has occurred. This does not mean that every person should be treated exactly the same as every other in every situation. Relevant variables are the key. It would not be acceptable to insist on the right to informed consent to one ethnic group but not to another. Ethnicity is not relevant to consent. In contrast, it would be proper to substitute parental informed consent for that of a child on the grounds that age and maturity are relevant characteristics.

These four principles are not the only ones valued in this field. Others that command high regard include conscientiousness, veracity, fidelity, honesty, confidentiality, and privacy.

Practitioners often face ethical dilemmas. Greenberg and Gold (1992) recommended applying values to decide morality when ethical principles conflict and present an ethical dilemma. Values, simply put, are estimations of worth. The Society for Public Health Education (SOPHE) suggested that, in the event of collision among responsibilities, the health educator's primary duty lies where the principles of self-determination and enhancement of freedom of choice is primary. This admonition, although providing a useful guideline, still does not provide the sort of strict boundary we often seek. See Box 5.2 for examples.

---

## Box 5.2   Ethical Dilemmas

The following are some examples of dilemmas that health educators/promoters face in real-world practice. Some alternative actions are suggested, and others may be applicable. What are the ethical responsibilities of a professional in these situations? What ethical theories and principles apply? What would you do?

- The school health team—including nurse, teacher, and counselor—have discovered that the teen pregnancy rate in some European countries is considerably lower than that in the United States. Contraceptives, especially condoms, are readily available in these nations, and comprehensive sexuality education is a part of the school curricula. However, school policy prohibits dispensing contraceptives, even in the school health clinic, and the family life education program stresses emphasis on abstinence with little mention of contraception.

**Alternatives for action:**

1. Educate students individually about contraception and refer them to sources of free condoms.
2. Openly challenge the school policy by teaching contraception in family life courses.

3. Petition the Board of Education to revisit its policy after seeking community support.
4. Assume the policy is the will of the community and implement it.

- A university faculty member working on a graduate admissions committee must recommend students for entry into a master's degree program in health education. While reviewing applications and conducting interviews of candidates for the final space, the faculty member notices that one of the two remaining applicants, an outstanding candidate named Joan, is the daughter of a high school classmate. Another applicant named Mary with equally outstanding credentials, is very overweight.

**Alternatives for action:**

1. Report the acquaintance with Joan's parent to the committee chair and ask for guidance on the course of action.
2. Withdraw from the committee decision.
3. Eliminate Mary as a poor role model, which would leave only Joan. Familiarity with Joan's parent is moot.
4. Recommend Joan for admission out of loyalty to an old friend.

## Developing Codes of Ethics in Health Education

Over forty years ago, Kleinschmidt and Zimand (1953) expressed a concern for ethics in health education by declaring, "It is very important that the health educator consider seriously what he is doing to the minds of people when he undertakes to influence them." If this was a clarion call for a code of ethics, it went unheeded until 1976, when SOPHE developed its code of ethics (SOPHE, 1976), which was revised in 1983. The code is a combination of standards and principles, thus indicating desirable traits professionals should have, such as honesty and competence, but it contains no specific rules of conduct. Therefore, it left individuals to their own professional judgment as to how to conduct themselves in particular work situations (Taub et al., 1987).

In 1994, the American Association for Health Education adopted its Code of Ethics for Health Educators, for which SOPHE's 1983 Code of Ethics served as a basis. The AAHE code, though similar to the SOPHE, is tailored more toward the needs of professionals whose interests are in the school health setting.

Despite the efforts of SOPHE and AAHE, there was no profession-wide code of ethics until the Coalition of National Health Education Organizations took the initiative. The efforts of CNHEO resulted in the first unified code of ethics for health educators, the Code of Ethics for the Health Education Profession, which was ratified in 1999. (This breakthrough document is presented in Appendix A.)

## Issues Addressed in the Codes of Ethics

The codes of ethics focused on several issues, each of which is discussed below. Although this text cannot cover the entire range of possible ethical issues that may arise during a practitioner's career, interested readers may wish to investigate the following specific areas further: health behavior change (O'Connell & Price, 1983; Read & Russell, 1985), the mission of health education (Penland & Beyrer, 1981), research/scientific inquiry/publishing (Breckon, Harvey, & Lancaster, 1998; Iammarino et al., 1989;

Vitello, 1986), the selection and employment of health educators (Barnes, Fors, & Decker, 1980; Penland & Beyrer, 1981), topical areas (Fennell & Beyrer, 1989), and the teaching of ethics (Patterson & Vitello, 1993).

**Informed Consent and Choice**   Behavior change in the absence of choice should be uncomfortable for health promoters. Of course, a certain level of persuasion or even coercion may be acceptable if the benefit to the client or society is great. However, health promoters must determine if their students/ clients are being unfairly coerced to act or not act. This is a basic freedom-of-choice issue requiring both informed consent and voluntary action in the absence of coercion.

Actions to reduce the behaviors that harm individual health must be done, in the vast majority of cases, under the illumination of informed consent. Hochbaum (1980) stated,

> In programs which address themselves to problems which affect only the health of the individuals and do not seriously affect the health of others there should be maximal respect for the individual's right to adopt or not to adopt recommended behaviors. The more seriously individual behavior threatens the health and welfare of others, however, the more the health educator is justified and even obligated to turn to more forceful means that may go so far as to support legal or other coercion.

Although this admonition came before the currently adopted codes of ethics, it provides useful guidance regarding consent and coercion.

Faden (1987) indicated that public health campaigns can be categorized as persuasive or manipulative, based upon the degree to which they respect individual autonomy. Persuasive campaigns are the least coercive, attempting to induce change by appealing to reason. Manipulative campaigns attempt to reduce individuals' options by controlling information. This may be done by deception or emotional appeal, psychological manipulation (such as subliminal suggestion), flattery, guilt, or feelings of obligation. It is easy to see how the line between

**justice**   the ethical principle that every person should be treated fairly and similarly

persuasion and manipulation, as well as that between respect and disrespect for autonomy, can be blurred, especially in light of the fact that most school-based and public health programs are governmental in nature. Government has a responsibility to protect and promote the public's health. However, the ethical health educator will reflect seriously upon the nature and justification of program components before embarking upon any course that might be described as manipulative.

Nongovernmental health promotion programs have a far weaker foundation for utilizing coercive measures. Use of subliminal messages; appeals to guilt, emotion, or peer pressure; and deception in commercial marketing of health promotion programs and services, whether proven effective or not, raise serious ethical concerns. Withholding or distorting information about expected short- or long-term benefits, costs, and side effects may be unethically coercive, robbing the consumer of the requisite informed consent and, thus, violating ethical standards.

### Acting on Health-Related Issues

The CNHEO code of ethics notes that "Health educators accept the responsibility to act on issues that can adversely affect the health of individuals, families, and communities." The SOPHE and AAHE codes also contain language holding health educators responsible for advocating for healthful change and legislation, speaking out on issues about public health, and encouraging actions and social policies that support benefits over harm.

However, the implementation of this responsibility may be limited by several conditions. First, practitioners must give precedence to protecting individuals' right to choose their own behaviors. Second, health promoters must consider the relative importance of the health problem and what benefits can be gained from their actions. Third, practitioners also must evaluate the demands of the effort in terms of time and personal energy, as well as their enthusiasm for investing that effort. Frequently, deciding to become involved in a substantial issue, such as limiting smoking in public places or requiring motorcycle riders to wear helmets, requires that the health educator look at the likelihood of a successful outcome.

### Privacy of Clients, Students, and Research Subjects

The privacy and dignity of students/clients and research subjects can be violated inadvertently. In teaching or in justifying programs, a health educator may refer to an individual case without mentioning the client/student by name, but still allow the person to be identified by describing the case. From an ethical perspective, we should not even request information about clients/students that is unnecessary, and when personal information is no longer needed, it should not be kept. Privacy includes the right to decide how much and what personal information to share with others (Greenberg & Gold, 1992).

Confidentiality should be guarded closely in research settings. Personal information that is unnecessary to the research should not be gathered, stored, or maintained. When respondents are told that their privacy and confidentiality will be upheld, the practitioner must keep that promise. Often, this becomes an issue when illegal activity, such as alcohol consumption by juveniles or drug abuse, is disclosed. This information must remain confidential. If the public, including participants in any research project, could not feel secure in the confidentiality of their responses, the entire process of self-reporting behaviors and, therefore, the research process, would be compromised.

### Quality of Instruction and Services

Common decency and all of the professional codes of ethics require educators to provide the highest quality instruction and services possible. The CNHEO code makes it clear that "health educators use strategies and methods that are grounded in and contribute to development of professional standards, theories, guidelines, statistics, and experience." Teachers should be current in the subject matter of their discipline and committed to presenting it in ways untainted by their own undisclosed biases.

As part of providing quality service and instruction, the health educator is bound to disclose the potential outcomes of proposed services or programs—including both benefits and consequences.

The profession-wide code of ethics holds that health educators are committed to rigorous evaluation of both program effectiveness and the methods used. A professional can be assured that his or her methods are achieving the desired ends (i.e., acquisition of skills and knowledge and changes in behavior by the target audience) only through effective evaluation. In addition, those who render services, including instruction, should be subject to objective evaluation by peers, supervisors, and students/clients—and that evaluation should be scrupulously unbiased.

**Equality**  Health educators are bound by considerations of equality. Discriminating against any student or program participant based upon irrelevant characteristics is both illegal and unethical. Tests and other evaluation instruments are meant to discriminate, not on irrelevant variables, but on variables such as ability to organize and communicate one's ideas, knowledge, and analytical skills.

Likewise, discrimination in hiring, promotion, retention, work assignments, and admission policies based upon nonprofessional attributes is unethical. By the same token, it is an ethical violation for an individual to accept a position for which he or she is less qualified than another applicant, knowing that he or she was the recipient of discriminatory benefit.

The Code of Ethics for the Health Education Profession makes several references to equality. It requires that health educators model and encourage nondiscriminatory standards of behavior in their interactions with others. It further requires sensitivity to social and cultural diversity in planning and implementing programs. Finally, the code requires that selection of students for professional preparation programs be based upon equal opportunity for all and academic and professional qualifications.

**Obligation to the Profession**  Ethical obligations to our profession take many forms. The way health educators/promoters respond to these obligations shapes the profession's reputation in the eyes of other professionals and with the lay public. Professionalism is displayed in our willingness to expose discriminatory practices and incompetence and to criticize unethical practices when we perceive them and in our commitment to avoid conflicts of interest and maintain professional competence.

Although the CNHEO code does not specifically mention it, the health educator is duty-bound to report and criticize all observed unethical practices. This could include an individual colleague's failing to attend his or her classes or failing to award grades fairly and equitably. It could be as far-reaching as a professional organization practicing unprofessionally, such as providing the name of an author of a manuscript to a reviewer for a journal when the review process is supposed to be anonymous. Even though repercussions may be brought to bear upon the person reporting the incidents, ethics makes it incumbent upon all of us to prevent and respond to unethical behavior.

Health educators are ethically responsible to maintain professional competence by continued study and education in the rapidly advancing field of health-related knowledge. This continuing study can take many forms. Many universities offer coursework or workshops with excellent, up-to-date information on the practice of health education. Health educators are strongly urged to join professional organizations. Attending meetings and serving on committees are professional responsibilities that provide occasion for growth. These organizations offer many opportunities—including conventions, workshops, and journals—for continuing improvement in knowledge and skills. Members are given the opportunity to present their own ideas and research in journals and by presentations at conferences. Many professional, technical, and lay journals provide excellent up-to-date information. Health educators should stay abreast of new developments by reading and serving on review panels for journals.

**Research**  Many professional health educators/promoters conduct research as a part of their occupational responsibility. Research should be conducted in accordance with recognized scientific and ethical standards. Although a thorough discussion of those standards is beyond the scope of this text, a few of them, such as informed consent and confidentiality, have been addressed. Universities that conduct research on human subjects have committees that review such research to ensure that it does no harm to participants and protects their privacy.

Because so much pressure is placed on professionals to publish in refereed journals, researchers must take credit only for work they have actually done. If others contribute to the work, all codes of ethics require the author to credit those contributors. Iammarino and colleagues (1989) suggested that, before initiating the project, issues such as authorship, ownership of data, and subsequent use of data be resolved in a carefully constructed agreement. This agreement should address responsibilities of each party, forms of acknowledgement, authorship and order of authorship, access to and appropriate use of data, and expectations regarding future writing.

Authors sometimes engage in the unsavory practices of plagiarism, fragmentation, or duplication. **Plagiarism**, the unauthorized use of the works or ideas of others without proper credit or permission, constitutes theft and, therefore, is a crime. **Fragmentation** may be an effort to inflate a resume by breaking down data from a study into several parts. In the case of **duplication** (submitting a manuscript to more than one journal simultaneously), most journals require a written statement to the effect that a submitted manuscript does not constitute duplication. This is done to avoid unnecessary reviewer and editorial staff time and, thus, higher publication costs. These three practices are all highly unethical.

## Enforcing a Code of Ethics

The weakest point of virtually all codes of ethics is the enforcement mechanism. A code of ethics is a guideline for behavior that, in many instances, requires that judgment be applied fairly and effectively. Even after adoption of the profession-wide code of ethics, no organization requires health educators to swear allegiance to that code. Deciding to adhere to the code of ethics becomes, oddly enough, a matter of ethics.

A number of approaches to enforcement are possible. Each has its inherent weaknesses. One approach could entail the utilization of a quasi-governmental agency. Just as states have certification requirements for teachers, they could have requirements of ethical practice for health promoters and educators. Charges of ethical violations could be adjudged by a panel of colleagues and private citizens. Of course, a single agency might have difficulty covering health educators in the school, public health, medical, and worksite arenas. In addition, states may not adopt a common code of ethics upon which to base decisions. Such an agency would also add more bureaucracy, in the form of independent staff and budget, to state services that already are inefficient in many cases.

Another approach (Greenberg & Gold, 1992) would have the professional organization appoint committees to review charges of unethical conduct. The American Psychological Association utilizes this manner of enforcement. Committees could recommend sanctions, such as expulsion from the organization, suspension of the right to practice, decertification, or rescinding the license to practice. Unfortunately, the final three sanctions are not practical at this time, because no professional health education organization grants the right or license to practice and no certification awarded by any organization is currently required to practice. The future of this strategy is unclear, but it has been suggested that the National Commission for Health Education Credentialing take on such a function. This new responsibility would serve the purpose of credentialing health educators as Certified Health Education Specialists. The credential, however, is not required currently for practice in any national sense, although some states have entertained legislation requiring the CHES for positions identified as "health education." It is a long step from NCHEC's current status to having the legal power to discipline members of the profession.

Public opinion is a rudimentary form of enforcement. Professions depend upon public confidence. When news reports shed light upon violations of one's own code, public confidence in both the individual and the profession is undermined.

When the day-to-day work of the professional is considered, compliance with a code of ethics may come down to a matter of voluntary self-monitoring. Certainly, when a charge of violation is brought directly to a professional, he or she may have the opportunity to resolve the charge. If no official body exists to deal with charges, self-monitoring may be the most appropriate means of dealing with claims of ethical violations. Health educators/

promoters presently are left to their own individual discretion to apply a code of ethics. Their professional career may depend on how well they do so.

Perhaps one of the most valuable steps health educators can take is to examine their feelings about ethical issues periodically. They have a responsibility to become aware of ethical perspectives in their discipline, to devote considerable energy to conscious decision making about ethics and its implications. "Unexamined and unchallenged assumptions about what is good, just, and true predisposes to moral blundering in the pursuit of high purpose" (Carlyon, 1975).

# STANDARDS OF EDUCATION

Health education is different from other subject areas in education, and it presents challenges that are not common to other disciplines. Its emphasis on attitudes, lifestyle, and behavior change make it unique among academic disciplines. Because individuals, especially youths, are often apathetic and sometimes antagonistic about health and safety, motivating people to make intelligent decisions is quite a challenge. In addition, health is bound up in cultural and social patterns of thinking and doing —patterns that involve attitudes, feelings, and behaviors. Educators must be sensitive to cultural differences. The challenges are intensified in that health information changes constantly. Science gives us new information that, at times, contradicts yesterday's ideas of truth. Health educators/promoters must remain current with health information.

Health instruction is often controversial. Discussing areas such as death and dying, human sexuality, HIV/AIDS and other sexually transmissible diseases, tobacco, suicide, and violence can elicit emotional reactions from pupils, family, and community. Yet, these are integral parts of health education that should be included in programs. Effective planning; age-appropriate curricula, materials, and terminology; written guidelines; and respect for students' questions and parents' concerns can help diffuse many of the inevitable objections.

These and other issues have led to the search for identifiable competencies that health educators should master and the relative importance of these competencies. These competencies become the standards for the education of health educators/promoters.

## Identification of Competencies

Identifying **competencies** is important at all strata of the profession, and nowhere is it more important than at the level of professional preparation. The Role Delineation Project formed a foundation for identifying competencies, and the work of others points out alternative ways of addressing the problem.

Although the nature of a person's education and training is important regardless of how we come to the profession, a certain level of proficiency in selected competencies must be attained if the individual is to be successful in meeting his or her responsibilities. Two mechanisms to enforce this would be (1) Professional preparation and credentialing to establish standardized qualifications for entry into the profession and (2) formalized entry routes for employment.

Most professionals would agree that some general skills are necessary to health educators, including

— ability to communicate clearly in writing and orally

— ability to apply theories of learning and behavior

— ability to plan for orderly formal educational experiences and to use "teachable moments" for health instruction

— ability to develop appropriate materials for education

---

**plagiarism**   the unauthorized use of the works or ideas of others without proper credit or permission

**fragmentation**   breaking down data from a study into several parts (the "least publishable unit") for the purpose of increasing the number of publications in which the study results can appear

**duplication**   submitting a manuscript or its essence to more than one journal simultaneously

**competencies**   acceptable levels of skill proficiency required to carry out activities

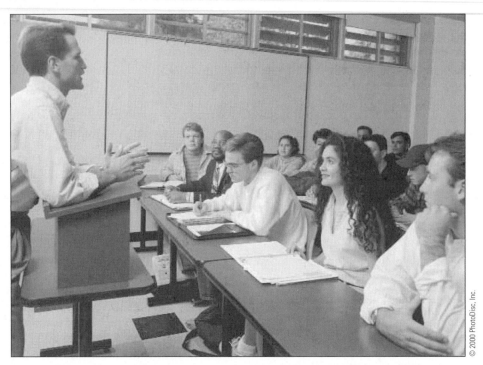

Acquiring the competencies to practice successfully is the main focus of the professional preparation of future health educators/promoters.

— ability to work with people of various educational backgrounds and social and cultural groups

— familiarity with a variety of sources of current health information and the ability to access information and resources

— ability to think critically

— ability to understand research and evaluate research findings

**The Role Delineation Project**    In 1978, a contract between the National Center for Health Education and the Bureau of Health Professions Division of Associated Health Professions (in the Department of Health and Human Services) was signed to specify the responsibilities, functions, **skills**, and knowledge required of entry-level health educators; to define entry-level into health education; and to identify levels of supervision required for entry-level personnel (Henderson, McIntosh, & Schaller, 1981). The work has come to be known as

the Workshop on Commonalities and Differences or, more often, the Role Delineation Project.

The major assumption behind the foundation of the project was that responsibilities, functions, requisite skills, and knowledge of health educators are common to all health educators, regardless of setting or constituency. Thus, all the competencies the Role Delineation Project identified apply to school health educators, community health educators, patient educators, and any others who identify themselves as health educators. Previously, professional preparation programs could operate from a variety of assumptions and goals, based on the belief that health educators working with different populations and in different settings function in disparate ways and apply different skills. The Workshop on Commonalities and Differences helped begin a trend to enforce a large measure of conformity on the preparation of health educators.

The Role Delineation Project led to the formation of the National Task Force on the Preparation and Practice of Health Educators; in 1985, the task force published *A Framework for the Development of Competency-based Curricula for Entry Level Health Educators,* which contained seven responsibilities and related competencies. In 1988, the same task force changed its incorporation papers and became the National Commission on Health Education Credentialing, Inc. (NCHEC). NCHEC published the seven responsibilities and competencies in *A Competency-Based Framework for Professional Development of Certified Health Education Specialists* (1996).

The responsibilities and competencies in this framework are used as a basis for accreditation of undergraduate teacher preparation programs through the National Council on Accreditation of Teacher Education (NCATE). They are also used to accredit undergraduate community health programs through SOPHE/AAHE Baccalaureate Program Approval Committee (SABPAC). Because of NCATE's and SABPAC's adoption of the competencies, a number of institutions have revised their professional preparation curricula to come into compliance (McMahon, Bruess, & Lohrmann, 1987; Waishwell et al., 1996).

The primary purpose of NCHEC itself is the certification of health educators. It bases its certification examination of individual health education specialists upon the seven responsibilities and competencies detailed in the 1996 document.

In 1999, AAHE, NCHEC, and SOPHE published *A Competency-Based Framework for Graduate-Level Health Educators* (1999). This document identified 3 new areas of graduate responsibility, 2 new competencies, and 43 new sub-competencies to be applied to graduate level professional preparation. (The responsibilities and competencies appear in Appendix B.)

The Competency Update Project was initiated in 1998. Its purpose is to evaluate the currentness of the responsibilities and competencies, to revalidate where appropriate, and to identify necessary new responsibilities, competencies, and sub-competencies for both entry-level and advanced health educators.

## An Approach for Classroom Teachers

Some specialists conclude that the responsibilities and competencies for entry-level health educators contained in the NCHEC framework are probably oriented more toward the responsibilities and competencies necessary for professionals in the public and community health settings. Many competencies required of the classroom teachers are missing.

During the 1980s and early 1990s, comprehensive (coordinated) school health education gained recognition as a national priority. This acknowledgment came from major health and education organizations such as the Carnegie Council on Adolescent Development (Carnegie Corporation of New York, 1989); the American Medical Association and the National Association of State Boards of Education (National Commission on the Role of the School and the Community in Improving Adolescent Health, 1990); American Association of School Administrators (1990); and the U.S. Centers for Disease Control (U.S. Public Health Service, 1990).

National surveys identified lack of teacher training as one of the most significant obstructions to effective implementation and delivery of school health education (ABT Associates, 1980; Metropolitan Life Foundation, 1985). The Joint Committee of the Association for the Advancement of Health Education (now the American Association for Health Education) and the American School Health Association (Joint Committee, 1992) was formed to address this situation by delineating responsibilities and competencies for the health instruction preparation of elementary school teachers (see Box 5.3). In 1999, AAHE published responsibilities and competencies needed by all middle-level classroom teachers (see Box 5.4).

Although these two sets of competencies do not include those for teachers in high school, the work of the committees produced welcome results for school health educators. The emphasis on classroom instruction, curriculum provision, planning lessons, and evaluation of instruction is the essence of classroom teaching. The responsibilities and competencies are modeled after *A Framework for the Development of Competency-based Curricula for Entry Level Health Educators* (National Task Force on the Preparation and Practice of Health Educators, 1985), but it also recognizes that a specific

**skills**  abilities to do or to apply something in order to carry out activities

## Box 5.3   Health Instruction Responsibilities for Elementary (K–6) Classroom Teachers

**Responsibility I:** Communicating the concepts and purposes of health education.

**Competency A:** Describe the discipline of health education within the school setting.

*Subcompetencies:*
1. Describe the interdependence of health education and the other components of a comprehensive school health program.
2. Describe comprehensive school health instruction, including the most common content areas.

**Competency B:** Provide a rationale for K–6 health education.

**Competency C:** Explain the role of knowledge, skills, and attitudes in shaping patterns of health behavior.

**Competency D:** Define the role of the elementary teacher within a comprehensive school health program.

*Subcompetencies:*
1. Describe the importance of health education for elementary teachers.
2. Summarize the kinds of support needed by the K–6 teacher from administrators and others to implement an elementary school health education program.
3. Identify available quality continuing education programs in health education for elementary teachers.
4. Describe the importance of modeling positive health behaviors.

**Responsibility II:** Assessing the health instruction needs and interests of elementary students.

**Competency A:** Utilize information about health needs and interests of students.

**Competency B:** List behaviors and how they promote or compromise health.

**Responsibility III:** Planning elementary school health instruction.

**Competency A:** Select realistic program goals and objectives.

**Competency B:** Identify a scope and sequence plan for elementary school health instruction.

**Competency C:** Plan elementary school health education lessons which reflect the abilities, needs, interests, developmental levels, and cultural backgrounds of students.

**Competency D:** Describe effective ways to promote cooperation with and feedback from administrators, parents, and other interested citizens.

**Competency E:** Determine procedures which are compatible with school policy for implementing curricula containing sensitive health topics.

**Responsibility IV:** Implementing elementary school health instruction.

**Competency A:** Employ a variety of strategies to facilitate implementation of an elementary school health education curriculum.

*Subcompetencies:*
1. Provide a core health education curriculum.
2. Integrate health and other content areas.
3. Incorporate topics introduced by students into the health education curriculum.
4. Utilize affective skill-building techniques to help students apply health knowledge to their daily lives.
5. Involve parents in the teaching/learning process.

**Competency B:** Incorporate appropriate resources and materials.

*Subcompetencies:*
1. Select valid and reliable sources of information about health appropriate for K–6.
2. Utilize school and community resources within a comprehensive program.
3. Refer students to valid sources of health information and services.

**Competency C:** Employ appropriate strategies for dealing with sensitive health issues.

**Competency D:** Adapt existing health education curricular models to community and student needs and interests.

**Responsibility V:** Evaluating the effectiveness of elementary school health instruction.

**Competency A:** Utilize appropriate criteria and methods unique to health education for evaluating student outcomes.

**Competency B:** Interpret and apply student evaluation results to improve health instruction.

Source: From "Health Instruction Responsibilities and Competencies for Elementary (K–6) Classroom Teachers," by the Joint Committee of the Association for the Advancement of Health Education and the American School Health Association, 1992, *Journal of School Health*, 62(2), pp. 76–77. Reprinted by permission of American School Health Association, Kent, Ohio.

**Box 5.4**   Responsibilities and Competencies for Teachers of Young Adolescents

| | |
|---|---|
| **Responsibility 1:** | Communicate the essential purposes of school health education. |
| *Competency A:* | Describe the role of health education in middle level curriculum. |
| *Competency B:* | Provide a rationale for health education for young adolescents. |
| *Competency C:* | Explain the role that knowledge, skills, attitudes/dispositions play in shaping health behaviors in young adolescents |
| **Responsibility 2:** | Collaborate with health education specialists in assessing the health behaviors of young adolescents. |
| *Competency A:* | Identify health needs, risks, and protective factors for young adolescents. |
| *Competency B:* | Assess the effects of reinforcing factors that influence the health behaviors of young adolescents (e.g., family, peers, media and the environment) |
| *Competency C:* | Identify the needs of young adolescents for their healthy development. |
| **Responsibility 3:** | Participate in school wide, cross-curricular planning that focuses on the healthy development of adolescents. |
| *Competency A:* | Consider the results of assessment of students' health needs when planning curriculum and instruction. |
| *Competency B:* | Plan ways to include life skills that are important for young adolescents' healthy development. |
| *Competency C:* | Utilize school and community resources in plans for health instruction across disciplines. |
| **Responsibility 4:** | Actively participate in the health education of young adolescents. |
| *Competency A:* | Reinforce health-related knowledge, life skills, and health-enhancing attitudes and beliefs in non-health specific curriculum and instruction. |
| *Competency B:* | Employ strategies that celebrate diversity and promote social health and well-being. |
| *Competency C:* | Utilize developmentally appropriate strategies when addressing sensitive health issues (e.g., family life education, HIV/AIDS education, death and dying education). |
| *Competency D:* | Apply strategies that actively engage young adolescents in learning health-related skills. |
| **Responsibility 5:** | Participate in evaluating the effectiveness of health education for adolescents. |
| *Competency A:* | Assess the health behaviors of young adolescents through formal and informal measures. |
| *Competency B:* | Assess the health literacy of students in collaboration with the health education specialist. |
| *Competency C:* | Utilize a variety of assessment resources for evaluation of program effectiveness. |
| **Responsibility 6:** | Work collaboratively with all professionals in implementing a coordinated school health program. |
| *Competency A:* | Contribute to a nurturing and health-promoting school health environment that supports students' capacity to learn. |
| *Competency B:* | Define the role of middle level teachers within coordinated school health programs. |
| *Competency C:* | Serve as a role model by exhibiting positive health behaviors and participating in faculty/staff wellness opportunities. |
| *Competency D:* | Collaborate with family members, school personnel, and community health professionals within a team approach to prevent and remediate health problems. |
| *Competency E:* | Advocate for and implement school policies that foster the health, wellness, and safety of young adolescents. |
| **Responsibility 7:** | Serve as a resource person to young adolescents regarding their healthy development. |
| *Competency A:* | Collaborate with the health education specialist in identifying effective health education resources that promote the healthy development of young adolescents. |
| *Competency B:* | Help students locate reliable sources of information that promote healthy development. |
| *Competency C:* | Refer students with special health needs to appropriate health services (e.g., school nurse, counselor, or social worker) |
| *Competency D:* | Communicate with family members about ways to work together to promote the healthy development of their children. |
| **Responsibility 8:** | Serve as an advocate for school health education and the well being of young adolescents. |
| *Competency A:* | Advocate for health literacy that enhances the healthy development of young adolescents. |
| *Competency B:* | Work collaboratively with families, school administrators, and other school personnel to improve the crucial interrelationships among health literacy, health behaviors, effective learning, and quality of life. |

Source: From *Responsibilities and Competencies for Teachers of Young Adolescents: In Coordinated School Health Programs for Middle Level Classroom Teachers*, by the American Association for Health Education, 1999, Reston, VA. Reprinted with permission of American Alliance for Health, Physical Education, and Dance/American Association for Health Education.

set of competencies applicable to elementary and middle-school classroom teachers is unlike competencies necessary in other health education settings.

## SHAPING LEGISLATION

Health educators/promoters often play a vital part in the legislative process. For example, on a national level issues such as health care reform, tobacco, family-planning programs, and funding of education programs have been in the forefront. On the local and state levels, professionals have been involved in issues relating to education reform, including development of standards and assessment tools. They also have been vocal on issues such as mandatory seat belt use, motorcycle helmets, services for AIDS patients, clean air efforts, smoking restrictions, and water quality.

Educators often are called upon as experts in the writing of legislation. They also testify before legislative committees and other bodies in an effort to assist government in developing the best laws possible. Professionals frequently organize group efforts to affect the passage or defeat of legislation. These may include letter-writing campaigns, rallies, or phone-ins to legislators.

Some professions are licensed by the states. These include physicians and nurses. License requirements may be a matter of law or regulation. Although not typically licensed, teachers must attain state certification, a function usually managed by the state department of education. The standards for certification are often created by the state board of education or the state department. Professionals should take an active part in updating the requirements for licensing and certification. Generally, there are no legally mandated requirements for health educators/promoters outside the school setting, but efforts are being made in some states to require the Certified Health Education Specialist credential.

In addition to the work of individuals, professional organizations work on behalf of their members to influence legislation. Many publish position papers on bills and issues. They usually employ lobbyists to help educate legislators and make sure that the profession's position is heard.

## FREEDOM FROM LAY CONTROL

Health education/promotion is largely free from control by people outside the profession, especially in matters of addressing unethical practice. An exception to this statement is the school health educator whose practice is governed by other educators, such as principals and curriculum supervisors and by lay boards of education.

Much of the control of practitioners of health education/promotion is exerted by peers. Educators in clinical settings are required to conform to the standards of state licensing boards. These boards are generally composed of professionals, although there usually is some consumer membership.

Research and publication is largely a peer-reviewed process. Much research is funded and monitored under the grants process. Usually grant applications are reviewed by professionals in the field and monitored by the grant source, often by peers.

The establishment of a certification (CHES) process in 1988 may someday be seen as a turning point in the control of health education practice. Certification may eventually represent control of entry into the profession based on academic background and possession of a core set of competencies. It may even be utilized as a method of censuring unethical practice. However, the CHES is currently voluntary and is not generally required by law or regulation, and the National Commission for Health Education Credentialing, Inc., is not advocating the use of the certification as a method of disciplining unethical behavior.

## STRENGTH OF IDENTITY

A professional maintains a strong identification with his or her profession. The profession becomes his or her life's work or calling and he or she believes in the indispensability of the profession. Part of this process is what Siegel (1968) called **professional socialization**, the process by which recruits into a profession develop values, attitudes, and beliefs that support their roles as practitioners. Although public recognition is one aspect of professional socialization, the public probably does not yet have as clear an image of a health educator as that it might of a physician, lawyer, or teacher. However, one can identify with the health education profession and demonstrate the commitment that follows that identification in several ways.

## Scholarly Productivity

This refers to research and publication in scholarly journals (although for teachers and professors, this "scholarly productivity" term should include teaching). The most effective way for any profession to respond to changing needs of its clients and identify and verify new techniques of addressing those needs is through the scientific process of research. The publication of one's research findings in peer-reviewed journals helps to establish one's identity with the profession. Similarly, one can publish perspective or opinion papers that share ideas or points of view on issues of professional interest.

## Service Activities

Many professionals exhibit their identity with the profession through service activities. Most communities need people with health education/promotion expertise to share their knowledge and skills. For example, community health organizations, schools, and places of worship often offer opportunities for service.

## Professional Organizations

The professional organizations present uncommon opportunities for identification with the profession. They serve a unique function in the socialization of health educators/promoters through an informal collegial network and student membership. Many organizations provide formal employment services and job banks. Most are managed and governed by members of the profession. Professionals can serve as directors, committee members, or other functions. Professional organizations also offer opportunities to present papers at conferences and conventions and to publish papers in journals, compendiums, and books. Membership in professional organizations is considered to be a minimal step in professionalism. Several professional organizations are

described here. (Contact information is listed in Appendix E.)

### Coalition of National Health Education Organizations
The coalition, established in 1972, has as its primary mission the mobilization of the resources of the health education profession in order to expand and improve health education, regardless of the setting. To achieve this mission, it (CNHEO, 1996) does the following:

— facilitates national communication, collaboration, and coordination among member organizations

— provides a forum for the identification and discussion of health education issues

— formulates recommendations and takes appropriate action on issues affecting member interests

— serves as a communication and advisory resource for agencies, organizations, and persons in the public and private sectors on health education issues

— serves as a focus for the exploration and resolution of issues pertinent to professional health educators

The eight professional organizations that make up the coalition are identified below.

### Society of State Directors of Health, Physical Education and Recreation
(CNHEO member) The mission of SSDHPER is to provide leadership in facilitating and promoting initiatives to achieve national health education goals and objectives. The society promotes effective school programs and practices that involve collaboration with parents and community groups to encourage healthy and active lifestyles. It maintains a network for professional development and a forum for sharing knowledge,

---

**professional socialization**   the process by which recruits into the profession develop values, attitudes, and beliefs that support their roles as practitioners

ideas, and strategies for implementing quality programs at national, state and local levels (CNHEO, 1999).

Membership includes state education agency directors and coordinators of state programs in comprehensive school health and physical education, and categorically funded programs such as HIV/AIDS prevention, safe and drug-free schools, and nutrition education.

## Society for Public Health Education, Inc.

(CNHEO member) SOPHE is the only professional organization devoted exclusively to public health education and health promotion. Its purpose is to promote, encourage, and contribute to the advancement of people's health through education. It encourages research, high standards of professional preparation and practice, and continuing education. SOPHE has a membership of 4,000 in eighteen chapters.

It publishes *Health Education and Behavior* six times a year, *Health Promotion Practice* and *SOPHE News and Views* quarterly (SOPHE, 1997). It holds an annual meeting in conjunction with the American Public Health Association and a mid-year scientific meeting each summer.

## Association of State and Territorial Directors of Health Promotion and Public Health Education

(CNHEO member) ASTDHPPHE has a membership of 66, made up of one area level director of public health education or health promotion or equivalent from each state, territory, and Indian Health Service. The purposes of the association are as follows (AASTDHPPHE, 1999):

— to serve as a channel through which directors of public health education programs of states and territories of the United States may exchange and share methods, techniques, and information for the enrichment and improvement of public health education programs

— to establish position statements and make recommendations on legislation and public policy related to and having implications for public health education

— to participate, with the Association of State and Territorial Health Officials, in promoting health and preventing disease

— to identify methods of improving the quality and practice of education, public health education, and health promotion

— to elicit the cooperation and coordination with those national, public, private, and voluntary agencies related to public health programs

— to provide a forum for continuing education opportunities in public health education and health promotion

ASTDHPPHE and the Centers for Disease Control and Prevention co-sponsor the National Conference on Health Education and Health Promotion.

## American Association for Health Education

(CNHEO member) The American Association for Health Education is an association of the American Alliance for Health, Physical Education, Recreation, and Dance. It is the oldest and largest health education organization, boasting a membership of 7,500 current and retired professionals and students. The purpose of AAHE is to advance the profession and serve health educators and other professionals who strive to promote the health of all people (AAHPERD, 1999). The organization attains its mission through a comprehensive approach that encourages, supports, and assists health professionals concerned with health promotion through education and other systematic strategies.

AAHE provides technical assistance to legislative and professional bodies engaged in drafting legislation and related guidelines and provides leadership in promoting policies and evaluative procedures that will result in effective health education programs. It is involved in accreditation of professional preparation programs. AAHE serves professionals in health care, communities, agencies, businesses, schools, and higher education. Publications include *Journal of Health Education* six times a year, *HE-XTRA* five times a year and a variety of books. The alliance holds a convention annually.

## American School Health Association

(CNHEO member) Founded in 1927, the American

School Health Association is a membership organization for professionals in schools who are committed to safeguarding the health of school-aged children and youth. The membership of 3,000 includes health educators, physical educators, administrators, counselors, dentists, physicians, school nurses, school food service personnel, and students in 56 countries. The mission of ASHA is to protect and improve the well-being of children and youth by supporting comprehensive school health programs (ASHA, 1997). The association provides advocacy for children and youth, professional education, public education, and research.

ASHA publishes the *Journal of School Health* ten times a year, *Pulse*, a quarterly newsletter, and a variety of resource materials. It holds an annual national convention. It also conducts a number of workshops; develops advocacy kits for school personnel; conducts peer training in health advocacy; and provides technical assistance to local school districts in curriculum development, needs assessment, program planning, and evaluation.

## American Public Health Association  APHA, founded in 1872, is the oldest of the organizations discussed in this chapter. The association brings together researchers, health service providers and members of other occupations in a unique, multidisciplinary environment of professional exchange. APHA has a membership of over 50,000 and represents the major disciplines in public health through its sections. The sections allow members to pursue specific professional interests while providing technical and scientific functions for association activities (APHA, 1999).

APHA's School Health Education and Services Section (CNHEO member) works independently, with other association substructures, and with external organizations to improve early childhood, school, and college health programs. Its purpose also includes interpreting the functions and responsibilities of health agencies to daycare, preschool, school, and college personnel; interpreting early childhood, school, and college health education and service objectives to other public health personnel and assisting them in integrating the objectives in their community; providing a forum for discussion of practices and research in early childhood, school,

and college health; encouraging the provision of health promotion programs within the school and college settings that address the needs of children and school personnel; and encouraging among interested members the study and discussion of procedures and problems in early childhood, school, and college health services, health education, and environmental health programs. The section has approximately 380 members and publishes a newsletter twice a year (CNHEO, 1996).

The Public Health Education and Health Promotion Section (CNHEO member) has a membership of approximately 3,600. Its mission is to be a strong advocate for health education, disease prevention and health promotion directed to individuals, groups, and communities and to set, maintain, and exemplify the highest ethical principles and standards of practice on the part of all professionals and disciplines whose primary purpose is health education, disease prevention, and/or health promotion. The section's purposes include being a strong advocate for health education, disease prevention, and health promotion; to encourage the inclusion of health education, disease prevention, and health promotion activities in all of the nation's health programs; to improve the quality of research and practice; and to provide networking opportunities for people whose professional interests and training are relevant (CNHEO, 1996).

APHA publishes *American Journal of Public Health* six times a year, *Nation's Health* eleven times a year, and books on public health topics.

## American College Health Association (CNHEO member) The American College Health Association has 2,500 individual members and 925 institutional members. The purpose of ACHA is to provide an organization in which institutions of higher education, other organizations, and interested individuals may work together to promote health in the broadest aspects for students and all members of the college community. Its mission is to be the principal advocate and leadership organization for college and university health. ACHA provides advocacy and representation, education, research, service and communication. ACHA has ten membership sections, including the Health Education Section, which are defined by the disciplines of college health (ACHA,

1999). Most members are associated with the health service facilities on their respective campuses.

ACHA has eleven affiliate organizations, each of which conducts an annual meeting. ACHA publishes *Journal of American College Health* and the newsletter *Action* six times a year. It also produces a variety of publications on policy, programming and law, and educational resource materials.

### International Union for Health Promotion and Education

IUHPE is a global association with membership from more than eighty countries organized through six regional offices. It is dedicated to improving world health through education, community action, and the development of healthy public policies. It works in close cooperation with the World Health Organization, the United Nations Educational, Scientific and Cultural Organization, and the United Nations Children's Fund (IUHPE, 1998). It publishes the journal *Promotion & Education* and sponsors an international conference every three years. There are approximately 2,000 members.

### Association for Worksite Health Promotion

AWHP is a not-for-profit network of worksite health promotion professionals dedicated to sharing the best-of-practice methods, processes, and technologies (AWHP, 1999). It has approximately 3,000 members, including health educators, human resource directors, wellness directors, physical and occupational therapists, dietitians, and exercise physiologists. There are regional chapters in the United States, Canada, and the United Kingdom. The association advocates for worksite health promotion to business and government. It also supports professionals through education and providing resources to those in the field. AWHP also supports research.

AWHP publishes a quarterly journal titled *Worksite Health*, a bi-monthly newsletter called *Action*. In addition, it has prepared several publications for those interested in worksite health promotion.

### Eta Sigma Gamma

Eta Sigma Gamma is the national health education honorary society, which focuses on its student members. Chapters are located on many college and university campuses.

The principal purpose of ESG is to elevate the standards, ideals, competence, and ethics of professionally trained men and women in and for the Health Science discipline (ESG, 1999). ESG is responsible for processing health education entries for the U.S. Department of Health and Human Services' Secretary's Award for Innovation in Health Promotion.

ESG produces *The Health Education Monograph Series*, its journal *The Health Educator*, and *The Vision*, its newsletter. Each publication is distributed twice a year.

### National Wellness Association

The NWA is an international, non-profit professional membership organization. It is a division of the National Wellness Institute, Inc. The mission of NWA is to serve members with information, resources, services, professional development, and networking opportunities to promote wellness. NWA publishes the newsletters *Health Issues Update, Wellness Management, Health Promotion Practitioner*, and *The Art of Health Promotion;* it also publishes the journal *American Journal of Health Promotion*. It provides the *NWA Job Opportunities Bulletin* and an on-line job connection link to job openings nationwide (NWA, 1999).

### Canadian Public Health Association

CPHA is a national not-for-profit association composed of health professionals from over 25 health disciplines (CPHA, 1998). It represents public health in Canada with links to the international public health community and is active in supporting and conducting health and social programs both nationally and internationally. CPHA encourages and facilitates measures for disease prevention, health promotion and protection, and public policy on health. It has a history of facilitating the development of public health goals for Canada, identifying public health issues, and advocating for policy change. Areas of interest include disease surveillance and control, health promotion, and equity and social justice. CPHA publishes *Canadian Journal of Public Health* and various newsletters (including *CPHA Health Digest*) and materials.

All professional associations provide methods for health educators/promoters to keep abreast of changing issues and maintain a grasp of contemporary developments in theory and practice. Opportunity for students and professionals to contribute to the field is immeasurably enhanced by professional associations. The ability of organizations to coalesce concerns and advocate for issues is an important part of development of a professional culture.

## KEY POINTS

1. There are three essential characteristics of a profession—a service mission, a unique body of knowledge, and a prolonged period of training—and at least six related characteristics.

2. Individuals enter the profession of health education/promotion from several types of academic programs. The length of training required for entry is not agreed upon.

3. One of the final steps in establishment of a profession is a code of ethics. The Coalition of National Health Education Organizations has adopted a profession-wide code of ethics.

4. Four ethical theories have been applied to the practice of health education/promotion: natural law, utilitarianism, paternalism, and distributive justice.

5. Accepted competencies drive the standards of education for health education/promotion.

6. A number of professional organizations provide opportunities for the individual to identify with the profession.

7. Health education/promotion is best described as an emerging profession.

## REFERENCES

ABT Associates. (1980). *School health education evaluation.* Cambridge, MA.

American Alliance for Health, Physical Education, Recreation and Dance. (1999). *AAHE: General overview* [On-line]. Available: www.aahperd. org/aahe/aahe-about.html

American Association for Health Education. (1999). *Responsibilities and competencies for teachers of young adolescents: In coordinated school health programs for middle level classroom teachers.* Reston, VA.

American Association for Health Education, National Commission for Health Education Credentialing, Inc., Society for Public Health Education. (1999). *A competency-based framework for graduate-level health educators.* Allentown, PA: NCHEC.

American Association of School Administrators. (1990). *Healthy kids for the year 2000: An action plan for schools.* Arlington, VA: American Association of School Administrators.

American College Health Association. (1999). *ACHA online* [On-line]. Available: http://acha.org/index.htm

American Public Health Association. (1999). *About APHA* [On-line]. Available: http://apha.org/about/basic. html

American School Health Association. (1997). *About ASHA* [On-line]. Available: http://www.ashaweb.org/ profile/

Association for the Advancement of Health Education. (1994). Code of ethics for health educators. *Journal of Health Education, 25*(4), 197–200.

Association for Worksite Health Promotion. (1999). *Welcome to AWHP on line* [On-line]. Available: http:// www.awhp.org/default/Default.htm

Association of State and Territorial Directors of Health Promotion and Public Health. (1999). *About ASTDHPPE* [On-line]. Available: www. astdhpphe.org/aboutastdhppe.html

Barnes, S., Fors, S., & Decker, W. (1980). Ethical issues in health education. *Health Education, 11*(2), 7–9.

Bayles, M. (1981). *Professional ethics.* Belmont, CA: Wadsworth.

Beauchamp, T.L., & Childress, J.F. (1989). *Principles of biomedical ethics.* New York: Oxford University Press.

Breckon, D.J., Harvey, J.R., & Lancaster, R.B. (1998). *Community health education: Settings, roles, and skills for the 21st century* (4th ed.). Gaithersburg, MD: Aspen.

Callahan, D. (1982). Should there be an academic code of ethics? *Journal of Higher Education, 53*(3), 335–344.

Canadian Public Health Association. (1998). *General information* [On-line]. Available: http://www.cpha.ca

Carlyon, W. H. (1975). *Science, ethics and health education: Dilemmas in doing good.* Unpublished manuscript.

Carnegie Corporation of New York, Carnegie Council on Adolescent Development, Task Force on Education of Young Adolescents. (1989). *Turning points: Preparing American youth for the 21st century.* Washington, DC.

Coalition of National Health Education Organizations. (1996). *Directory: Coalition of national health education organizations, U.S.A.* Columbia, MO.

Coalition of National Health Education Organizations. (1999). *Society of State Directors of Health, Physical Education and Recreation* [On-line]. Available: http://www.med.usf.edu/~kmbrown/ NCHEO.htm

Cottrell, R.R., Girvan, J.T., & McKenzie, J.F. (1999). *Principles & foundations of health promotion and health education.* Boston: Allyn & Bacon.

Deeds, S.G. Cleary, M.J., & Neiger, B.L. (Eds.). (1996). *The certified health education specialist: A self-study guide for professional competency* (2nd ed.). Allentown, PA: NCHEC.

Eta Sigma Gamma. (1999). *ESG history* [On-line]. Available: http://www.cast.ilstu.edu/temple/esghis.htm

Faden, R. (1987). Ethical issues in government sponsored public health campaigns. *Health Education Quarterly, 14*(1), 27–37.

Fain, G.S. (1992). *Ethics in health, physical education, recreation, and dance. ERIC* [On-line]. Available: http://www.ed.gov/databases/ERIC_Digests/ed342775.html

Fennell, R., & Beyrer, M.K. (1989). AIDS: Some ethical considerations for the health educators. *Journal of American College Health, 38*(3), 145–147.

Greenberg, J., & Gold, R. (1992). *The health education ethics book.* Dubuque, IA: Wm. C. Brown.

Greene, W.H., & Simons-Morton, B.G. (1984). *Introduction to health education.* New York: Macmillan.

Henderson, A.C., McIntosh, D.V., & Schaller, W.E. (1981). Progress report of the Role Delineation Project. *Journal of School Health, 51*(5), 373–376.

Hochbaum, G. (1980). Ethical dilemmas in health education. *Health Education, 11*(2), 4–6.

Iammarino, N.K., O'Rourke, T.W., Pigg, R.M., & Weinberg, A.D. (1989). Ethical issues in research and publication. *Journal of School Health, 59*(3), 101–104.

International Union for Health Promotion and Education. (1998). *Mission* [On-line]. Available: http://www.ldb.org/iuhpe/mission.htm

Joint Committee of the Association for the Advancement of Health Education and the American School Health Association. (1992). Health instruction responsibilities and competencies for elementary (K–6) classroom teachers. *Journal of School Health, 62*(2), 76–77.

Kleinschmidt, H., &. Zimand, S. (1953). *Public health education—Its tools and procedures.* New York: Macmillan.

Livingood, W.C. (1996). Becoming a health education profession: Key to societal influence—1995 SOPHE presidential address. *Health Education Quarterly, 23*(4), 421–430.

McMahon, J.D., Bruess, C.E., & Lohrmann, D.K. (1987). Three applications of the role delineation project 1985 curriculum framework. *Journal of School Health, 57*(7), 274–278.

Metropolitan Life Foundation. (1985). *Healthy me—school health education survey.* New York.

National Commission for Health Education Credentialing, Inc. (1996). *A competency-based framework for professional development of certified health education specialists.* Allentown, PA.

National Commission on the Role of the School and the Community in Improving Adolescent Health. (1990). *Code blue: Uniting for healthier youth.* Alexandria, VA: National Association of State Boards of Education.

National Task Force on the Preparation and Practice of Health Educators. (1985). *A framework for the development of competency-based curricula for entry level health educators.* New York: National Commission for Health Education Credentialing.

National Wellness Association. (1999). *More about NWA* [On-line]. Available: http://www.wellnesswi.org/nwa

Newman, D.L., & Brown, R.D. (1996). *Applied ethics for program evaluation.* Thousand Oaks, CA: Sage.

O'Connell, J.K., & Price, J.H. (1983). Ethical theories for promoting health through behavioral change. *Journal of School Health, 53* (8), 476–479.

Patterson, S.M., & Vitello, E.M. (1993). Ethics in health education: The need to include a model course in professional preparation programs. *Journal of Health Education, 24*(4), 239–244.

Penland, L.R., & Beyrer, M.K. (1981). Ethics and health education: Issues and implications. *Health Education, 12*(4), 6–7.

Pigg, R.M. (1994). Ethical issues of scientific inquiry in health science education. *The Eta Sigma Gamma Monograph Series, 12*(2), iii.

Read, D., & Russell, R. (1985). Is behavioral change an acceptable objective for health educators? *The Eta Sigma Gamma Monograph Series, 4*(1), 9–61.

Shireffs, J.A. (1984). The nature and meaning of health education. In L. Rubinson & W.F. Alles (Eds.), *Health education: Foundations for the future.* Prospect Heights, IL: Waveland.

Siegel, H. (1968). Professional socialization in two baccalaureate programs. *Nursing Research, 17*(5), 403–407.

Simons-Morton, B.G., Greene, W.H., & Gottlieb, N.H. (1995). *Introduction to health education and health promotion* (2nd ed.). Prospect Heights, IL: Waveland.

Society for Public Health Education, Inc. (1976). SOPHE code of ethics. *Health Education Quarterly, 3*(1), 79.

Society for Public Health Education, Inc. (1997). *SOPHE snapshot* [On-line]. Available: www.sophe.org/AboutSOPHE/AboutSOPHE.htm

Taub, A., Kreuter, J., Parcel, G., & Vitello, E. (1987). Report of the AAHE/SOPHE joint committee on ethics. *Health Education Quarterly, 14*(1), 79–90.

Thomasma, D.C. (1979). Human values and ethics: Professional responsibility. *The Journal of the American Dietetic Association, 75*(5), 533–536.

U.S. Public Health Service. (1990). *Healthy people 2000: National health promotion and disease prevention objectives.* Washington, DC: Government Printing Office.

Vitello, E.M. (1986). Ethical issues: Questions in search of answers. *Health Education, 17*(5), 39–42.

Waishwell, L., Morrow, M.J., Micke, M.M., & Keyser, B.B. (1996). Utilization of the student portfolio to link professional preparation to the responsibilities and competencies of the entry level health educator. *Journal of Health Education, 27*(1), 4–9.

Wikler, D.I. (1978). Coercive measures in health promotion: Can they be justified? *Health Education Monographs, 6*(4), 223–241.

Wilensky, H.L. (1964). The professionalization of everyone? *American Journal of Sociology, 70*(2), 137–158.

# Settings for Health Education and Health Promotion

Health promotion/education—defined here as a planned process with specific objectives of establishing behavior, increasing knowledge, changing attitudes, or making environmental changes to support healthy lifestyles and communities—can be found in almost every setting imaginable. Multiple settings allow health promotion/education to reach the greatest number of people in convenient, cost-effective ways. Settings, which represent channels for delivering programs and access to specific populations, usually have pre-existing communication systems for diffusion of programs, and they facilitate development of policies and organizational change to support positive health practices (Mullen et al., 1995). Although a practitioner's specific duties may vary from setting to setting, many of the skills needed to carry out the responsibilities of health promoter/educator are similar across many settings (the relative emphasis may vary). However, professional preparation programs usually prepare practitioners to work in specific environments. The primary content areas that come into practice may also differ by setting, largely because of the mandate of the organization and the needs of the target population. (The setting most commonly associated with health education is the school. The complex and multifaceted modern school health program will be dealt with in detail in Chapter 7.)

## HEALTH CARE SETTINGS

Health care settings include hospitals, free-standing medical care clinics, community clinics, home health agencies, managed care organizations (MCOs), weight loss clinics, sports medicine clinics, and health spas. Patient education has typically been concerned with adherence to medical regimens, self-management of chronic conditions, and pretreatment instruction. More recently, patient education has become a cost control measure because it can reduce length of stay and amount of treatment required by a patient. Breckon and associates (1998) wrote about this phenomenon:

> Concurrent with cost-containment measures, health education shifted emphasis to health promotion, with health promotion specialists seeing education as one of several emphases. Moreover, the wellness movement gave more emphasis to promoting higher levels of wellness for apparently healthy people. Weight reduction, cessation of smoking, aerobic exercise, and other programs came into prominence. Many people demanded such services and health care providers responded to this consumer demand.

Client education is now seen as one of the most important roles for all health care providers (DeAmicis, 1997). In 1972, the American Hospital Association passed "A Patient's Bill of Rights" (shown in Box 6.1), mandating health education as a right of all clients. The Health Maintenance Organization Assistance Act of 1973 also required

## Box 6.1     A Patient's Bill of Rights

### INTRODUCTION

Effective Health Care requires collaboration between patients and physicians and other health care professionals. Open and honest communication, respect for personal and professional values, and sensitivity to differences are integral to optimal patient care. As the setting for the provision of health services, hospitals must provide a foundation for understanding and respecting the rights and responsibilities of patients, their families, physicians, and other caregivers. Hospitals must ensure a health care ethic that respects the role of patients in decision-making about treatment choices and other aspects of their care. Hospitals must be sensitive to cultural, racial, linguistic, religious, age, gender, and other differences as well as the needs of persons with disabilities.

The American Hospital Association presents *A Patient's Bill of Rights* with the expectation that it will contribute to more effective patient care and be supported by the hospital on behalf of the institution, its medical staff, employees, and patients. The American Hospital Association encourages health care institutions to tailor this bill of rights to their patient community by translating and/or simplifying the language of this bill of rights as may be necessary to ensure that patients and their families understand their rights and responsibilities.

### BILL OF RIGHTS*

1. The patient has the right to considerate and respectful care

2. The patient has the right to and is encouraged to obtain from physicians and other caregivers relevant, current, and understandable information concerning diagnosis, treatment, and prognosis.

    Except in emergencies when the patient lacks decision-making capacity and the need for treatment is urgent, the patient is entitled to the opportunity to discuss and request information related to the specific procedures and/or treatments, the risks involved, the possible length of recuperation, and the medically reasonable alternatives and their accompanying risks and benefits.

3. The patient has the right to make decisions about the plan of care prior to and during the course of treatment and to refuse a recommended treatment or plan of treatment or plan of care to the extent permitted by law and hospital policy and to be informed of the medical consequences of this action. In case of such refusal, the patient is entitled to other appropriate care and services that the hospital provides or transfer to another hospital. The hospital should notify patients of any policy that might affect patient choice within the institution.

4. The patient has the right to have an advance directive (such as a living will, health care proxy, or durable power of attorney for health care) concerning treatment or designating a surrogate decision maker with the expectation that the hospital will honor the intent of that directive to the extent permitted by law and hospital policy.

    Health care institutions must advise patients of their rights under state law and hospital policy to make informed medical choices, ask if the patient has an advance directive, and include that information in patient records. The patient has the right to timely information about hospital policy that may limit its ability to implement fully a legally valid advance directive.

5. The patient has the right to every consideration of privacy. Case discussion, consultation, examination, and treatment should be conducted so as to protect each patient's privacy.

6. The patient has the right to expect that all communications and records pertaining to his/her care will be treated as confidential by the hospital, except in cases such as suspected abuse and public health hazards when reporting is permitted or required by law. The patient has the right to expect that the hospital will emphasize the confidentiality of this information when it releases it to any other parties entitled to review information in these records.

7. The patient has the right to review the records pertaining to his/her medical care and to have the information explained or interpreted as necessary, except when restricted by law.

8. The patient has the right to expect that, within its capacity and policies, a hospital will make reasonable response to the request of a patient

(continued)

---

* These rights can be exercised on the patient's behalf by a designated surrogate or proxy decision-maker if the patient lacks decision-making capacity, is legally incompetent, or is a minor.

**Box 6.1**    A Patient's Bill of Rights (continued)

for appropriate and medically indicated care and services. The hospital must provide evaluation, service, and/or referral as indicated by the urgency of the case. When medically appropriate and legally permissible, or when a patient has so requested, a patient may be transferred to another facility. The institution to which the patient is to be transferred must first have accepted the patient for transfer. The patient must also have the benefit of complete information and explanation concerning the need for risks, benefits, and alternatives to such a transfer.

9. The patient has the right to ask and be informed of the existence of business relationships among the hospital, educational institutions, other health care providers, or payers that may influence the patient's treatment and care.

10. The patient has the right to consent to or decline to participate in proposed research studies or human experimentation affecting care and treatment or requiring direct patient involvement, and to have those studies fully explained prior to consent. A patient who declines to participate in research or experimentation is entitled to the most effective care that the hospital can otherwise provide.

11. The patient has the right to expect reasonable continuity of care when appropriate and to be informed by physicians and other caregivers of available and realistic patient care options when hospital care is no longer appropriate.

12. The patient has the right to be informed of hospital policies and practices that relate to the patient's care, treatment, and responsibilities. The patient has the right to be informed of available resources for resolving disputes, grievances, and conflicts, such as ethics committees, patient representatives, or other mechanisms available in the institution. The patient has the right to be informed of the hospital's charges for services and available payment methods.

The collaborative nature of health care requires that patients, or their families/surrogates, participate in their care. The effectiveness of care and patient satisfaction with the course of treatment depend, in part, on the patient fulfilling certain responsibilities. Patients are responsible for providing information about past illnesses, hospitalizations, medications, and other matters related to health status. To participate effectively in decision making, patients must be encouraged to take responsibility for requesting additional information or clarification about their health status or treatment when they do not fully understand information and instructions. Patients are also responsible for ensuring that the health care institution has a copy of their written advance directive if they have one. Patients are responsible for informing their physicians and other caregivers if they anticipate problems in following prescribed treatment.

Patients should also be aware of the hospital's obligation to be reasonably efficient and equitable in providing care to other patients and the community. The hospital's rules and regulations are designed to help the hospital meet this obligation. Patients and their families are responsible for making reasonable accommodations to the needs of the hospital, other patients, medical staff, and hospital employees. Patients are responsible for providing necessary information for insurance claims and for working with the hospital to make payment arrangements when necessary.

A person's health depends on much more than health care services. Patients are responsible for recognizing the impact of their lifestyle on their personal health.

## CONCLUSION

Hospitals have many functions to perform, including the enhancement of health status, health promotion, and the prevention and treatment of injury and disease; the immediate and ongoing care and rehabilitation of patients; the education of health professionals, patients, and the community; and research. All these activities must be conducted with an overriding concern for the values and dignity of patients.

HMOs to provide health education (although no requirement for professional preparation of the provider was included). The Joint Commission on Accreditation of Healthcare Organizations in 1992 established standards within hospitals requiring that, throughout the patient's stay, the client (and, as appropriate, his/her significant other[s]) receive education specific to the client's health care needs, including instructions on how to obtain follow-up care after discharge. This is especially important in light of shortened hospital stays, patients being discharged "sicker," and increasing family- and self-care needs.

Potter and Perry (1993) identified three main purposes of health education: promotion of health and illness prevention; restoration of health when one becomes ill; and maintenance of health while coping with chronic, long-term conditions. The health care delivery system has historically focused its health education on the latter two of these purposes. Because cost containment has become a dominant priority, the system should focus on health promotion and disease prevention to degrees never before attempted.

When health education is delivered in health care settings, the educator must assess several factors to understand the client's (usually an adult) health beliefs and practices. The American Public Health Association recommends that health care providers, especially managed care organizations, conduct baseline assessment and periodic reassessment of members' knowledge, attitudes, cultural practices, behaviors, and literacy levels to design appropriate health education programs (Belote, et al., 1999). Factors include many internal and external variables; examples are listed in Box 6.2.

## Hospitals and Managed Care Organizations

Hospitals initially saw health promotion as a way to generate income and a means of lowering costs. Where they had previously only delivered care to sick or injured people, they began to provide care for well consumers. New services such as health clubs, fitness centers, eating disorder centers, and aquatic centers became more commonplace. Some health care organizations constructed facilities of

---

| Box 6.2 | Client Variables in Patient Education |

**Developmental state**   emotional growth and development that affect behavioral patterns; age-related barriers to learning, such as sensory and cognitive impairments

**Intellectual background**   knowledge about illness and bodily functions; educational background; past experiences

**Learning style**   methods preferred for learning; reading level

**Self-concept issues**   client's perception of how the illness affects activities or lifestyle

**Emotional and spiritual factors**   religious values; stress; life changes

**Family characteristics**   family access to health care services; family educational levels; willingness to assist client; stability of marital or intimate relationships

**Socioeconomic factors**   occupation and occupational environment; social network; need for assistance with providing tools and equipment involved in education plan

**Cultural environment**   values and customs that may affect beliefs and practices

Sources: From *Fundamentals of Nursing: Concepts, Process, and Practice*, by B. Kozier, G. Erb, K. Blaise, & J. Wildinson, 1995, Redwood City, CA: Addison-Wesley *Nursing and Fundamentals of Nursing*, by P. Potter & A. Perry, 1993, St. Louis: Mosby YearBook.

---

their own; some contracted with nearby commercial facilities. Many hospitals hired professionally trained health educators. Some hospitals have since eliminated some programs, because poor management led to increased costs.

Recently, health care providers began to form regional or national consortia to contain costs. They developed contracts with employees and insurance companies. These networks became MCOs when they began to determine which services would be provided as necessary and covered services. Managed care organizations are designed to address the medical needs of employee groups and their families.

The role of managed care organizations is controversial. Many authorities, including some physicians, feel that MCOs are more concerned with profit than with the patient. Often physicians are overruled in their choice of treatment by company personnel who have never seen the patient and, in some cases, are not doctors. Many MCOs have reduced the frequency of some covered preventive services and routine examinations in an effort to cut costs. Where possible, surgery is done on an outpatient basis. Patients are often sent home from hospitals much earlier and "sicker" than before, with perplexing treatment regimens to follow. MCOs' basic philosophy seems to be to reduce short-term costs. The fact that most insurance does not cover, and hospitals may not offer, health education suggests that reducing short-term costs has priority over greater long-term savings.

Into this environment steps the health promoter, whose position is often administrative rather than educative. Medical specialists often do the actual education. Health education/promotion specialists are more likely to be involved in planning, implementing, and evaluating programs. Often health educators carry titles such as patient education manager and bear responsibility for design and evaluation of specific programs and for the acquisition, development, and distribution of educational materials (Giloth, 1993), with attendant duties to include staff training, needs assessment, program evaluation, budgeting, and reporting. Whatever the title, health educators must be able to address management, in its own language, and document their benefits to the organization.

Although professionals with degrees in health education or health promotion may find employment in hospitals or managed care facilities, those who want to specialize in patient education may have to complete a program in nursing or some other medical specialty. The skills of the health educator do not receive the level of respect in MCOs that they have in other settings, but this may change in the future. Sheinfeld Gorin and Arnold (1998) listed the following future challenges for these managed care entities:

- Broaden their programs to encompass a wider variety of health promotive services. (This applies particularly to health maintenance organizations.)

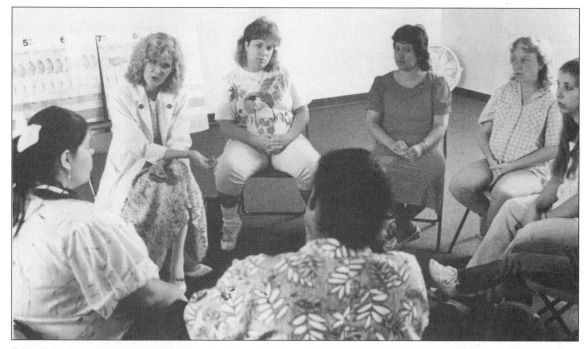

Education of pregnant women about diet, smoking, and other drug use may alter behavior and increase the likelihood of delivering a healthy baby.

- Increase development of new managed care options for vulnerable groups in the population who currently lack access to adequate health care.
- Grow employee assistance and community health programs to assist marginally employed and unemployed workers.
- Target programs to ethnic and racial minority populations.

These challenges imply an increase in community outreach by hospitals. Already many offer health and fitness programs to community members, often as memberships. In the future, they will expand these offerings, targeting vulnerable populations in the business community.

MCOs, with their emphasis on cost control, should place more attention and resources on health education. The American Public Health Association encourages MCOs to designate at least six percent of a member's premium for prevention and health promotion programs and adequate staffing by trained health educators (Belote, et al., 1999). For the time being, the programs that command the most acceptance in hospitals and MCOs are those that can lower costs and generate revenue. Programs that prepare patients to deal with outpatient procedures, minimize admissions and readmissions, deal with problems that affect a large number of people, can be done inexpensively, and can demonstrate cost savings are accorded priority.

## Primary Care Settings

The first provider that a patient meets in a medical setting is the **primary care** clinician. In this encounter, the clinician can identify problems and treat them before more serious illnesses develop. The primary care provider is responsible for addressing most of the patient's health care needs. This allows the provider to develop a relationship with the patient, including assessing the family and community factors that play a role in the health of the individual.

The health care site, particularly one that provides comprehensive services, provides a number of opportunities for health education. Ideally, the activities of the health care site are focused on health promotion and disease prevention, with primary care services that enable behavior change

provided under one roof. This makes it a natural place for health education. Health care providers generally are trusted by patients and communities to be knowledgeable and reliable sources of information on health topics and are thus well suited to be providers of health education (Mullen et al., 1995). Primary care physicians agree that part of their responsibility is to educate their patients about healthy behaviors, risk factors, and benefits of a healthy lifestyle (Russell & Roter, 1993). However, a 1996 survey of Massachusetts primary care physicians showed that two-thirds reported little confidence in helping patients change behaviors (Wechsler et al., 1996).

Fortunately, the health center, with its multidisciplinary team, has other professionals available to assist physicians, nurse practitioners, and physician assistants in fulfilling this responsibility. Often, health educators develop interventions, meet individually or in groups with patients, and provide other necessary services to patients and health care providers. The person may be identified as the health educator but professionally trained in another discipline, such as nursing or social work. (Visser, Thurmond, & Stinson, 1998). This is a weakness of this approach unless the individual has acquired additional schooling in health education to develop the necessary competencies.

Health care centers often serve diverse populations. The centers are often very culturally competent, having a provider team that reflects the ethnic background and languages of the population being served. Providers understand the cultural contexts from which their patients come and are trained to be culturally aware and sensitive (Visser, Thurmond, & Stinson, 1998). This makes it easier for minorities, who are often underserved and vulnerable, to obtain the services, including health education, that are offered by the centers. For instance, while bringing a child for a check-up or routine immunization, a single mother can attend a parenting class knowing that her child is being cared for by center staff.

Evidence supports the significant contributions made by health education in the health care setting to the treatment and care of patients with chronic disease (Steckler et al., 1995). This evidence suggests that a more intense role for health education

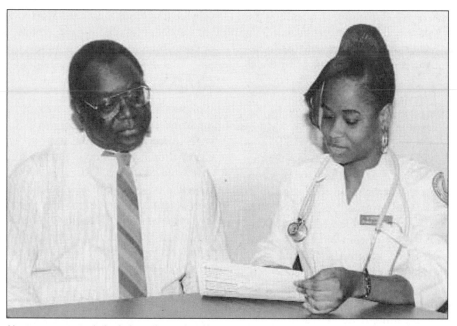

Nurses occupy a vital role in patient education.

would be beneficial to patients. However, insurers do not usually reimburse for health education services.

The private physician and office staff can play a large role in the promotion of health through education. Many practice within the MCO framework, but remain independent in their interactions with patients. Good physicians deliver health education as a part of routine interaction with patients. Those in large group practices often employ health educators or nurses with academic preparation in patient education.

## Other Health Care Environments

One of the most accessible settings for health education is the pharmacy. Most people are comfortable going to their pharmacist for information about prescription and nonprescription medications. Many pharmaceutical companies have developed pamphlets to help consumers understand drug interactions, side effects, and proper use of medications. These are usually available from the pharmacists' counter. In addition, most pharmacy chains produce printouts with similar information applicable to the specific drug being purchased.

Fitness centers are located throughout the United States. The growth of this industry is a result of consumer demands and clever advertising. The cost and quality of the equipment, services, and counseling at fitness centers vary greatly. At times the staff is more interested in selling a lengthy membership contract than in helping the consumer develop an individual fitness plan. The consumer should investigate the center thoroughly before signing a contract. Through diligent information gathering, the consumer can find a center that can meet his or her needs at a reasonable fee. Hospital-based fitness centers are usually good choices. They offer counseling by certified personnel, programs tailored to physicians' recommendations for the individual, and, by comparison to private fitness centers, at lower cost and shorter contract length. They rarely exert pressure to join.

Although nursing homes constitute ideal settings to target health promotion programs (Taylor-Nicholson et al., 1990), this potential has been

**primary care**   the provision of integrated, accessible health care services by clinicians who are accountable for addressing a large majority of personal health care needs, developing a sustained partnership with patients, and practicing in the context of family and community (Murphy, 1996)

neglected until recently. Encouraging nursing home residents to practice healthy behaviors increases the lifespan and quality of life. The key factors in improved mental and physical functioning for the elderly are social connectedness, exercise, and engaging in productive activities (Seeman et al., 1994, 1995). Emotional support is also critical (Center for Advancement of Health, 1998). These are obvious objectives for a nursing home health promotion program. A number of studies have reported that enhanced physical and mental health status is consistent with an increase in sense of control (e.g., Langer & Rodin, 1976; Avorn & Langer, 1982). The feeling that one's health is influenced by one's own behavior affords a sense of control over one's own welfare. This feeling of control has been demonstrated to affect physiologic processes (Rodin, 1986; Krantz et al., 1981) and it influences people to take better care of themselves, seek health-related information, and comply more frequently with medical instructions (Rodin, 1986). Indeed, health promotion programs should have been introduced in nursing homes long ago.

Senior citizen centers have become popular gathering places for retired persons. The centers usually provide nutritious meals; social activities, including trips and dances; classes; and exercise groups. The opportunities for health promotion are abundant.

## WORKSITES

Worksite health promotion grew out of industrial medicine and hygiene programs. These programs were concerned with first aid, medical care, and Occupational Health and Safety Administration–mandated programs. Programs focused on medical surveillance, environmental hazards (such as toxic components), or employee safety (Breckon, Harvey, & Lancaster, 1998). Gradually the programs expanded to the level of a wellness orientation and then included the health of workers' families. Rosen (1991) observed,

> Healthy people make healthy companies. And healthy companies are more likely, more often, over a longer period of time, to make healthy profits and to have healthy returns on their investments. So healthy people and healthy relationships are at the very core of success in business . . .

Pelletier (1993) reviewed 24 studies of worksite health promotion conducted between 1991 and

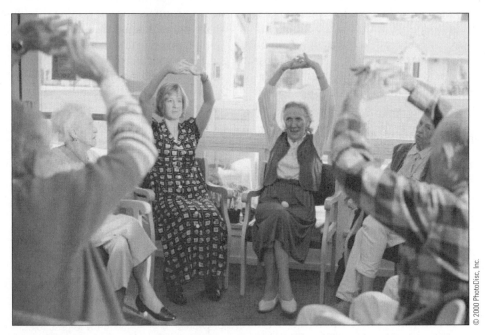

Exercise groups are popular activities at many senor centers. They offer opportunities for social interaction and physical activity.

1993. He found that 23 evidenced positive health outcomes, and every one indicated cost benefits.

Nationally, employers devote approximately 95 percent of health benefit expenses to treating illnesses. In contrast, only 15 percent of the working age population is ill at any given time, and the remaining 85 percent are either well or at risk of developing future illness. Overall health benefit expenses could be significantly decreased by shifting more resources to preventive care and health promotion efforts (Association for Worksite Health Promotion, 1999). Achieving the three chief goals of worksite health promotion—(1) assess health risks, (2) reduce those health risks that can be reduced, and (3) promote socially and environmentally healthy lifestyles (Chenoweth, 1998)—could certainly reduce overall benefit expenses.

Worksites are relatively new entries in the realm of health promotion locations. Most started in the mid-1970s. Yet there has been remarkable growth in worksite health promotion. By 1996, 89 percent of employers had some type of managed health initiative in place (Hewitt Associates, 1996), in comparison to 66 percent in 1985. Few programs are

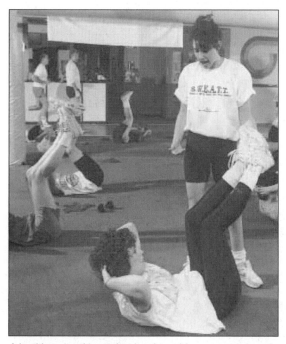

A health promotion professional provides encouragement and instruction to program participants.

comprehensive. Common activities include job hazards/injury prevention, exercise/physical fitness, smoking cessation, stress management, blood pressure and cholesterol control, and programs and policies on alcohol and other drug use. More comprehensive programs include assessment and screening, self-help activity plans, and educational programs. Some employers have implemented financial incentives/disincentives such as asking employees who continue unhealthy habits to pay a greater share of the costs of personal health care. Others have provided environments conducive to participation, such as jogging and cycling trails, nonsmoking policies, and cafeteria and vending machine modifications. Some of the motivations for this trend are listed in Box 6.3.

Many employers have developed **employee assistance programs**. EAPs originally helped employees deal with alcohol and other drug problems, primarily because these problems affected job performance. They have been expanded to address problems that can seriously threaten the health or well-being of employees or their families, including marital, legal, or financial problems; depression and other emotional concerns. EAPs may include lifestyle change approaches, family support, and counseling. Some employers contract with outside social workers or therapists; some employ licensed professionals. Health educators working in EAPs may plan and conduct programs and manage external contracts for health promotion.

Productive health promotion programs coordinate with other programs within the company and with community resources. In large companies, the occupational safety and health program monitors environmental hazards, trains workers in safety practices, and attempts to ensure compliance with regulations. Health promotion programs can work with the occupational safety and health program to encourage a supportive environment for health promotion. Such programs may suggest reorganizing the physical work setting and developing healthy corporate policies. They also encourage employee

**employee assistance program**  initiative for the purpose of helping employees cope with health problems that affect work

## Box 6.3 Why Businesses Offer Worksite Health Promotion

1. **Absenteeism.** Half of all unscheduled absences are due to minor ailments. To battle these ailments, companies offer medical self-care programs to employees and dependents.

2. **Accessibility.** The workplace is usually a convenient setting for offering educational and motivational programs to many people at once.

3. **Aging workforce.** As American workers age and experience more health problems, many employers are implementing age-appropriate interventions to slow the effects of aging and detect problems earlier.

4. **Competition.** Concern about retaining employees is prompting companies to provide health club subsidies and other perks to improve morale and increase retention.

5. **Health insurance premiums.** Employer-paid health insurance premiums for employees and dependents have risen nearly 1,000 percent since 1960. This statistic alone is enough to move many companies to action. More and

more employers are finding WHP (worksite health promotion) to be the best option for combating the huge costs of insurance premiums.

6. **Image.** Many corporate leaders realize that successful WHP programs boost a company's image among workers, community, and industry peers.

7. **Keeping up with growing national interest.** Nationwide interest in personal health enhancement is reflected in today's print and electronic media coverage. Companies that want to be perceived as innovative pacesetters cannot afford to ignore such trends.

8. **Productivity.** Because healthy employees generally outperform unhealthy employees, more companies are offering health promotion programs to increase overall productivity.

9. **Workers' compensation costs.** Customized WHP programs are successful in many case-management and return-to-work efforts (thus reducing time away from work).

Source: From *Worksite Health Promotion, 6,* by D.H. Chenoweth, 1998, Champaign, IL: Human Kinetics. Reprinted by permission of the publisher.

participation in planning and implementing the programs.

The health promoter/educator must be able to "sell" a program to management. O'Donnell (1994) identified three primary motivators for employers to invest in health promotion: reduced medical care costs, enhanced productivity, and enhanced image of the company. There is certainly good evidence of the economic benefits associated with worksite health promotion programs, including a meta-evaluation of approximately thirty major evaluation studies (Chapman, 1996), a review of outcome studies (Pelletier, 1993), and research conducted in 1987 and 1995 that indicated, "A significant difference exists in the cost of medical care by health risk status" (Milliman & Robertson, 1995). Reduced absenteeism, increased productivity, decreased turnover, decreased insurance costs, and decreased disability payments make health promotion attractive to employers (Breckon, Harvey, & Lancaster, 1998). Table 6.1 presents information on return on investment of several worksite programs. It should be understood that these data do not guarantee an overall reduction in future health care

costs. As more retirees demand more services, workers stay on the job longer and require more health care, and the overall demand for health care increases, actual costs may increase as well.

An additional benefit is increased worker satisfaction and morale. Most employees appreciate the

## Table 6.1 Return on Investment in Worksite Health Programs

| Company | Dollars Saved Per $1.00 Invested |
|---|---|
| Coors | $6.15 |
| Bank of America | 6.00 |
| Kennecott Copper | 5.78 |
| Equitable Life Insurance | 5.52 |
| Travelers Insurance | 3.40 |
| Blue Cross/Blue Shield of Indiana | 2.50 |
| DuPont | 2.05 |

Source: From *Economic impact of worksite health promotion* [On-line], Fitwell, Inc., 1998. Used by permission. Available: http://www.fitwellinc.com/noframe/hlthpro.htm

efforts of companies to protect and improve the health of staff and their families; they also appreciate the convenience of the program. This becomes both a retention and recruiting tool.

The complexity of a good worksite health promotion program requires acceptance and support on many levels. This includes a supportive environment (among both management and employees), an orderly management process, and maintenance of a consistent level of awareness. Figure 6.1 demonstrates the intricacy of implementing the comprehensive worksite program. (Of course, not all programs will be as complete as depicted in the figure.)

In cultivating a new program, health promoters may use several helpful ideas to gain support and acceptance among employees. First, programs should be offered at convenient times near normal working hours and on days preferred by employees. They should be available to all shifts. In advertising, positive, catchy titles and short personal testimonies can be attractive. Incentives such as lotteries, prizes

for reaching goals, and competition are often effective at reaching potential participants.

Once the program is in place, the program director must keep the workers involved in the program. Many participants drop out for a number of reasons, including lack of interest, lack of time, inconvenience, and lack of creativity on the part of program directors. The ability to continue program participation requires organization, administrative support, motivation and reinforcement, and programming that meets participants' needs (Bensley, 1991). Positive incentives may include lower insurance premiums, recognition and awards, membership in a fitness club, coupons and gift certificates, and token prizes such as T-shirts and caps. Helping employees set realistic goals broken into reachable short-term objectives will keep participants motivated. Visual depictions, such as maps signifying distance covered by walkers in a "coast-to-coast" challenge with rewards for reaching landmarks, or bar graphs depicting minutes of exercise, distance

**Figure 6.1** Three levels of the comprehensive worksite health promotion program

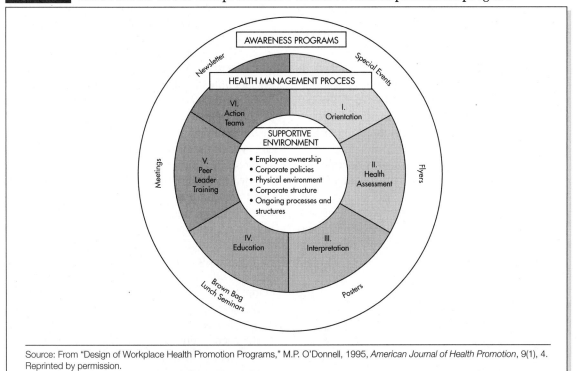

Source: From "Design of Workplace Health Promotion Programs," M.P. O'Donnell, 1995, *American Journal of Health Promotion*, 9(1), 4. Reprinted by permission.

jogging, or repetitions in the weight room help drive participants.

**Health risk appraisals** (HRAs), systematic collections of information—including individual and family health history, risk factors, and health-related behaviors—can provide valuable incentives to employees. A number of HRAs are on the market, many of which construct an estimated life expectancy or numerical risk score for each individual. HRAs are useful as kickoff events for programs aimed at changing individual behaviors as well as for assessing needs. They can help generate individual health promotion plans and therefore assist in keeping participants involved.

Health educators employed in worksite health promotion programs need administrative skills and should be able to plan, implement, and evaluate programs. The ability to function in an atmosphere of organizational and policy change is essential. They should also be content specialists. They often conduct classes or clinics and, therefore, need a foundation in adult learning theory. Many professional groups foresee more career opportunities in corporate wellness, including exercise physiologists, nurses, nutritionists, sociologists, and health psychologists. This increases competition for positions in the field, making it important to have adequate preparation for health promotion specific to the worksite. Anspaugh, Dignan, and Anspaugh (2000) identified study in business and marketing, adult education, personnel management, budget development, counseling theories, behavior change techniques, and traditional health promotion curriculum as important areas of study for worksite health promoters.

As the population ages, the proportion of retirees will increase. Industry will consider wellness programs for retirees. This will increase the quality of life for people who have served the industry and cut health care expenditures. There may be a growing partnership between labor unions and community health organizations.

# COMMUNITY/PUBLIC HEALTH AGENCIES

Community health agencies include those that are funded by taxation and mandated by law (called **public health agencies**) and voluntary agencies funded primarily by citizen donations, endowments, and grants. Both perform a host of health promotion functions, including education and providing information relating to primary prevention, detection and treatment of disease, family assistance and support groups, research, and legislative advocacy. They are adept at providing **community health education**.

Voluntary health agencies play a larger role in community health in the United States than in most other countries (Breckon, Harvey, & Lancaster, 1998). These agencies often focus on a specific set of conditions (such as diseases like cancer, pulmonary disease, or diabetes) or issues (such as human sexuality, domestic abuse, or substance abuse). They frequently carry out patient education. They may also be active in issues such as environmental health, homelessness, smoking, public safety, and the health of special populations, such as migrant workers. They generally have a small paid professional staff and are governed by a board of directors, the members of which have acute interest in the activities of the agency. Volunteers are the backbone of these organizations; they are often trained to apply their empathy, understanding, compassion, and enthusiasm to help other people live with a damaging medical condition or alter their lifestyle. For example, the American Cancer Society offers Fresh Start, a smoking cessation program staffed by volunteers, to businesses and schools. The American Red Cross offers courses to develop individual skills in child care and babysitting, cardiopulmonary resuscitation, first aid, and water safety.

Health educators in voluntary health agencies often are engaged in fund-raising, community action, public education, and professional inservice education. They may be charged with recruiting, training, retaining, and documenting volunteers. Health educators may seek external funding through grants. They usually conduct needs assessment, develop or supervise the development of programs, implement programs, evaluate them, and report on their success. The professional in the voluntary health agency must be multi-skilled and flexible.

Public health agencies and departments help to execute the government responsibility for doing for the people as a whole what individuals cannot do for themselves. They may be established on any of several levels: federal, state, county, groups of counties, or city.

Local health departments provide direct constituent services. Most state and federal health departments primarily serve other agencies, including local health departments.

Public health agencies employ health educators whose work in public health agencies is quite diverse. Professionals may work as consultants for educational components of programs in and out of the department. They may cooperate with departments of education and schools to develop educational materials and resources for instruction. They may deliver health education/promotion services in worksites, schools, public health clinics, or in outreach programs designed for target groups in the community. Their work often requires them to support public health nurses, environmentalists, epidemiologists, and staff planners.

Public health educators plan, implement, and evaluate educational activities that cut across all lines—racial, income, age, and gender. They also conduct public relations activities and market programs. Media, politics, and advocacy are all part of job performance. They work with members of the community to identify health and social needs so that, together, they can develop programs to meet those needs.

Because health education is the job of everyone in a public health department, especially on the local and county levels, health educators are in something of a quandary. Some administrators believe that a specialist in health education is unnecessary. Fortunately, most administrators understand the unique role that health educators play in public health.

Community/public health agencies are called upon frequently to reinforce the reasons for and benefits of regulations or environmental controls through health education. They often must educate decision makers, including legislators. For instance, a campaign of public education might be launched about the risks of drunk driving or environmental tobacco smoke before the legislation to strengthen drunk driving laws or to restrict smoking in public places is introduced. When taxes on tobacco products are raised, states have utilized health promotion to clarify the economic reasons for the taxation, publicize the health effects of smoking, and communicate the promise to use the increased revenue for programs acceptable to the majority of people, such as tobacco education in schools.

## COLLEGES AND UNIVERSITIES

In recent years, the number and quality of health promotion programs on campuses of higher education has grown. Hundreds of U.S. colleges and universities have some type of wellness program. The philosophy behind colleges' embarking on health promotion is the institution's mission to support the growth and development of the individual student intellectually, socially, and physically. Helping the student develop habits that promote wellness optimizes his or her growth and development. These programs may also be directed at faculty and staff and at the community in which the institution is located.

College and university health service programs have become similar to health care settings. They usually have physicians or nurses on duty to care for minor health problems. More recently, they have employed health educators, whose functions include

**health risk appraisal**   questionnaires used to estimate individuals' health risks by comparing behaviors and current health status to those of a cross section of healthy people who are the same age and gender as the user

**public health agencies**   community agencies created by government and funded by taxes for the purpose of protecting, improving, and maintaining the health of the citizens

**community health education**   the application of a variety of methods that result in the education and mobilization of community members in actions for resolving health issues and problems which affect the community. These methods include, but are not limited to, group process, mass media, communication, community organization, organization development, strategic planning, skills training, legislation, policy making and advocacy (1990 Joint Committee on Health Education Terminology, 1991)

patient education. They also cooperate with academic college departments to provide preventive programs for students. These may take place in classes, dormitories, assemblies, student organizations, or campus media. Health service personnel sometimes arrange for faculty and people from the outside community to cooperate in planning, developing, and implementing programs, which are often directed toward specific topics such as HIV/AIDS, contraception and safer sex, exercise, weight control, relationships, safety, and alcohol and other drugs. Sometimes they coordinate peer education programs. These are excellent opportunities for students who aspire to be health educators to obtain some valuable experience.

Programs for faculty and staff are also gaining popularity. These are basically worksite health promotion programs. Colleges and universities have the advantage of already having facilities (such as classrooms, gymnasiums, weight rooms, pools, and tracks), equipment (such as stationery bicycles, implements to measure components of fitness, and sports equipment), and expertise (faculty who

specialize in exercise physiology, physical education, and health education).

Many institutions have wellness centers on campus, some with fully certified staff, flexible hours, and facilities and equipment. These centers provide opportunity for formal, planned programs and for individual participation with little supervision. Like the worksite health promotion program, they may begin with administration of an HRA and health screening, followed by assistance in setting goals and prescription of a program tailored to meet the individual's goals. They have been offered for faculty and staff, students, and community members. This is looked upon as a way of building a bond between the community and the institution. If services and facilities meet their needs, community members gladly pay fees to enjoy them. However, regardless of whether the program serves only students or employees or the community or all three groups, adequate assessment of participants is necessary, and the proper medical supervision should be provided if indicated. Only properly trained personnel should be employed in the program to

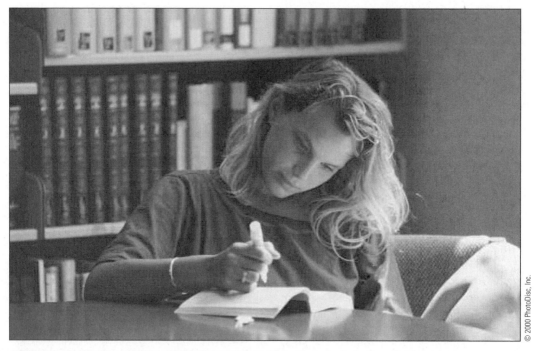

© 2000 PhotoDisc, Inc.

College and university wellness centers offer many benefits to students, including relief from the stress associated with the pressures of college life.

maintain the program's credibility and reduce legal liability.

# THE FAITH COMMUNITY

Religious organizations may be significant settings for health promotion in the near future. Many affluent places of worship already have recreation facilities that could easily be transformed into health promotion centers. In fact, many colleges, schools, summer camps, daycare centers, hospitals, and indigent service providers are church-related.

The religious community appears to be mobilizing and focusing on health promotion. Attention to the effects of stress, including biochemical and immunological effects, have brought religion and medicine closer together. The popularity of holistic and alternative therapies have also contributed to this new focus. A variety of studies have shown that religiosity improves immunity to communicable diseases, reduces the incidence of chronic and degenerative disease, improves the survival rate of surgery patients, increases social interaction, increases a sense of humor, reduces stress, increases hope, reduces death anxiety of older people, and generally makes people happier and healthier (Breckon, Harvey, & Lancaster, 1998).

Houses of worship are excellent opportunities to reach senior citizens. Church attendance is higher among seniors, and they require more health care than other groups. Many can be helped enormously by the activities and services of health promotion.

The Interfaith Health Program (1997) described a plan for selecting and training congregational health promoters and listed six characteristics of health promoters in the faith community:

— They have an ability to listen to the community.

— They possess natural leadership skills.

— They are respected by the community.

— They actively participate in collective solution processes.

— They evidence a concern for health and well-being of others.

— They understand that health is more than a medical issue.

Health educators/promoters may soon find many sources of employment within these settings. However, anyone considering such a job should investigate the goals and belief structures of the organization thoroughly. Religious beliefs are not likely to be altered and, when they form the basis for the organization's existence, the health promoter must be careful to learn about them and not violate or challenge them.

# THE MILITARY

The armed services have always been interested in the nutritional and physical fitness of personnel in order to ensure readiness and the ability to perform efficiently. The military is, therefore, a good environment for health promotion. Collins and Custis (1993) wrote that the military is implementing programs so that health promotion

> 1) supports . . . total organizational efficiency by optimizing the performance of its human resources, 2) promotes and supports policy development and management efforts to contain escalating costs of the Department of Defense's corporate health benefits program.

This is similar to the reasons that other managers support worksite health promotion. In addition, service personnel, most of whom are young, lapse into many of the risk behaviors that befall other young people, including smoking, excessive drinking, aggressive conduct, and reckless sexual behavior. This makes them an even more urgent target for health promotion.

Just as the reasons for health promotion in military settings resemble those in other worksites, the role of health educators/promoters will not differ significantly. Practitioners might view the military as a community of workers and dependents who interact with others. The military has its own system of health care as well as extensive facilities and equipment; they provide opportunities for patient education and the plethora of programs available at worksites, recreation centers, and fitness centers.

It is unclear whether the health promotion personnel will come from the civilian environment or from enlisted or civil service personnel. It does appear that the military is making more of a commitment to health promotion, which will provide new opportunities for health educators/promoters.

## KEY POINTS

1. Health promotion/education takes place in a variety of settings. Multiple settings allow health promotion/education to reach the greatest number of people.

2. Health care facilities offer excellent opportunities for health education/promotion. Patient education is attractive because it can become a cost control measure while helping patients manage their own chronic conditions and adhere to medical advice.

3. Health centers are staffed with multi-disciplinary teams, including health educators. They often serve diverse populations in culturally sensitive ways.

4. Worksites are relatively new locales in health promotion. However, they offer significant opportunities to assess health risks of employees, reduce those health risks, and promote socially and environmentally healthy lifestyles.

5. There are three primary motivators for employers to implement worksite health promotion programs: reduced medical costs, enhanced worker productivity, and enhanced image of the company.

6. The role of health educators in public and community health agencies varies greatly and is more established by practice than in many other settings.

7. Health promotion programs on college and university campuses offer services to students, faculty, staff, and community members. They are linked with academic programs and health service programs.

## REFERENCES

American Hospital Association. (1972). *A patient's bill of rights*. Chicago.

Anspaugh, D.J., Dignan, M.B., & Anspaugh, S.L. (2000). *Developing health promotion programs*. Boston: McGraw-Hill.

Association for Worksite Health Promotion. (1999). *The benefits of worksite health promotion* [On-line]. Available: http://www.awhp.org/default/whatis.html

Avorn, J., & Langer, E.J. (1982). Induced disability in nursing home patients: A controlled study. *Journal of the American Geriatric Society, 30*(3), 397–400.

Belote, A., Giloth, B., Auld, E., Gottlieb, N., & Smith, S. (1999, September). Providion of health education within managed care organizations. *The Nation's Health* 13–15.

Bensley, Jr., L.B. (1991). Schoolsite health promotion: Ways of sustaining interest. *Journal of Health Education, 22*(2), 86–89.

Breckon, D.J., Harvey, J.R., & Lancaster, R.B. (1998). *Community health education: Settings, roles and skills for the 21st century* (4th ed.). Gaithersburg, MD: Aspen.

Center for the Advancement of Health. (1998). Getting old: A lot of it is in your head. *Facts of Life: Issue Briefings for Health Reporters*, [On-line] *3*(2). Available: www.cfah.org/website2/fol3-2.htm

Chapman, L.S. (1996). *Proof-positive: Analysis of the cost-effectiveness of worksite wellness*. Seattle: Summex Corporation.

Chenoweth, D.H. (1998). *Worksite health promotion*. Champaign, IL: Human Kinetics.

Collins, B.S., & Custis, S.H. (1993). Health promotion in a sinking military. *Military Medicine, 158,* 386–389.

DeAmicis, P. (1997). The impact of health beliefs on adult client education. *Journal of Health Education, 28*(1), 13–17.

Fitwell, Inc. (1998). *Economic impact of worksite health promotion* [On-line]. Available: http://www.fitwellinc.com/noframe/hlthpro.htm

Giloth, B.E. (1993). Developing effective patient education management structures. In B.E. Giloth (Ed.), *Managing hospital-based patient education*. Chicago: American Hospital Publishing.

Hewitt Associates. (1996). *Health promotion initiatives/managed health provided by major U.S. employers in 1996.* Lincolnshire, IL.

Interfaith Health Program, The Carter Center. (1997). *Starting point: Empowering communities to improve health—A manual for training health promoters in congregational coalitions.* Atlanta.

Joint Commission on Accreditation of Healthcare Organizations. (1992). *Accreditation manual for hospitals.* Chicago.

Kozier, B., Erb, G., Blaise, K., & Wildinson, J. (1995). *Fundamentals of nursing: Concepts, process, and practice.* Redwood City, CA: Addison-Wesley Nursing.

Krantz, D.S., Glass, D.C., Contrada, R., & Miller, N.E. (1981). *The five year outlook in science and technology, National Science Foundation.* Washington, DC: Government Printing Office.

Langer, E., & Rodin, J. (1976). The effects of choice and enhanced personality responsibility. *Journal of Personality and Social Psychology, 34*(2), 191–198.

Milliman & Robertson, Inc. (1995). *Health risks and their impact on medical costs.* Brookfield, WI.

Mullen, P., Evans, D., Forster, J., Gottlieb, N., Kreuter, M., Moon, R., O'Rourke, T., & Strecher, V.J. (1995). Settings as an important dimension in health education/promotion policy, programs, and research. *Health Education Quarterly, 22*(3), 329–345.

Murphy, P. (1996). Primary care for women: Health assessment, health promotion, and disease prevention services. *Journal of Nurse Midwifery, 41*(2), 83–91.

1990 Joint Committee on Health Education Terminology. (1991). Report of the 1990 Joint Committee on Health Education and Terminology. *Journal of Health Education, 22*(2), 97–108.

O'Donnell, M.P. (1994). Employers' financial perspective on health promotion. In M.P. O'Donnell & J.S. Harris (Eds.), *Health promotion in the workplace* (2nd ed.). Albany, NY: Delmar.

Pelletier, K.R. (1993). A review and analysis of health and cost-effective outcome studies of comprehensive health promotion and disease prevention programs at the worksite: 1991–1993 Update. *American Journal of Health Promotion, 8*(1), 50–62.

Potter, P., & Perry, A. (1993). *Fundamentals of nursing.* St. Louis: Mosby YearBook.

Rodin, J. (1986). Aging and health: Effects of the sense of control. *Science, 233*(4770), 1271–1276.

Rosen, R. (1991). *The healthy company: Eight strategies to develop people, productivity, and profits.* Los Angeles: Tarcher.

Russell, N.K., & Roter, D.L. (1993). Health promotion counseling of chronic disease patients during primary care visits. *American Journal of Public Health, 83*(7), 979–982.

Seeman, T.E., Berkman, L.F., Charpentier, P.A., Blazer, D.G., Albert, M.S., & Tinetti, M.E. (1995). Behavioral and psychological predictors of physical performance: MacArthur studies of successful aging. *Journals of Gerontology, Series A, Biological Sciences and Medical Sciences, 50A*(4), M177–183.

Seeman, T.E., Charpentier, P.A., Berkman, L.F., Tinetti, M.E., Guralnik, J.M., Albert, M., Blazer, D., & Rowe, J.W. (1994). Predicting changes in functioning in a high-functioning elderly cohort: MacArthur studies of successful aging. *Journals of Gerontology, Series A, Biological Sciences and Medical Sciences, 49*(3), M95–106.

Sheinfeld Gorin, S., & Arnold, J. (1998). *Health promotion handbook.* St. Louis: Mosby.

Steckler, A., Allegrante, J.P., Altman, D., Brown, R., Burdine, J.N., Goodman, R.M., & Jorgensen, C. (1995). Health education interventions strategies: Recommendations for future research. *Health Education Quarterly, 22*(3), 307–328.

Taylor-Nicholson, M.E., Brannon, D., Mahoney, B., & Bucher, J. (1990). Assessing the need for health promotion programs in nursing homes. *Health Education, 21*(3), 23–28.

Visser, L., Thurmond, L., & Stinson, N. (1998). Health education: A "primary" component to the delivery of comprehensive primary care. *Journal of Health Education, 29*(5), S-10–S-14.

Wechsler, H., Levine, S., Idelson, R.K., Schor, E.L., & Coakley, E. (1996). The physician's role in health promotion revisited—A survey of primary care practitioners. *New England Journal of Medicine, 334*(15), 996–998.

# Coordinated School Health Programs

Even though health education takes place in a multitude of settings—hospitals, clinics, voluntary health agencies, and worksites— the most appropriate place for health education remains the school, the only institution that has the opportunity to coordinate the health education of other sectors of society. The great educator Horace Mann said more than a century ago,

> In the great work of education, then, our physical condition, if not the first step in point of importance, is the first in order of time. On the broad and firm foundation of health alone, can the loftiest and most enduring structures of the intellect be reared. (Kime, Schlaadt, & Tritsch, 1977)

School health instruction within a complete school health program is a fundamental part of the overall mission of education for a number of specific reasons:

1. Pupils spend a major part of their young lives in school. We owe it to our children to safeguard their health as a means of ensuring their fitness to learn and helping them make decisions that will enhance their health.

2. A coordinated, planned, sequential health education program represents an efficient means to improve both the health and education of Americans (Kolbe, 1993) by helping youth develop health-enhancing behaviors.

3. In many cases, we can influence healthy living habits and attitudes in children before they establish habits that are detrimental to health.

4. Compared to other settings, schools offer the best opportunity to provide high-quality health instruction and the best environment to contribute to the health of children.

5. Health is a "basic," addressed in the *Cardinal Principles of Secondary Education* (Commission on the Reorganization of Education, 1918/1928)—just as important as the development of fundamental mathematics or language skills. Actually, the objectives of comprehensive school health education are related closely to other cardinal principles: worthy home membership, citizenship, worthy use of leisure time, and ethical character (Seffrin, 1990).

6. Children who engage in health-enhancing behaviors perform better academically. There is a direct relationship between health and academic excellence.

Support for the coordinated school health program (CSHP) is substantial. A scientifically valid poll conducted for the American Cancer Society in 1994 showed that support for comprehensive school health education (as CSHP was called in 1994) is present among parents, adolescent students, and administrators. Administrators, screened to include only those who had general responsibility for overall school district curriculum, indicated that they believe in the importance of teaching about health to school children. All three groups, including 85 percent of the administrators, strongly believe that

CSHP is of equal or greater importance compared with other subjects taught in school. All three groups, including 90 percent of administrators, believe that health information and skills are just as useful, if not more useful, than other subjects, such as English, mathematics, and science. Some 80 percent of adolescents and 74 percent of parents believe health should be afforded at least as much, if not more, instructional time than other subjects taught in school. An astounding two-thirds of general school district administrators, who are most familiar with the overall school curriculum, share this opinion (The Gallup Organization, 1994).

A national survey of public opinion about school health education conducted by The Indiana University Center for Survey Research indicated wide public support for school-based health education (Torabi & Crowe, 1995). The study used trained personnel to select and interview a representative sample of 1,005 adults during October and November 1993. When asked to what extent they agree or disagree with the statement "School health education can reduce health problems of students such as drug use, poor nutrition, AIDS, and tobacco use," 56 percent agreed strongly and 32 percent agreed somewhat. Respondents with higher education backgrounds were significantly more likely to believe that health education can reduce health problems in children. The respondents were asked, "How does a health education course compare with other science courses?" More than 20 percent said health education is "more important" than other science courses, and about 70 percent indicated "equally important." When asked, "Who is responsible for the health education of students?" about 80 percent said that it is the responsibility of both schools and parents.

Many national organizations and federal agencies have published support for a coordinated (comprehensive) school health program, among them:

National Commission on the Role of the School and Community in Improving Adolescent Health (1990)

National Commission on Children (1991)

National PTA (1992)

Both houses of Congress (U.S. House of Representatives, Select Committee on Children, Youth and Families, 1992; U.S. Senate, Subcommittee on Oversight of Government Management, Committee on Governmental Affairs, 1992)

The World Health Organization, United Nations Educational, Scientific, and Cultural Organization, and United Nations Children's Emergency Fund (1992)

The U.S. Department of Health and Human Services (1991), along with the hundreds of organizations who helped develop the Year 2000 Objectives for the nation's health, acknowledged the role of school health programs. The following statement in *Healthy People 2000: National Health Promotion and Disease Prevention Objectives* supports and describes school health:

> Health education in the school setting is especially important for helping children and youth develop the increasingly complex knowledge and skills they will need to avoid health risks and maintain good health throughout life. Quality school health education that is planned and sequential for students in kindergarten through 12th grade, and taught by educators trained to teach the subject, has been shown to be effective in preventing risk behaviors. Quality school health education addresses and integrates education, skills development, and motivation on a range of health problems and issues (e.g., nutrition, physical activity, injury control, use of tobacco, alcohol and other drugs, sexual behaviors that result in HIV infection, other sexually transmitted diseases, and unintended pregnancies) at developmentally appropriate ages. . . . The content of the education is determined locally by parents, school boards, and other members of the community.
>
> Other aspects of the school environment can also be important to school health. State and local health departments can work with schools to provide a multi-dimensional program of school health that may include school health education, school-linked or school-based health services designed to prevent, detect, and address health problems, a healthy and safe environment, physical education, healthful school food service selections, psychological assessment and counseling to promote child development and emotional health, school site health promotion for faculty and staff, and integrated school and community health promotion efforts.

Again in the year 2000, the Department of Human Services and the hundreds of organizations and individuals who served in the development of the *Healthy People 2010* objectives for the nation accentuated the importance of school health programs. Fourteen objectives address various components of school health programs. The objectives include providing school health education on six behaviors; achieving proper nurse-to-student ratio; providing oral health services at school health centers; elimination of weapons on school property; providing tobacco-free school environments; acceptance of disabled students in regular classes; providing healthy school meals and snacks; providing head, face, eye, and mouth protection; requiring that students participate in daily physical education; requiring physical activity in physical education; providing access to school physical activity facilities; offering employee health promotion at the worksite; and increasing high school completion rates.

# THE LINK WITH ACADEMIC PERFORMANCE

The sixth reason listed above for instituting school health programs is currently most critical. American students score poorly on standardized measures of educational achievement in comparison with their counterparts of thirty years ago. They also score lower in science and mathematics than their peers in most western industrialized nations. In response to this trend, many states are implementing so-called "accountability" platforms, which typically take the form of standardized examinations in "core" course work such as mathematics, language arts, history, and science.

In some cases, course work that is not included in the examinations, such as health education, is neglected in the classroom. This practice puts students at risk on a number of levels. The link between academic performance and health is acknowledged by many authorities (see Box 7.1). Educational reforms will be effective only if students' health and well-being are identified as contributors to their academic success (Marx, 1998). This would suggest that implementation of a thorough school health program would lead to greater academic achievement.

No data exist to demonstrate the efficacy of the coordinated health program in improving student health and achievement. However, a review of a few documented positive effects of some of its eight individual components demonstrates the potential for collective gains:

- School health education can positively change students' health behaviors and attitudes (Dusenbury & Falco, 1995; Gold, 1994; Kirby et al., 1994) as well as their knowledge and skills (Errecart et al., 1991; Walter, Vaughan, & Wynder, 1989).

- School health education is a cost-effective public health measure (Rothman et al., 1993).

- School-based health centers can increase student attendance at school and reduce suspensions and dropout rates (Dryfoos, 1994).

- School nutrition services can relieve short-term hunger and improve students' scores on standardized tests (Meyers et al., 1989; National Research Council, 1989; U.S. Department of Health and Human Services, 1988, 1991).

In fact, school health programs could become one of the most efficient means the nation could employ to prevent major health problems. By preventing health problems in the young and in the adults they become, school health programs also could help improve educational outcomes, reduce the spiraling costs of health care, and thus improve economic productivity (Kolbe, 1993). The relationships among student health, health education, and academic performance will be visited again and again.

In 1994, the Secretary of Health and Human Services and the Secretary of Education released a joint statement announcing a new level of cooperation between their two departments and affirming the importance of school health programs in accomplishing education goals. The following points were emphasized in the joint statement (U.S. Departments of Education and Health and Human Services, 1994):

- America's children face many compelling educational and health and developmental challenges that affect their lives and their futures.

- To help children meet these challenges, education and health must be linked in partnership.

- School health programs support the education process, integrate services for disadvantaged and disabled children, and improve children's prospects.

- Reforms in health care and in education offer opportunities to forge the partnerships needed for our children in the 1990s.

- Education Goals 2000 and *Healthy People 2000* provide complementary visions that, together, can support our joint efforts in pursuit of a healthier and better-educated nation for the next century.

# COST CONTAINMENT

A seventh (unlisted) benefit of school health education was revealed in a recent analysis (CDC, 1997a) that estimated that, for every dollar spent on high-quality, multicomponent health education delivered in a school, society saves more than $13 (other studies place it as high as $14—see Box 7.3). Some of these savings come in direct costs, such as medical treatment for preventable diseases, addiction counseling, alcohol-related motor vehicle injuries, and drug-related crime. Others come in the form of indirect cost reductions, such as lost productivity

**Box 7.1**    The Links Between Health and Academic Performance

There is an inextricable link between students' health and their ability to learn.
—World Health Organization, 1996

Students who are hungry, sick, troubled, or depressed cannot function well in the classroom, no matter how good the school. . . . [Schools must] improve academic performance through fostering health and fitness of young adolescents, by providing a health coordinator in every middle school, access to health care and counseling services, and a health-promoting school environment.
—Carnegie Council on Adolescent Development, 1989

In the larger context, schools are society's vehicle for providing young people with the tools for successful adulthood. Perhaps no tool is more essential than good health. . . . Poor health interferes with learning; good health facilitates it.
—Council of Chief State School Officers, 1991

School health programs offer the opportunity for us to provide the services and knowledge necessary to enable children to be productive learners and to develop the skills to make health decisions for the rest of their lives.
—National School Boards Association, American Association of School Administrators, American Cancer Society, National School Health Education Coalition, 1995

To help children meet these [educational, health, and developmental] challenges, education and health must be linked in partnership. . . . Health, education, and human service programs must be integrated, and schools must have the support of public and private health care providers, communities, and families. . . . School health programs support the educational process, integrate services for disadvantaged and disabled children, and improve children's health prospects.
—U.S. Department of Education and U.S. Department of Health and Human Services, 1994

From an educator's perspective, it's important for schools to be concerned with a child's health because healthy children are more effective learners. For parents, it is very reassuring to know that their local school is concerned not only with reading and writing, but is also looking out for their child's health and well-being.
—William Casey, District Superintendent, Brooklyn, New York (Making the Grade, 1997)

Clearly, no knowledge is more crucial than knowledge about health. Without it, no other life goal can be successfully achieved. Therefore, we recommend that all students study health, learning about the human body, how it changes over the life cycle, what nourishes it and diminishes it, and how a healthy body contributes to emotional well being.
—Ernest Boyer, President of the Carnegie Foundation for the Advancement of Teaching, 1983

because of premature death and social welfare expenditures associated with teen pregnancy.

The same analysis found that every dollar invested in effective tobacco education saves society an estimated $18.80 in health care and other costs caused by smoking. Each dollar invested in preventive programs to reduce alcohol and other drug use saves an estimated $5.69. Each education dollar to prevent too-early and unprotected sexual behaviors saves $5.10.

## A Carefully Planned Approach

Some basic philosophical guidelines have been asserted (A Point of View, 1992). School health education should

— emphasize "broad-based constructive action in the shaping and reshaping of human lives for better health, rather than . . . the acquisition of knowledge about health"

— display a "broad curricular scope and methodological diversity, rather than . . . focus on narrow topical coverage or limited methodology"

— be "dynamic and evolving, not static and fixed"

— be flexible enough to alter structure because "experiences and research point out improved ways to accomplish the goal"

— invite "participation in design and delivery from all actors in the school and community, including students, employees and citizens"

In order to conform to these guidelines, school health education cannot be haphazard, as many efforts have been, but rather a well-planned curricular endeavor practiced and evaluated realistically by trained professionals. Figure 7.1 resembles the jumbled and disorganized situation in many school districts. Much more effective would be a

**Figure 7.1** An Example of a Haphazard System

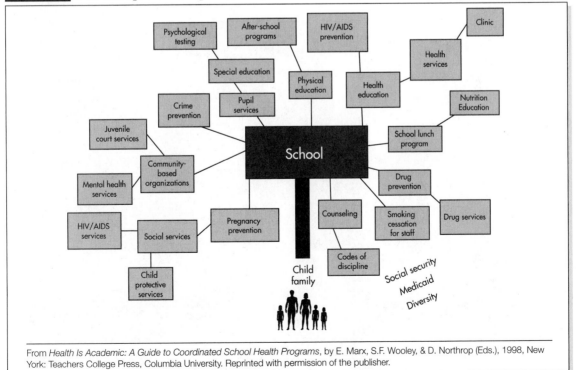

From *Health Is Academic: A Guide to Coordinated School Health Programs*, by E. Marx, S.F. Wooley, & D. Northrop (Eds.), 1998, New York: Teachers College Press, Columbia University. Reprinted with permission of the publisher.

comprehensive program from kindergarten through high school graduation that covers a variety of appropriate learning experiences suitable to the grade level. Effective health education—like any educational effort—is based upon a realistic assessment of pupil needs, interests, and capabilities. Community and parental values and interests also should be implicit to health education programs.

**Why "Coordinated"?**  The Institute of Medicine's Committee on Comprehensive School Health Programs in Grades K–12 (Committee, 1997) adopted this provisional definition of the *comprehensive* school health program:

> An organized set of policies, procedures and activities designed to protect and promote the health and well-being of students and staff which has traditionally included health services, healthy school environment and health education. It should also include, but not be limited to physical education; food and nutrition services; counseling, psychological and social services; health promotion for staff; and family/community involvement.

Recently, over 300 health education professionals were polled on the question of using "coordinated" rather than "comprehensive" to describe the school health program. The profession, as a whole, accepted that "coordinated school health program" (CSHP) was a more appropriate term and that label has been adopted.

## CHARACTERISTICS OF THE CSHP

The CSHP promotes wellness and motivation for health maintenance and improvement. Although this philosophy implies prevention of disease and disability, prevention takes a secondary position to the concept of overall wellness. In this way it focuses on the key risks to health and learning.

The CSHP offers educational opportunities for the family and community members. This is justified because the school is a part of the community and therefore is obligated to provide services for its members. By providing educational activities for the family and community at large, the school can gain valuable support for the CSHP. This often strips away many of the misconceptions surrounding health education and eliminates a good deal of the opposition from people who do not understand the nature of the CSHP. Support from family,

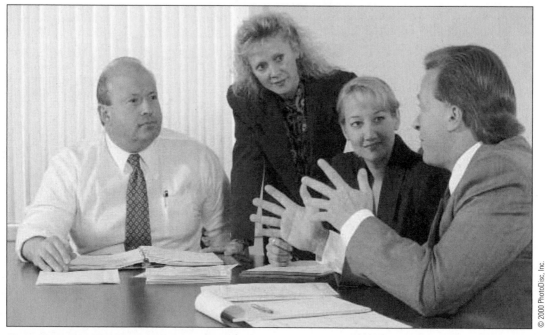

© 2000 PhotoDisc, Inc.

The school health coordinating council is a building-level body composed of school personnel, parents, students, representatives of the community organizations, and other interested parties.

friends, and adults within the community is crucial to success.

Coordination and leadership are necessary to ensure that the program operates effectively. A number of models can be effective. The most traditional is the **school health coordinating council**, set up in individual schools. In this model a council made up of teachers, the school nurse, physicians, parents, students, voluntary health agencies, the health department, and other interested parties provides direction to the health program. The functions of this council include identifying health and safety problems in the school, studying them, and making recommendations to the administration for solutions. These functions have been expanded in recent years to include outreach to the community, such as arranging for speakers, providing necessary materials the school district does not supply, and securing support from outside the school.

Planned and ongoing inservice programs are provided by the district or the state department of education for teachers and key school personnel, including the principal, the nurse, and curriculum specialists. This allows people who are planning and delivering instruction and services to stay current and continue to improve their skills.

The CSHP requires continual assessment and evaluation to determine if the objectives are met. Aspects to be evaluated include student gains in knowledge, improved attitudes, and changes in behavior; the process of implementing the curriculum; the currentness of curriculum and materials; and parent, student, and community perceptions of the program's value.

# NATIONAL HEALTH EDUCATION STANDARDS

School health curriculum development and instruction and assessment of student performance can be built upon the National Health Education Standards, developed by the Joint Committee on National Health Education Standards (1995). The standards are designed to promote **health literacy**, which is the individual's capacity to obtain, interpret, and understand basic health information and services and the competence to use the information

and services in ways that enhance health. The health-literate person is a critical thinker and problem solver, a responsible, productive citizen, a self-directed learner, and effective communicator.

These standards are not a federal mandate, nor do they define a national curriculum. They are intended to serve as a framework to organize health knowledge and skills into curricula at the state and local levels and to improve the teaching of health education. Teachers and policymakers can use the standards to design curricula, to allocate instructional resources, and as a basis for assessing student achievement and progress. They may guide local school districts, teachers, institutions of higher education, national organizations, state education agencies, and parents who are interested in improving health education. The standards identify what knowledge and skills students should obtain, yet are broad and flexible enough so the explicit means of accomplishment are left to teachers and curriculum specialists.

For students, they clarify what is expected. The national standards identify knowledge and skills that can be assessed. Each standard is accompanied by a rationale statement and performance indicators to be attained by the end of grades 4, 8, and 11. This allows for easy application in curriculum development, classroom application, and evaluation. Box 7.2 contains the standards (Appendix C contains the standards along with their rationale statement and performance indicators).

The Council of Chief State School Officers and the State Collaborative on Assessment and Student Standards (1999) have developed assessment measures, performance tasks, and performance events for the National Health Education Standards. They

**school health coordinating council**    body of concerned community members that serves as a liaison with the outside environment, ensuring support and establishing links between the school health program and outside community

**health literacy**    the capacity of individuals to obtain, interpret, and understand basic health information and services, and the competence to use the information and services in ways that enhance health

have also developed a portfolio assessment model to measure student progress toward the standards. States that join the CCSSO-SCASS consortium can have access to sufficient assessment resources to conduct assessment at state and local levels. Professional development materials are also being developed.

Health education that is based on the national standards contributes to the mission of education by encouraging students to use technology to access information and to use language arts, science, and mathematics skills in a health context. Moreover, standards-based health education provides students opportunities to learn and practice speaking and

---

**Box 7.2**  National Health Education Standards

1. Students will comprehend concepts related to health promotion and disease prevention.
2. Students will demonstrate the ability to access valid health information and health-promoting products and services.
3. Students will demonstrate the ability to practice health-enhancing behaviors and reduce health risks.
4. Students will analyze the influence of culture, media, and technology, and other factors on health.
5. Students will demonstrate the ability to use interpersonal communication skills to enhance health.
6. Students will demonstrate the ability to use goal-setting and decision-making skills to enhance health.
7. Students will demonstrate the ability to advocate for personal, family, and community health.

This represents the work of the Joint Committee on National Health Education Standards. Copies can be obtained through the American School Health Association, American Association for Health Education, or the American Cancer Society.

Source: *National Health Education Standards: Achieving Health Literacy*, by the Joint Committee on Health Education Standards, 1995, Atlanta: American Cancer Society.

---

listening skills as well as conflict resolution skills that they need to function effectively in school, in social settings, at home and, later, in the workplace. (Lohrmann & Wooley, 1998).

## COMPONENTS OF THE CSHP

Allensworth and Kolbe (1987) suggested a model with eight components that has come to represent the CSHP. The model is depicted in Figure 7.2.

If the eight components of the CSHP are to be organized and integrated, some locus must provide leadership, coordination, and management to ensure that the independent elements of the school health program become interdependent partners. The exact model for this leadership may vary from state to state and from district to district.

Among the different styles and systems of leadership, advisory boards, coordinating councils, individual leaders, and work teams have all provided leadership successfully. Davis and Allensworth (1994) identified the following prerequisites of effective leadership and management:

- **program familiarity**, including some familiarity with all eight components
- **programmatic vision** of the power of CSHP to create an environment in which health behaviors can change
- **leadership and management skills** to perform tasks such as preparing budgets, distributing health promotion work plans and policy statements, providing direction and supervision to others, conducting performance evaluations, and providing promotions or other awards
- **sufficient time** as measured by outcomes, although the program manager needs an agreed-upon portion of job time assigned for management
- **program planning and evaluation skills** necessary to understand what to do and how to get it done, as well as to evaluate others and the program
- **awareness of resources** such as voluntary health organizations, public health departments, medical schools, professional societies, business, and others who might assist in the CSHP

**Figure 7.2**   The Coordinated School Health Program

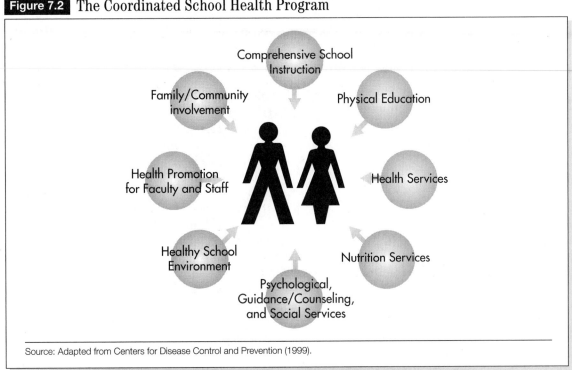

Source: Adapted from Centers for Disease Control and Prevention (1999).

• **communication skills,** both oral and written, that are needed to achieve the potential of the program

Public schools are regulated by individual states. Legislation affecting the school health program varies among the states. Laws regarding health services and school environment usually are mandated; their provisions specify what *must* be done. Examples of mandated legislation include safe maintenance and inspection of buildings and grounds, proper sanitation, and quality of food service. Laws regarding instruction, especially health instruction, are more often permissive; they specify only what *may* be done. Although most of the states now have laws mandating comprehensive health instruction, state governments do not necessarily enforce implementation, leaving it to the local decision-makers. Providing properly prepared teachers, time in the school day, and quality materials so that comprehensive health instruction and the other components of the CSHP can be implemented requires a supportive board of education and aggressive leadership.

## Component 1: Comprehensive School Health Instruction

This component is the foundation of the coordinated school health program. The 1990 Joint Committee on Health Education Terminology (1991) defined it as follows:

> **Comprehensive school health instruction** refers to the development, delivery, and evaluation of a planned curriculum, preschool through 12, with goals, objectives, content

**comprehensive school health instruction** the development, delivery, and evaluation of a planned, sequential preschool–12 curriculum (with goals, objectives, content sequence, and specific classroom lessons) that includes, but is not limited to, the following major content areas: community health, consumer health, environmental health, family life, mental and emotional health, injury prevention and safety, nutrition, personal health, prevention and control of disease, substance use and abuse

sequence, and specific classroom lessons which includes, but is not limited to, the following major content areas: community health; consumer health; environmental health; family life; mental and emotional health; injury prevention and safety; nutrition; personal health; prevention and control of disease and substance use and abuse.

McKenzie and Richmond (1998) defined the term "comprehensive school health education" as follows:

Classroom instruction that addresses the physical, mental, emotional, and social dimensions of health; develops health knowledge, attitudes, and skills; and is tailored to each age level. Designed to motivate and assist students to maintain and improve their health, prevent disease, and reduce health-related risk behaviors.

Hochbaum (1982) said that the ultimate goal of school health education is

to endow children with an *enduring* sense of the value of health and with the knowledge, attitudes, and motivations that would make them opt for healthful living practices years after they have left school—the rest of their lives.

Few health educators would disagree.

Instruction must be a planned and sequential K–12 (possibly starting at preschool) curriculum, based upon student needs, current and emerging health concepts, and societal issues. Curricula are usually mandated by the state or the school district. First, the **scope** of the program—the total range of subject areas or health topics selected to represent the body of knowledge of the discipline (Pollock & Middleton, 1994)—must be selected. The National Health Education Standards (Joint Committee on National Health Education Standards, 1995) provide an excellent framework upon which to build such a curriculum.

After defining the scope, the order of organizing elements must be determined. This is the **sequence** of the curriculum. Merely repeating the same concepts and information throughout the grades is not productive. The sequence may be vertical or horizontal. Scope and sequence should demonstrate both progression and continuity. Care must be taken to emphasize the dimensions of health—physical, mental, social, spiritual, and emotional—in both scope and sequence lest the curriculum degenerate to simply imparting a set of facts.

The basis for study is the integration of and dynamic relationships among physical, mental,

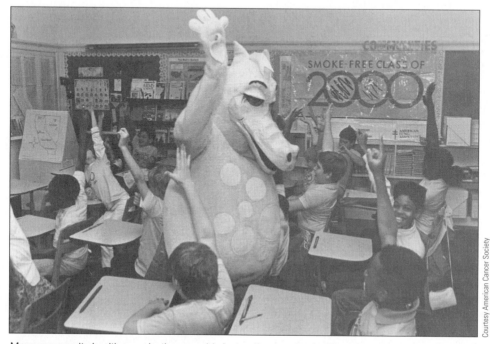

Many community health organizations provide instruction in schools. Here, a health educator dresses as a smoke-free dragon to promote a smoke-free class—an example of primary prevention.

Courtesy American Cancer Society

emotional, spiritual, and social dimensions of health. The widely recognized health education content areas—community health, consumer health, environmental health, family life, mental and emotional health, nutrition, personal health, prevention and control of disease, injury prevention and safety, and substance use and abuse—are addressed with reference to the dimensions of health. Growth and development may be included as a content area. Although specific content may change from time to time, these broad areas are useful in planning curriculum and instruction. The specific content and methodology of instruction must be adapted to meet the needs, interests, and maturity of the student at each grade level.

Health teaching differs from other teaching in important ways. It is one of the few curricular areas that emphasizes the person over the subject matter. Rather than present facts to memorize, health instruction approaches and engages the learner on a personal level. If presented by a skilled teacher, it fosters individual growth and introspection. After experiencing well-planned and implemented health instruction, students should know more about themselves. However, even though it focuses on content basic to complete development of the student, motivating learners is often difficult, because children are usually incapable of attaching health risks to themselves. In addition, no other area of study in elementary school depends so heavily on positively influencing attitudes and behavior. These are inextricably bound to cultural and social patterns of thinking and doing, requiring the teacher to be especially aware of cultural differences. A unique feature of health instruction is the constantly changing nature of health information. Teachers must be alert to changing "truths" and prepare students for scientific change.

## Goals of Health Instruction
One major goal of health instruction is the advocacy of health as an instrumental value, one that focuses on beliefs of how people ought or ought not to behave. Complementing health are the values of responsibility, honesty, worthy citizenship, and quality of life (Lohrmann, Gold, & Jubb, 1987). Valuing health means behaving in ways that promote health.

Accepting responsibility for one's actions and well-being, honesty in communication, and working toward the common good (the health of the community) demonstrates that a person values health.

A second goal of health instruction is to provide students with skills, attitudes, and knowledge that will empower them to make choices and decisions that promote health. These choices are manifested in their actions. Health instruction should offer opportunities to practice and apply these skills and knowledge. The rationale for the focus on skills is derived from health education theory (Wooley, 1995; Lohrmann, Gold, & Jubb, 1987; Kolbe et al., 1981) and is supported by research that has demonstrated the effectiveness of skills-based curricula in influencing students' health attitudes and practices (Kirby et al., 1994; Dusenbury & Falco, 1995; Botvin et al., 1995). Examples of skills include problem-solving, critical and scientific thinking, self-assessment, self-management, self-discipline, and skills related to refusal.

A third goal is to cultivate students' ability to obtain, evaluate, and use new health-related information. This is important because the supply of new information broadcast, printed, and used in advertisements is endless. A person has to be able to separate the valid from the invalid and utilize accurate, beneficial information in everyday life.

The Joint Committee on National Health Education Standards designed standards that meet these three goals. Applying the national standards, the thoughtful curriculum designer and teacher can plan lessons that will allow students to reach these goals.

## The Coursework
The coursework is coordinated with other subjects. Although a separate course in health instruction is needed, especially at the middle and high school levels, health instruction should be coordinated with most, and integrated into some other, subject areas. Just as the language arts have promoted "writing across the

**scope** the total range of subject areas or health topics selected to represent the body of knowledge of the discipline

**sequence** order of the organizing elements to be taught in a curriculum

curriculum," certain parts of health education can be promoted as "health across the curriculum." Language arts classes can write compositions on topics such as the appeal of advertising. Mathematics courses can conduct surveys and utilize health data as examples, problems, and graphing exercises. Likewise, social studies, science, and consumer and family studies classes can include health-related exercises in a number of creative ways. This coordination and integration necessitates continuing education and staff development for health educators and teachers in other disciplines.

Because most of the major health problems facing young people are grounded in a number of factors, a single message delivered by one teacher is not enough to change behavior. Consistent and repeated messages delivered by several teachers, the school staff, peers, and parents can be more effective at altering behavior (Bremberg, 1991). As we seek to integrate health education into other disciplines, however, we must be careful not to relinquish

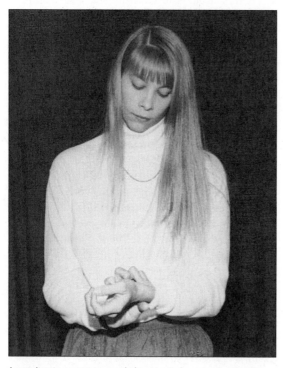

Learning to measure one's heart rate is an example of a skill learned in physical education class with application to health class. It may also be reinforced in science class.

the identity and uniqueness of health education as a discipline.

Effective curricula share eight characteristics (Lohrmann & Wooley, 1998); they

- are research based and theory-driven;
- include basic, accurate information that is developmentally appropriate;
- use interactive, experiential activities that actively engage students;
- provide students an opportunity to model and practice relevant social skills;
- address social or media influences on behaviors;
- strengthen individual values and group norms that support health-enhancing behaviors;
- are of sufficient duration to allow students to gain the needed knowledge and skills; and
- include teacher training that enhances effectiveness.

In addition, school health education should display a broad curricular scope and methodological diversity; emphasize broad-based constructive action in the shaping and reshaping of lives for better health, rather than only the acquisition of knowledge about health; and be dynamic, flexible, and evolving (A Point of View, 1992).

### Successful Approach
Gold (1994) reviewed the science base for health education and identified some major studies that document effectiveness. He then proposed the following lessons, winnowed from a review of the scientific health education literature:

- Significant improvements in outcomes are achieved with attention to multiple-risk behaviors, rather than focusing on separate categorical behaviors.
- School health instruction based on skills training, peer involvement, social learning theory, and community involvement has the greatest impact.
- Environmental variables influence the prevalence and consequences of behavior choices.

- Social support affects all phases of behavior change.

- Significant benefits can come from the active and appropriate engagement of parents and families in prevention programs.

- Appropriate attention must be paid to literacy and to social, cultural, gender, and ethnic diversity in program planning.

- Teacher training is required for effective educational programs.

- Relapse prevention efforts are necessary to sustain behavior changes.

The instructional program appears to have undergone a change in focus in the 1990s (Allensworth, 1994; DeGraw, 1994; English, 1994). To a large degree this change continues. School health instruction is moving from providing health information encompassing the traditional ten content areas to a focus on needs-driven and health-enhancing behaviors and skills that influence lifestyle changes. The instructional model is shifting from health content instruction in a classroom to a health promotion model that involves a variety of strategies by an interdisciplinary–interagency team. Instead of teaching skills in isolation through categorical areas, more instructors focus on teaching generic skills—such as problem-solving, refusal skills, assertiveness and media analysis—that promote health-enhancing behaviors.

Evidence shows this approach is successful. The Centers for Disease Control and Prevention (CDC, 2000) reported that rigorous studies show that health education effectively reduces the prevalence of health risk behaviors among young people. For example,

- Planned, sequential health education resulted in a 37 percent reduction in the onset of smoking among seventh-grade students.

- The prevalence of obesity was decreased by half among girls in grades 6–8 who participated in a school-based intervention program.

- Among students who were enrolled in a school-based life skills training program, 44 percent fewer used tobacco, alcohol, or marijuana one or more times per month than those not enrolled in the program.

The School Health Policies and Programs Study (SHPPS), a national study of U.S. secondary schools (Kann et al., 1995), provided insight as to the status of comprehensive health education programs. SHPPS found that

- 97 percent of middle/junior high and senior high schools require instruction in health topics and many provide instruction through a required course

- required health courses last one semester in 44 percent of all middle/junior high schools and senior high schools and for an entire school year in 20 percent of these schools

- the topics most likely to be included in such courses are alcohol and other drug use prevention (90 percent), HIV prevention (86 percent), tobacco use prevention (86 percent), disease prevention and control (84 percent), nutrition and healthy eating (84 percent), STD prevention (84 percent), human growth and development (80 percent), human sexuality (80 percent), personal health (79 percent), and physical activity and fitness (78 percent) (Collins et al., 1995)

Few schools offer truly comprehensive school health instruction. Health education is often not taught at every grade. Frequently, the duration is less than necessary to affect student health practices. Far too often, it is taught by teachers who lack professional preparation in health education. The American Association for Health Education addressed these and other issues in its position statement, which is shown in Box 7.3.

## Component 2: Healthy School Environment

Henderson (1994) stated,

> The outcomes of education are dependent upon the willingness and ability of the learner to participate in the education process. The location and physical facilities of the school, its learning resources, support services, staff and administrators are the underpinnings of teaching and learning; they influence the outcomes of the process.

## Box 7.3    Comprehensive School Health and Instruction: American Association for Health Education August 1999

**A STATEMENT OF POSITION:**

A planned, sequential curriculum in health education from pre-primary through grade 12 is necessary to help attain the objective of education: an educated populace whose health permits continued productivity throughout the lifespan. School health education is one component of the comprehensive school health education program which includes the development, delivery, and evaluation of a planned instructional program and other activities for students pre-school through grade 12, for parents and for school staff, and is designed to positively influence the health knowledge, attitudes, and skills of individuals. Comprehensive school health instruction refers to the development, delivery and evaluation of a planned curriculum, pre-school through grade 12, with goals, objectives, content scope and sequence and specific classroom lessons. These lessons should include, but are not limited to, instruction in ten content areas: community health, consumer health, environmental health, family life, mental and emotional health, injury prevention and safety, nutrition, personal health, prevention and control of disease and substance use and abuse. Examples of logical subtopics under these content areas include: violence prevention, cultural diversity, global health, eating disorders, and HIV infection. Comprehensive health instruction programs should include appropriate instructional strategies to enable students to achieve the National Health Education Standards.

Additionally, provisions should be made for reinforcement of health instruction with other subject matter areas. The curriculum should be developed by school personnel and curriculum directors who work in collaboration with parents, community health professionals and consultants from the state and national levels.

The following factors should shape school health education:

1. Instruction intended to motivate health maintenance and promote wellness, not simply to prevent disease.

2. A planned, sequential pre-school through 12 curriculum based upon students' needs and interests as well as emerging health concepts and community issues.

3. Activities designed to develop critical thinking and decision-making skills related to health behavior.

4. Opportunities for all students to demonstrate health-related knowledge, attitudes and practices.

5. Clearly articulated goals and objectives that describe the nature and character of the curriculum.

6. Well-planned evaluation procedures built into the program.

7. Individuals charged with teaching health education at any grade level be adequately prepared in health education.

8. An effective program management system similar to those found in other academic disciplines.

9. Sufficient resources to deliver the program and keep it updated.

Additionally, to be effective, school health instruction should specifically:

1. Be taught as one portion of the larger coordinated school health program.

2. Be taught by pre-serviced and regularly in-serviced teachers at the elementary level who have been grounded in the instructional responsibilities and competencies of the health education profession and by certified/licensed health education teachers at the middle and high school levels. In addition to state teacher certification/licensure, at appropriate levels teachers should be Certified Health Education Specialists (CHES) who are credentialed as a result of demonstrating competencies based on criteria established by the National Commission for Health Education Credentialing, Inc.

3. Be taught for a minimum of 50 hours per school year.

4. Be based upon curricula that have been formally evaluated and determined to be effective for improving health knowledge, attitudes, and behaviors and health literacy.

(continued)

**Box 7.3**  Comprehensive School Health and Instruction:
American Association for Health Education August 1999 (continued)

5. Be taught in classes of reasonable enrollment conducive to instructional strategies that promote the development of health promoting skills. Twenty-five students per class is the maximum number suggested.

6. Be free of gender bias and be multiculturally-sensitive.

7. Be formally evaluated in the same manner as other core subject areas.

Further, successful participation in a school health instruction program should be a requirement for passing into the next grade at the middle school level and a requirement for receiving a high school diploma.

**RATIONALE:**

The majority of premature deaths and disabilities of people of all ages is related to poor health decisions and unhealthy behaviors/practices. The ultimate goal of school health instruction is to prevent premature deaths and disabilities by empowering children and youth with health literacy. Health enhancing practices can be successfully learned in school health education programs. Teaching school age children and youth to adopt positive health behaviors and practices should enhance our national well-being and economy. For every $1 spent on tobacco education, drug and alcohol education, and sexuality education, $14 were saved in avoided health care costs. This savings compares favorably with the cost-effectiveness of other prevention programs, such as childhood immunization.

Source: Position statements approved, 1999, *HE-XTRA, 24*(4), pp. 1+. Reprinted by permission of the American Alliance for Health, Physical Education, Recreation, and Dance/American Association for Health Education.

The school health environment is a broad component of the CSHP. It refers not only to a healthful physical and emotional environment but also to healthy school personnel and an overall healthy school day. This component, to some degree, depends upon the participation of local and state health departments to enforce legal codes and on community health organizations to provide a link between the school and the community. Even the most carefully planned health instruction program is hindered if it is practiced in an unhealthy environment. Therefore, the school health environment is a necessary component of CSHP. The overall purpose of the environment is to establish a positive, supportive, and safe climate for children, enabling them to feel good about being in school and enhancing opportunities for learning.

**Site Selection**    The school environment begins with site selection and design. Most states prescribe the type and amount of land to be used, size of rooms, number of restrooms, drinking fountains, and other construction specifications. School site selection should be based on the premise that the buildings and grounds are an integral part of the community (Rowe, 1987). Present and future needs should be considered.

Site selection and construction planning should include

- enough space for playgrounds
- adequate space for growth and adaptation
- acceptable water supply and sewage system availability
- access to traffic but away from main traffic arteries
- orientation of the building(s) in relation to sun, wind, and other environmental factors
- a large indoor space for play
- restrooms and drinking fountains inside classrooms or within sight of classroom door
- sinks with running water inside each classroom
- separate restrooms for teachers

and should take into consideration

- proximity to sources of noise, such as airports and highways, and other forms of pollution, including heavy industry or commercial districts
- proximity to landfills, dumps, incinerators

- potential for floods, earthquakes, and other natural disasters

Many of the same factors must be considered when existing schools are renovated or enlarged.

## Safety

The first priority of the school must be to provide a safe and healthy environment. This applies to students' routes to and from school and during the school day.

The playground is an important part of the school environment. It can contribute to children's emotional health or can be a virtual minefield of hazards. The playground should be planned by specialists, utilizing guidelines of the National Safety Council. Playgrounds account for the largest number of student injuries in elementary schools (U.S.

Congress, Office of Technology Assessment, 1995) and child care centers (Briss et al., 1994). Over 208,000 children are treated in emergency departments for playground injuries each year (Mack, Thompson, & Hudson, 1998).

The four primary risk factors in playground injuries are lack of appropriate surfacing, poorly maintained surfaces, lack of equipment maintenance, and height of the equipment (Mack, Hudson, & Thompson, 2000). The use of slip-resistant materials that cushion the shock of falls from slides, swings, and climbing apparatuses can reduce injuries (Children's Safety Network, 1997; Rowe, 1987). Because approximately 70 percent of all playground injuries involve a fall, the chance of injury increases with the height of equipment. Playground equipment should be inspected weekly and any repairs

Two important factors in playground safety are the height of equipment and the capacity of the surface below it to absorb force.

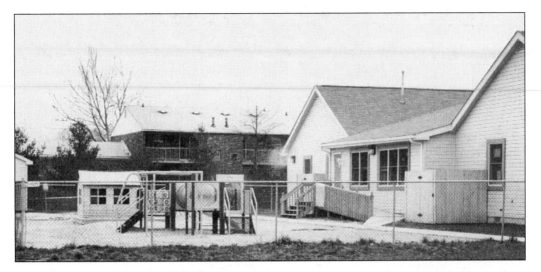

The fence and the proximity of the playground to the main building at this Head Start center provide security for the children.

made immediately. Playgrounds should be fenced and have a large shaded area. The possibility of student injury and accompanying litigation is great. The playground equipment most enjoyable to children is often the equipment that seems to impose the most risk.

It is acutely important to provide adequate adult supervision; comfortable seating for adults encourages this. Older and younger children should generally play separately. Pushing, grabbing, and other inappropriate behavior should be discouraged. The days when school playgrounds were havens for after-school and summer play are in the past. Now we recommend no unsupervised use of a playground after school hours.

Interscholastic and intramural sports and physical education activities contribute to an alarming number of injuries to school children. Athletic facilities and equipment should be well maintained. Uniforms and protective equipment should be sized properly. Coaches and physical educators should be trained in how to manage athletic injuries and administer first aid. They also should be alert for signs of excessive fatigue and the effects of heat. No athletic contest is worth serious and permanent injury. Many school districts now require the presence of a physician at all games and athletic team practices.

Safety procedures must be written and disseminated to each school employee. Appropriate versions of the safety document should be given to parents and children as well. The procedures should include specific instructions on dealing with hazards and emergencies. Teachers, not just the school nurse, should be trained in first aid, and first aid kits should be on hand and taken on field trips. The buildings and grounds should be inspected regularly for hazards. Accompanying inspectors as they examine playgrounds and equipment is an excellent learning opportunity for pupils.

Traffic safety is a vital element of school operation, because many injuries occur in transit to and from school. It also provides opportunities for teaching and learning. Proper signage and training of crossing guards is a matter of law, and school personnel should be involved.

School buses frequently are under school or district jurisdiction. Millions of children ride buses each day, so maintenance, operation, and safety policies are matters of life and safety. Although much of this is out of the hands of health educators, bus safety education is a practical part of health instruction. For example, children might be asked to write a safety policy booklet for the bus, incorporating rules they think are important. They might go on a bus inspection with the principal, examining the windows for loose glass; inspecting the seats for safe construction and exposed dangerous surfaces; identifying emergency exits; and examining fire extinguishers, safety belts (if required), first aid kits, and other features.

A number of sensible steps can be taken to improve safe school transportation:

- Provide well-developed and marked pickup and drop-off points at curbs.
- Mark pedestrian crosswalks clearly and have adult crossing guards at busy intersections.
- Prohibit parking where students are likely to cross streets.
- Use speed bumps and proper signage.
- Enforce speed limits.
- Provide separate entrances to schools for buses and cars, especially before and after school.
- Teach community members to adhere to and report violations of laws requiring traffic to stop when children are boarding or unloading from a school bus.
- Educate students to cross streets at intersections and walk facing traffic.
- Promote use of bicycle and motorcycle helmets.
- Promote bicycle safety at the elementary level and motorcycle safety and driver education courses at the secondary level.
- Carefully select, screen, and train school bus drivers.
- Provide modern, state-of-the-art features on school buses.
- Provide for discipline on buses and avoid overcrowding.
- Promote safety restraints on buses.
- Inspect buses regularly for mechanical and safety hazards.

## School Security
Certainly, protecting and promoting the health and safety of students, teachers, administrators, and staff are basic responsibilities of schools. Legally, schools act *in loco parentis*, that is, they take the place of parents in a distinct way. School security has become a major issue in modern society. Physical attacks, kidnapping, and weapons have become all too common in America's schools. During the 1996–97 school year, about 4,000 incidents of rape or sexual battery were reported in our nation's schools. There were 11,000 incidents of physical attacks or fights in which weapons were used and 7,000 robberies that year (National Center for Education Statistics, 1998). The 1997 Youth Risk Behavior Survey (CDC, 1999) reported that 8.5 percent of high school students had carried a weapon on school property during the thirty days preceding the survey. The survey also revealed that 4 percent of U.S. high school students had missed at least one day of school in the preceding month because they felt unsafe either being at school or going to or from school. This threat of violence has spread beyond large cities to suburban and rural areas, as witnessed by highly publicized murders in middle and high schools. The situation contributes to a sense of helplessness and having little or no control over one's life, which makes it difficult for pupils and teachers to concentrate on the teaching and learning for which schools exist.

A number of schools have employed police officers to patrol the grounds and halls and serve as resource officers. Some schools utilize metal detectors and locker searches. Many school administrators carry two-way radios. Some states have passed laws requiring possession of any object deemed to be a weapon or any action that could be considered an assault occurring on school property to be reported to police. Separate alternative schools have been established for students who are repeatedly disruptive or who are violent. Although no one solution to this repugnant situation is satisfactory in every school, a few ideas may be helpful.

A committee should be formed to address school security before injuries or threatening incidents occur. The committee should consist of teachers, school board members, parents, police officers, members of the school health council, and parties who command respect in the community, such as ministers. Because of the safety concerns involved, the health educator should be a member of the committee. Each building should be inspected to identify trouble spots. A policy complying with board and state policy, but specific to the school, should be developed. Even though schools should develop individual policies in accordance with their own problems, all policy statements should contain the following points:

- Any visitors who enter the building will go to the office first.
- Doors that may present problems will be locked from the inside.
- Halls and stairwells will be monitored during times of student traffic.
- No one will pick up a child from school or a bus without written permission from a parent or guardian.

Perhaps the most important thing we can do to reduce security problems is to reinforce the importance of the school to the community. The school was once the community focal point and meeting place. In many communities, court-ordered busing dampened the allegiance to the neighborhood school. Still, the school in the neighborhood can be a source of pride to the community. Civic groups can be invited to adopt the school. The school can host neighborhood block parties to build a sense of identification with nearby residents. When people take ownership in the school, they are less likely to damage it or to tolerate inappropriate behavior from others in their school.

A great deal has been made of the "drug-free school zone" initiatives. Signs announcing participation adorn many streets surrounding schools. Laws call for more severe penalties for possessing controlled substances in close proximity to schools. More and more school districts are adopting policies prohibiting the use of tobacco products on school property. Federal law prohibits smoking in school buildings. Schools, as part of the health services component, should assist smokers by offering and/or referring them to cessation programs.

## Emotional and Social Atmosphere of School

Educational objectives can be undermined or bolstered by the often intangible emotional or social climate of a school. Maslow (1986) suggested a way to reach emotionally and psychologically satisfying outcomes:

> The needs for safety, belongingness, love relations, and for respect can be satisfied only by other people, i.e., only from outside the person. This means considerable dependence on the environment.

Even though the family should play the primary role in meeting these needs, the school is and should be an obvious source of comfort to children. The school should be a positive, supportive, nurturing, productive environment that promotes social development and networking, self-strengthening independence, and personal responsibility. The emotional/social environment of the school is the set of expectations, interpersonal relationships, and experiences that contribute to students' development by way of their own feelings and sensibilities (Meeks, Heit, & Page, 1996).

The emotional atmosphere of the school and the classrooms is crucial to learning. Social experiences help shape the health attitudes, values, and practices of youth as they mature into adults (Henderson, 1994). All adults who work in the school should strive to make it a warm and friendly place where pupils feel welcome and comfortable. Teachers and staff should overtly recognize and value individual differences.

Children should be greeted by name when they approach a teacher, principal, secretary, and other school personnel. It means a great deal to a child to know that the custodian or a teacher down the hall knows his or her name. It means the child is an important part of the school. When a child is not addressed by name, the youngster often infers that he or she is not important enough for people to take the time to learn the child's name. Teachers and classmates should learn each others' names on the first day of school. A number of fun activities promote the learning of names. Individual worth is important to young children, and calling them by name is one way to promote individuality and self-esteem.

Teachers should have high expectations for student achievement and behavior. Schools, communities, and families that value academic achievement and set high standards for children have higher-achieving students (Henderson & Rowe, 1998). Teachers and others should consistently show respect for students and their work. They should deal with each student as a unique and valuable person and be familiar with the talents and interests of all the students.

Soon after the beginning of school, hallways and classrooms should be decorated with pupils' work. Bulletin boards are excellent places to display pupils' work. No pupil should be excluded. Everyone's efforts should be considered worthwhile.

Positive interpersonal interaction is important in creating a healthy emotional atmosphere. Every child's opinion is important and should be taken seriously. Each child should be encouraged to participate within the bounds of the activity in a climate that promotes trust, safety, cooperation, and mutual respect. Although taunting and teasing are almost impossible to avoid, these expressions should be discouraged when they are observed. They create a negative atmosphere and damage efforts to establish cooperation and equality. Active listening skills should be promoted.

Perhaps one of the most important elements of the emotional environment of the modern school is classroom management. Classroom rules should be few, sensible, easily understood, and articulated early on. They should be enforced immediately, consistently, and fairly. Teachers should use firmness, fairness, and friendliness as guiding principles in disciplining students.

The "assertive discipline" approach—wherein one establishes clear rules and expectations accompanied by rewards and punishments for compliance or noncompliance—may be a useful starting point for teachers who have difficult students or problems controlling their classrooms. More democratic methods are needed, however, if the goal is to enhance self-esteem and help students to become effective problem solvers.

Where students discipline themselves, they become more capable learners and problem solvers. One approach is to involve students in setting guidelines for classroom behavior and cooperatively enforcing them. Encouragement of discipline from within rather than discipline imposed by others should be a goal. This can be nourished by inviting students to behave in ways that assist others rather than harm the classroom atmosphere, by involving all students in classroom activities, and developing more positive student-teacher relationships.

Schultz, Glass, and Kamholtz (1987) summed up the issue of emotional health of a school:

> The emotional health of the school is a reflection of the well-being of the faculty, staff, and students. When individuals feel good about themselves they promote emotional health which effectively helps to create an

environment conducive to learning. Living and working in this environment perpetuates a healthy school climate.

Certain teaching techniques can be utilized to enhance the social-emotional climate of the classroom. Cooperative learning—placing children in small, heterogeneous groups—can improve self-esteem; establish positive interaction among students of different racial, ethnic, and social backgrounds (Johnson & Johnson, 1982); and also, in many cases, increase academic achievement (Johnson et al., 1981). Social skills training in sharing and conflict resolution techniques—such as apologizing, avoiding a fight, negotiating, and dealing with group pressure—can improve the emotional and psychological climate of the classroom and school.

**Sexual Harassment**    Sexual harassment, or unwanted sexual behavior, is a form of violence and a form of emotional attack. As such, it affects the emotional atmosphere of the school and requires security and supervision to prevent it and deal with its occurrence.

A survey commissioned by the American Association of University Women (Bryant, 1993) identified fourteen actions that constitute sexual harassment. A student has been harassed if someone

1. Made sexual comments, jokes, gestures, or looks

2. Showed, gave, or left the student sexual pictures, photographs, illustrations, messages, or notes

3. Wrote sexual messages/graffiti about the student on bathroom walls, in locker rooms, etc.

4. Spread sexual rumors about the student

5. Said the student was gay or lesbian

6. Spied on the student as the student dressed or showered at school

7. Flashed or "mooned" the student

8. Touched, grabbed, or pinched the student in a sexual way

9. Pulled at the student's clothing in a sexual way

10. Intentionally brushed against the student in a sexual way

11. Pulled the student's clothing off or down

12. Blocked the student's way or cornered the student in a sexual way

13. Forced the student to kiss him or her

14. Forced the student to do something sexual other than kissing

Results indicated that 81 percent of the students (girls 85 percent, boys 76 percent) had been sexually harassed. Sexual harassment at school begins early; 32 percent of students were harassed by grade 6 or lower, and a shocking 6 percent by grade 3. Eighteen percent of students were harassed by school employees.

Although students do not routinely tell adults about sexual harassment, the harassment had profound effects on students' academic life, causing many not to want to attend school, to pay attention less in class, or to receive lower grades. Emotions and feelings, such as self-consciousness, upset, and less confidence also resulted. Many students changed their seats, avoided certain areas of school, changed routes to school, or gave up attending a sport or activity.

School officials must take steps to prevent and stop sexual harassment. Failure to act constitutes negligence and violates a federal law, Title IX, which prohibits sexual harassment and sexual discrimination in schools. Recent Supreme Court decisions have clarified the conditions under which school districts can be held financially liable for sexual harassment by students and employees. Policies must be developed; made clear to students, employees, and parents; and strictly enforced. Programs must be initiated to educate all school personnel and students about sexual harassment, the law, and school policy. Where it occurs, school officials must take steps to deal with it. Counseling should be available for those who have been sexually harassed.

## Physical Environment

The physical environment of a school has tremendous impact upon students' perception of themselves, as well as their safety, well-being, and ability to learn. Some learning activities have great potential for harm to students. Science laboratories are an example. Blending, pipetting, plating, and centrifuging may generate aerosols that contain infectious germs (Rowe, 1987) or hazardous chemicals. Animals, plants, and microorganisms used in some science instruction can create biological hazards. Art activities such as pottery and making jewelry can expose students and teachers to lead, silica, and toxic pigments. Well-planned operations, careful disposal of waste, and proper handling and storage are necessary to ensure student and staff well-being. Industrial arts classes also pose safety and health risks to students unless they are supervised adequately and equipment is maintained properly. Likewise, gymnasiums and pools require diligent supervision and maintenance.

Almost one out of every two public school buildings in the United States contains an environmental hazard, such as asbestos, peeling lead-based paint, radon gas, lead-contaminated water, or biologically contaminated heating and ventilating systems (Kowalski, 1995). In certain buildings, air pollutants have produced what is referred to as "sick building syndrome." Contaminants from cleaning agents, art studios, copy machines, pesticides, tobacco smoke, and combustible gases from kitchens and laboratories are examples of air pollutants. Often, ventilation systems in older buildings permit cross-contamination from various parts of the building. When possible, repair and remodeling, such as roofing and painting, should be done in the summer when student traffic is less.

The physical environment of the school and classroom can contribute greatly to the learning process. Therefore, classrooms should be bright, colorful, and lively. Halls and classrooms should be well lighted. Illumination measured in foot-candles, should be 50–100 foot in general classrooms. Play areas require 30–50 foot-candles of illumination. Teachers should make sure that lighting is constant, with no glare, minimal shadowing, and no bright or dark areas caused by differences in light intensity from one area to the next. Any of these conditions should be remedied, because they detract from the learning environment, can cause eyestrain, and can lead to fatigue and tension.

Glare can be reduced by rearranging desks or computer stations, by closing window shades, and by a change in the teacher's position. Teachers should take pains to ensure that pupils are not bothered by glare, especially during video presentations. Desks should never face windows, because children are easily distracted.

A classroom with appropriate colors can directly affect feelings of safety and security. It also can produce desired emotions. For rooms with northern exposures, warm colors such as yellow are recommended; for southern exposures, cool colors such as light blue are suggested. Light pastels help to attain proper reflectance. Light colors are recommended for large areas (Redican, Olsen, & Baffi, 1993).

Temperature and humidity are important factors affecting students' and teachers' performance. In extremes, they can result in serious health consequences. The classroom should not be drafty. Children are affected more by temperature than adults are. Differences in metabolic rate and body fat cause children and adults to react differently to changes in room temperature. The primary consideration should be the children's comfort. This may become a problem during fall and spring in schools that have no air conditioning.

Students participating in physical education, athletics, band, or cheerleading should not be exposed to temperature extremes. Activities should be curtailed or rescheduled during times of temperature extremes. Students should be encouraged to replace fluids lost from perspiration. All too often, students suffer from heat stroke, especially during late summer and early fall practices.

Creating a safe and healthful school environment requires a cooperative effort among faculty, staff, students, parents, community health professionals, and state and local authorities. The school environment is the framework within which the other seven components of the coordinated school health program operate. Teachers, particularly health educators, should not miss the opportunity to use the school environment as a teaching/learning tool. Occasions arise to discuss sanitation, the role of color and emotions, safety hazards, and a multitude of other environmental factors.

## Component 3: School Health Services

**School health services** began at the end of the nineteenth century with physicians and nurses collaborating in the pre-antibiotic era to control communicable diseases and to keep children healthy and in school as much as possible (Zanga & Oda, 1987). Today, schools provide health services continuously. These encompass all procedures to promote, appraise, and protect the health of every child in the school. They are provided by physicians, nurses, dentists, teachers, counselors, dieticians, principals, and others. The rationale for school health services is clear and simple: If we receive a healthy child, we are obligated to return the child to the home in at least an equal state of health. Beyond that, we should take every opportunity to improve the child's current health and to enhance his or her chance for future well-being. School health services can reinforce the efforts of parents and the medical community in promoting the health of children.

Support for school health services is evident. The Education Goals for the Year 2000 (National Education Goals Panel, 1994) concentrated on coordination and collaboration of health, education, and social services for young people within and outside the school organization. Reports of the National Association of State Boards of Education (1996), the American Medical Association (1994), and National Commission on the Role of the School and the Community in Improving Adolescent Health (1990), the Carnegie Foundation (Carnegie Council on Adolescent Development, 1990), the Robert Wood Johnson Foundation (1995), the American Nurses Association (1991), and the National Nursing Coalition for School Health (1995) have advocated strengthening school health services. A survey of the American public found that 91 percent of respondents considered "servicing the emotional and health needs of students" an important function of schools (Elam & Lowell, 1995).

School health services, in partnership with community resources, can benefit children in a number of ways. Children and youth will

- come to school healthy and ready to learn, thus reducing barriers to their learning and enhancing their learning potential (Committee on Comprehensive School Health Programs in Grades K–12, 1997)

- be safe from major injuries caused by hazards or violence (Education Commission of the States, 1996)

- have a primary provider for preventive medical and dental services (Casamassimo, 1996; American Medical Association, 1994)
- receive needed nutrition and mental health, substance abuse, sexual abuse, and other counseling services (Knitzer, Steinberger, & Fleisch, 1990).

School health services should be integrated with the health instructional component. Certainly, a primary justification for health services in schools is that they contribute to the schools' educational goals. One way they do this is by using the nurse and other service providers as classroom resources. When services are rendered, they become opportunities for learning. Health service programs also can identify problems that can interfere with learning and sometimes provide solutions.

Members of the school health services team should work with members of the other components of the CSHP. The school physician can consult with the health teacher on a lesson about communicable disease. Physical education teachers can help the physical therapist design appropriate activities for students with physical limitations. Athletic trainers can work with nutrition services personnel to coordinate the dietary needs of athletes. School nurses can work with health and physical educators to coordinate staff wellness programs. Counseling, psychological, and social services personnel can participate in staff wellness. The health coordinator can use student health records to identify health problems related to the school environment and suggest corrective actions (Duncan & Igoe, 1998).

The schools' ability to reach children and youth who do not have access to the health care system and who are at highest risk for health problems and potentially life-threatening behaviors is unmatched (Schlitt, 1991). The advantages of school health service programs, according to Klein and Sadowski (1990) and Porter (Policy Studies Associates, 1992), are that they

- are equitable, by offering an entry point into the health care system for all children
- can provide a broad range of comprehensive, preventive services not reimbursed by most health insurance policies

- are confidential
- are user-friendly, because the services are provided in a trusting and familiar environment
- are convenient, making teens more likely to walk in
- are easily accessible and immediately available, requiring students to travel less to receive services
- have access to well-developed health record-keeping and tracking systems
- allow all children and youth an opportunity to participate in the health care system early in their lives and form good habits for their health and well-being

School nurses play a pivotal role in a number of school health services. As opposed to other nurses, the school nurse may not work under the supervision of a physician and is working in an educational setting rather than a medical one. The nurse also works with a mostly well population. Another hallmark of the school nursing profession is being overworked: The National Association for School Nurses recommends ratios of one nurse per 750 students in the general school population, one nurse per 225 mainstreamed students with special needs, and one nurse per 125 students with severe disabilities (Proctor, Lordi, & Zarger, 1993). According to the School Health Policies and Programs Study (SHPPS) (Small et al., 1995), only 14 percent of states have a student-to-nurse ratio requirement, although 38 percent of the states have recommendations.

Budgetary constraints have forced many school districts to augment school health services by employing school health assistants to work under close supervision of school nurses. School health assistants may provide first aid for minor injuries, administer medications, screen students for lice, perform clerical duties, and maintain immunization records (Fryer & Igoe, 1996).

The National School Health Survey (Davis et al., 1995) found that 85 percent of all public school systems offer some health services. SHPPS, examining service delivery for junior high/middle schools and

**school health services**   all procedures to promote, appraise, and protect the health of every child in school

high schools found that 74 percent of all school districts examined had a person responsible for directing or coordinating school health services (Small et al., 1995). Many schools do not have the financial resources to provide all of the services that should be included in a comprehensive school health services program. To overcome this shortage, many schools are sharing resources and personnel to provide more services to more students. They also are relying more on community support and partnerships. This sets up a three-tiered service system (based on the level of services being provided) that is shown in Figure 7.3

**Traditional Basic Care Model**  In the traditional basic care model, the predominant model in the United States, basic screening and health appraisal is the outstanding feature. Most of the actual provision of service is provided by the school nurse with school health assistants. Some districts employ physicians or use them as paid or volunteer consultants to deliver some services.

**Screening** is a preliminary low-cost appraisal technique to identify health problems needing referral and diagnosis by trained specialists. Screening identifies students who deviate from the average on one or more of a series of tests. It often is done by teachers, nurses, and trained volunteers. Health screening can take several forms. Various tests can be conducted separately or, more commonly, as a battery of tests administered in a single session. The latter is referred to as **multiphasic screening**. Regardless of the format, screening presents an opportunity for health instruction after administering the tests. When appropriate, teachers should discuss the nature of the test, what it was measuring and evaluating, and possible steps to mitigate deficiencies found.

Some examples of screening are those for vision, hearing, scoliosis, head lice, tuberculosis, overweight, and underweight. Screening also may include blood tests for certain illnesses in high-risk groups. It is possible, for example, to measure cholesterol level in about 3 minutes at low cost.

**Figure 7.3**  School Health Services

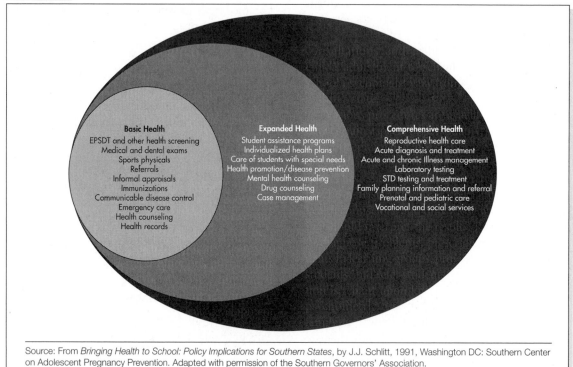

**Basic Health**
EPSDT and other health screening
Medical and dental exams
Sports physicals
Referrals
Informal appraisals
Immunizations
Communicable disease control
Emergency care
Health counseling
Health records

**Expanded Health**
Student assistance programs
Individualized health plans
Care of students with special needs
Health promotion/disease prevention
Mental health counseling
Drug counseling
Case management

**Comprehensive Health**
Reproductive health care
Acute diagnosis and treatment
Acute and chronic Illness management
Laboratory testing
STD testing and treatment
Family planning information and referral
Prenatal and pediatric care
Vocational and social services

Source: From *Bringing Health to School: Policy Implications for Southern States*, by J.J. Schlitt, 1991, Washington DC: Southern Center on Adolescent Pregnancy Prevention. Adapted with permission of the Southern Governors' Association.

In some schools, specially trained nurses perform Early and Periodic Screening, Diagnosis, and Treatment physicals for students with no other source of well-child health care. The focus of this federally funded screening program is on referral and treatment for identified health problems.

Comprehensive medical examinations are the best means of appraising a child's overall level of health and determining if immunizations are up to date. All fifty states require medical examinations as a condition of admission to kindergarten. Most school districts require additional examinations, although the number and regularity vary according to state and district policy. At a minimum, four regular physical examinations should be required during the K–12 school span.

The examination usually is done by the family physician, a health department physician, or a physician or nurse practitioner employed by the school district. Obviously, utilizing a physician makes the cost much higher than that of other forms of appraisal. Nevertheless, it provides the opportunity to establish a family doctor-patient relationship when none exists. For this reason, and because the family doctor is more qualified than anyone else to evaluate any change in the child's health status, the physician should conduct the examination.

Most school districts have their own form for the exam and the health history the physician fills out during the examination. The forms are kept in school records or the results are entered into the district computer.

Regular medical examinations have a number of purposes:

- They may identify problems that have not been identified through other appraisal techniques.

- They enhance the physician-patient relationship.

- They present the opportunity for the child and parent or guardian to get answers to important health questions.

- Particularly for adolescents, they usually provide reassurance that they are normal.

Dental decay is the most common health defect in school-age children. For this reason, a dentist or dental hygienist should conduct an examination of every child. This also presents an opportunity for young dentists to acquaint themselves with children and their families, so they may be willing to conduct examinations in school at a reduced fee. In some areas, public health dentists perform dental screenings. The dental examination provides an excellent opportunity for education about diet, flossing, brushing, and fluoride applications. Some school districts provide free fluoride applications for children who live in areas where drinking water is not fluoridated. Information should be sent home to parents, reinforcing dental education programs.

Informal appraisals of aspects of each child's health are an important part of school health services. Health care for young people is episodic and crisis-related. Opportunities for preventive health screenings are scarce for many children, for whom school health appraisals become the only source of early diagnosis. The purposes of appraisal are to

- locate pupils needing medical or dental treatment;

- locate pupils who need modified programs;

- locate pupils who need thorough medical examinations;

- notify parents and school personnel of the child's health status;

- help students and teachers make adjustments that promote the learning process;

- reduce illness, illness-related disabilities, and their associated costs; and

- serve as learning experiences for pupils.

To be effective, a teacher must be aware of the health status of the students and committed to working with students to maintain and improve health status (Meeks, Heit, & Page, 1996). The child's appearance, behavior, and functioning are key indicators of his or her health. Detecting changes in these

**screening**   preliminary appraisal technique that identifies health problems or deviations from the average

**multiphasic screening**   the use of various tests, conducted separately or in a single session, to identify health problems or deviations from the average indicators through the continuous observation by the classroom teacher can be the most critical part of the appraisal process. The classroom teacher is usually the person in the school who knows the child best. The teacher can compare the child's appearance and behavior not only to what is normal for the age group but also to what is normal for that child. Successful appraisal requires some teacher training.

The teacher should be alert for signs of communicable diseases, which include fatigue, flushed face, sleepiness, fever, and rash. A conscientious observer will notice discharge from the ears, inflamed watery eyes, sties, runny nose, enlarged glands, and stained teeth. The teacher can look for signs of hearing deficiency, such as turning the head to one side, cupping the ear, misunderstanding directions, or mispronouncing words frequently. The classroom teacher is often the first person to notice signs of vision problems, such as squinting or holding a book very close or unusually far away from the face. Other signs of physical problems include tiring easily, poor coordination, lack of interest in games or activities, and shortness of breath after moderate exercise.

Emotional problems may be indicated by a child's behavior change, such as from being outgoing to being withdrawn. Irritability, hyperactivity, being overly docile, or being unable to work with others could indicate emotional problems.

Occasionally the family does not notice speech difficulties, such as failure to pronounce certain consonants or stuttering. The teacher should not ignore these signs.

Signs of social problems—such as child abuse and neglect, drug use, or alcoholism in the family—often manifest themselves in children's behavior, appearance, stories they make up, pictures, or relationships with other children. In most states, adults, including teachers, are legally mandated to report signs of abuse or neglect.

Procedurally, the elementary school teacher should make an effort to observe each child during the day, giving attention to verbal and nonverbal behavior. Because children of low-income and disadvantaged families have a greater incidence of health problems, these children should get extra attention. Keeping notes on each child to identify patterns is a good practice. At no time should the teacher attempt to diagnose a health problem or to render medical care beyond basic first aid or emergency care. Any concerns should be referred to the appropriate professional, usually the school nurse or counselor.

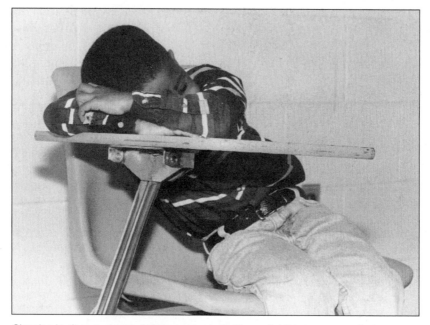

Sleeping in class or chronic fatigue can be indications of child abuse or neglect.

When a teacher suspects a health problem, the matter usually is referred to the school nurse. In many schools, the nurse sees any individual child infrequently and relies heavily on teacher referrals and comments. The teacher, observing the child on a daily basis, may be better able than the nurse to identify atypical behavior or appearance. Therefore, the teacher-nurse conference is an extremely important link between the child and the school's health care service.

In some cases, school medical records that contain results of screening and examinations provide information to the nurse regarding a child's condition. In others, notes from parents or physicians directed to the nurse describe medical conditions and appropriate care. Often, for the child to function at the highest level possible, communication between nurse and teacher is the key. For follow-up purposes, the teacher and the nurse should confer about students who return after long absences as well as those who were out because of infectious diseases. The nurse can help the teacher ease returning students back into classroom activities.

In some schools, nurses and teachers confer annually about students and their individual needs. In others, they confer only on a "need" basis.

A cumulative health record for each child should be stored at the school site or in the computer system so it is accessible to school personnel. This record can provide indispensable information regarding reports of teacher observations; screening; medical, dental, and psychometric exams; nurse's reports; immunization records; and a health care plan for students with disabilities. It can provide a valuable service to the child or parent when emergencies arise or when referral is indicated.

Most states (90.2 percent) and districts (99.7 percent) require schools to keep immunization records on file for each student. More than 84 percent of districts also require schools to keep medical emergency forms, and 81.7 percent require medical information cards. More than 94 percent of the states take action to increase the likelihood that school staff will detect and report cases of physical and sexual abuse (Small et al., 1995).

Health records should not contain any subjective statements or value judgments. The only diagnoses to be contained in the record are those by qualified professionals.

Health records should be maintained separately from academic and disciplinary records. Federal law requires that all written records from physicians

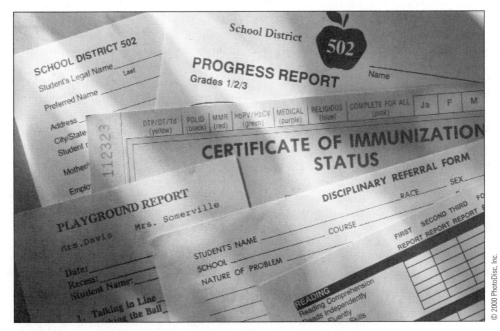

Maintaining immunization and other records is a basic school health service.

© 2000 PhotoDisc, Inc.

to schools receiving federal funds be open to parental inspection. Parents may review, challenge the accuracy of, or seek correction of a health record. Health records cannot be released to a third party without permission of a parent or guardian. Policy should indicate which individuals have access to health records, keeping in mind the child's right to confidentiality.

Emergency care is one of the most important health services in schools. Children frequently become ill or injured at school. Accidents are the leading cause of death in children. Children incur injuries on playgrounds, in buildings, and coming to and going from school. The school has a fourfold responsibility in emergency care and accident prevention:

- School personnel must prevent accidents by foreseeing hazards and correcting them.

- Schools must provide a good safety education as part of the health instruction program, including warnings about hazards that are not readily correctable. The goal is to establish safe habits in children, along with a philosophy that accidents are preventable and everyone has a responsibility to prevent them.

- The school must have a written plan for handling emergencies, including access to names, addresses, and telephone numbers of parents and guardians, as well as a responsible adult to contact when parents or guardians are not available. The plan should include the name of the family doctor, the hospital of preference, and any special medical problems the child has, such as allergies or chronic disorders.

- Several school employees, in addition to the school nurse, should be trained in first aid treatment, to lessen the consequences of injuries. First aid kits, cots or beds, and a quiet place for recovery should be a part of every emergency plan.

The plan should include provisions for transporting children to hospitals, if necessary. A policy should be in place for releasing the child to the care of an adult. Under no circumstances should a child be released to another adult without written permission of the parent or guardian.

School personnel should not administer medication without securing written permission from the parent unless it is deemed a life-threatening situation. Even over-the-counter remedies should be withheld unless written permission is given. A report of each incident should be on file in the school office.

On most days in most schools, some children come to school ill or become ill after arriving. At these times, decisions must be made to protect other pupils and school personnel. Alert teachers frequently identify sick children during routine observation. These are parts of communicable disease control.

Policies regarding infectious disease and exclusion of students should be well known to all personnel. Administrators have to be familiar with state laws and school district rules. By consulting pupil records, the nurse can contact parents, guardians, or other adults named on the record to come and take the child home or to a physician. Someone should follow up by calling about the child later in the day or the next day. The follow-up is important because it emphasizes the school's concern for the child and may provide information about a disease to which other children have been exposed. Policy should dictate the conditions under which a note from a physician is necessary for the child to return to school. Certainly, the teacher should observe returning children carefully for a few days for signs of relapse.

Parents should be encouraged to keep the child home if he or she is ill. Many children are allowed to come to school when they are sick because parents feel obligated to be on the job and cannot arrange child care.

The health educator can utilize cases of illness to educate parents about symptoms, means of transmission, prevention, and control of infectious diseases. Flyers sent home with children can be excellent sources of information for parents.

Although many of the basic strategies of communicable disease prevention discussed here are integral parts of the traditional basic care model, enhancing these services by placing them in the student assistance program and emphasizing preventive education make for a more expanded health program.

Other interventions provided by the basic model include sports physicals, individualized health care plans, administering of medicines, and provision of health counseling and patient education. Many states have legislated this type of school health services programming.

## Expanded School Health Services

The focus of child health has shifted from medical care to the promotion of health and prevention of disease. Problems such as substance use, stress disorders, and suicide can be ameliorated through health promotion interventions (Giordano & Igoe, 1991). The expanded health services program extends the range of services provided to students by the health service staff and public health and community mental health providers who often work part-time in the school (Schlitt, 1991). It can also work in concert with the community and family involvement component of the CSHP.

Student assistance programs have been inaugurated in schools as a result of the focus of the U.S. Department of Education on substance abuse prevention. These programs may be administered by the school or by an outside mental health agency contracted by the schools. It is recommended that an interdisciplinary school health service task force that would include parents be formed in the district. Student assistance programs sometimes provide alcohol and other drug abuse counseling as well as individualized health promotion. In addition to the conventional screening provided by school nurses, health hazard appraisal, fitness screening, developmental evaluation, and nutritional history could be added. From these evaluations, annual individualized health plans that emphasize disease prevention measures are developed. Instructional programs in health and safety, nutrition, and environmental health and safety could be integrated into the program.

Providing for the health of individuals with special needs is a responsibility in most schools. Students with special education needs frequently also have health and human services needs; schools are the logical settings to provide these services in an integrated fashion (Committee on School Health, 1993; Dryfoos, 1994; Lear, 1996; Santelli et al., 1996). Commitment to achieving minimum health standards for all social groups regardless of disability has become an integral part of school health services.

Schools are required by law to provide educational opportunities to all children no matter how severe their disabilities. Disabilities include mental retardation, learning disability, visual impairment, emotional disturbance, autism, and a wide range of physical disabilities. The Education for All Handicapped Children Act of 1975 (Public Law 94-142) became effective in September 1978 for ages 3–18 and was expanded to include ages 3–21 in September 1980. It requires that no child be excluded from a free appropriate public education because of what then was labeled "handicap"; that every child be assessed fairly on an annual basis to achieve proper placement and services; that every child be given an education that is meaningful to him or her, taking the handicap into account; that the handicapped child may not be separated inappropriately from non-handicapped peers; and that each child has the right to protest the school's decision about placement. Other provisions stipulate structural modification to ensure wheelchair access to buildings, classrooms, hallways, and restrooms. PL 94-142 quickly ignited the growth of special education programs of many kinds.

The clause requiring that children with disabilities be separated from their peers as little as possible into a "least restrictive environment" led to the so-called mainstreaming of children with disabilities into virtually every classroom and providing them with the best education possible in the integrated setting. One result is the placement of increasingly younger children with increasingly more serious medical problems into the education mainstream (Zanga & Oda, 1987). The value of this practice has been debated in many forums. This practice, in any case, has presented challenges to schools to design effective and fair policies to render services and educational opportunities to all children. This practice requires coordination not only between the nurse and the physician but also between the nurse and other members of the school health team, including guidance counselors, social workers, speech pathologists, and school psychologists. Teachers, in cooperation with school nurses and other health care practitioners, should utilize innovative methods of teaching to accommodate individual differences in children. They must have a positive attitude toward the student with disabilities in addition to the skills to teach that student.

The Education of the Handicapped Act Amendments of 1986 (PL 99-457) addressed the needs of preschoolers by requiring that states provide services for all eligible children ages 3–5 years. EHA provided funding to states to develop and implement statewide, comprehensive, multidisciplinary, interagency programs of early intervention for infants and toddlers with disabilities and their families. In 1990 the term "handicapped" was replaced by the term "disability" with the passage of the Individuals with Disabilities Education Act (PL 101-476).

Students with chronic health conditions or developmental delays require an assessment that is given to the school staff as an Individualized Education Plan. The school nurse should participate in the development of the IEP in many cases. An Individualized Health Plan is also developed for many children to organize and document the delivery of services, procedures, and technical assistance. Nursing assessments, diagnoses, interventions, and outcomes are included in the IHP. Knowledge of the disability, community resources, and the perceived needs of the child and his or her family are essential to developing an effective program for children with disabilities.

The IEP and the IHP can lead to classroom modification and environmental adjustments. They can also result in modified individual physical education programs. Federal legislation requires schools to provide special meals to children who have medical certification that disabilities restrict their diets.

## Comprehensive Health Services    Fifteen percent of Americans under the age of 18 do not have health insurance. The rate is higher among African-American (21.5 percent), Hispanic-American (34.2 percent), and poor (23.8 percent) children (U.S. Census Bureau, 1997). Many of these children have no regular source of health care. Historically, when other systems have proven inadequate, the public school system has stepped in to address the health needs of children and youth. School-based clinics

(school-based health centers or wellness centers) were initiated to render services for children and youths with unmet health care needs. The number of school-based clinics or wellness centers grew during the decades of the 1980s and 1990s. More than 1,200 school-based health centers are now in operation (Dryfoos, 1998). Of these, 41 percent are located in high schools, 32 percent in elementary schools, and 17 percent in middle schools (The George Washington University, 1997). There is strong evidence of utilization of clinics by needy children, with highest risk students most likely to make multiple visits (Dryfoos, Brindis, & Kaplan, 1996).

Many schools are choosing the less-centralized approaches offered by the school-linked clinic. In these plans, the clinic serves students from more than one school and students from elementary through secondary school. It may be located in one school or in the outside community with links to schools.

Many of the services discussed here are provided in both school-based and school-linked clinics. In addition, physicians and other health-care providers often rotate among a district's clinics. Where primary health care was once the mainstay of school clinics, many have become more comprehensive, offering mental health counseling, vocational services, and social services. At many clinics a counselor or mental health professional is available at all times. Clinic personnel have access to health records. Services can be comprehensive and self-contained, including testing, diagnosis, counseling, and treatment. At least 80 percent of school-based health centers provide injury treatment, physical exams, family planning counseling, medication dispensing, primary care, prescriptions, immunizations, pregnancy testing, and sports physicals (Making the Grade, 1997). In a well organized school-based clinic, the opportunities for services and instruction are endless. The clinic should not replace classroom instruction, but it can provide a useful supplement.

Both school-based and school-linked health centers can offer a variety of services. These may include health education, nutrition education, drug and substance abuse programs, mental health counseling, family counseling, sexuality education in a classroom setting, and routine sports physicals.

As early as 1968, the school-based health clinic was implemented in Cambridge, Massachusetts. The Cambridge school-based primary care program for children was initiated to operate under the auspices of the city's Department of Health and Hospitals. By 1976, five school-based clinics were established, providing pediatric care as well as accessibility to comprehensive health care. The program was designed so a single, integrated health service would follow the child from birth through adolescence. As a result of the program, immunizations rates rose dramatically, elevated blood levels of lead decreased significantly, and iron deficiency anemia in preschool-aged children dropped substantially.

In 1986, the General Assembly of Delaware funded four school-based wellness centers, allocating $100,000 to each yearly. Even in fiscally tight years, the level of funding has been maintained because of the general support the centers have received. New start-up funds were made available so that in the fall of 1999, school-based wellness centers performing many of the functions of clinics were open to students in 24 of the 30 state's high schools.

The U.S. Congress, through the Office of Technology Assessment (1991) attested to the usefulness of having health services available to school campuses by stating, "The most promising recent innovation to address the health and related needs of adolescents is the school-linked health or youth services center."

## Component 4: Physical Education

The relationship between health education and physical education has a complex history. As detailed in Chapter 4, health education had much of its origins in physical education. Today the two are recognized as separate disciplines. There is, however, mutual purpose in the two. Pate et al. (1987) explained that school-based physical education can and should serve as a primary intervention tool to enhance the health of children and youth; a health-oriented approach to physical education is supported by compelling, scientifically based logic.

Physical education, like health education, should be a planned, sequential K–12 curriculum. It should promote each student's optimal physical,

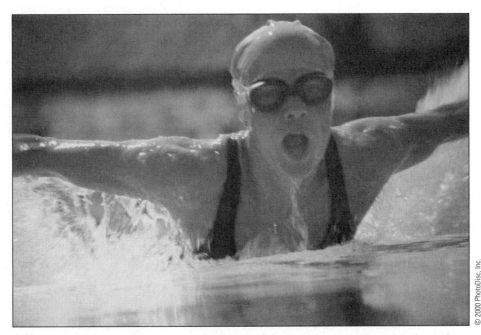

© 2000 PhotoDisc, Inc.

Swimming is an example of a health-oriented skill that can be taught in physical education and enjoyed throughout the lifespan.

mental, emotional, social, and spiritual development. It also should provide activities that students can enjoy throughout the lifespan, not just sports. Physical education should emphasize fitness, rhythms, dance, aquatics, and individual and dual sports. The SHPPS reported that 74.2 percent of all middle/junior high and senior high schools offer physical education classes including continuous exercise lasting 20 minutes or more, three times per week, and 37.9 percent provide opportunities for students to get 30 minutes of physical activity each day. It also revealed that 94 percent of states and 95 percent of school districts require some physical education (Pate, Small, et al., 1995).

Regular exercise is a well-established component of a healthy lifestyle. Indeed, regular physical activity is associated with lower risk of many health problems, including coronary heart disease and obesity. Adult health characteristics and behaviors seem to begin in childhood, suggesting that childhood exercise experiences may be important to adult habits. Because of their mutual origins, physical educators and health educators represent a huge resource to one another, which is highly compatible with the contemporary "preventive health" philosophy.

Many physical education programs have not embraced health promotion issues, choosing instead to maintain their concentration on competitive games and sports, especially team sports. The shift toward competitive sports begins as early as grades 3 and 4. These activities take valuable time to organize and often result in only a few students being truly active. For most participants, many sports activities are not usable in adulthood and, from a fitness perspective, are "time wasters." "Every effort should be made to encourage schools to require daily physical education in each grade and to promote physical activities that can be enjoyed throughout life" (USDHHS, 1996). This indicates that both a need and an opportunity exist to redirect the energy and philosophy of physical education practitioners to promote wellness. From a national viewpoint, the health-related approach to physical education that nourishes an interest and sense of self-efficacy in physical activities that students can enjoy throughout adulthood seems to be gaining a foundation in American schools.

Quality school-based physical education can contribute to the health of children and the adults they will become (American Heart Association, 1995; Pate, Pratt, et al., 1995). Physical education that emphasizes moderate to vigorous activity can increase students' knowledge about ways to be physically active (Arbeit et al., 1992), the amount of physical activity in physical education classes (Luepker et al., 1996), and students' physical fitness levels (Arbeit et al., 1992; VanDongen et al., 1995). This is especially important given that the number of students who regularly engage in physical activity decreases during adolescence (CDC, 1996a). Serving nearly all children, schools have a unique position to encourage lifetime physical activity.

Professional health educators have an excellent opportunity to collaborate with their colleagues in physical education. Efforts to measure fitness levels and plan programs to develop cardiorespiratory endurance, muscular strength and endurance, flexibility, and improved body composition in students can be enhanced by joint planning and cooperation. Health education and physical education curricula overlap when they explore the health benefits

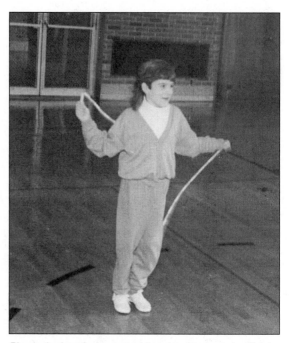

Physical education can provide enjoyable opportunities to develop cardiovascular endurance.

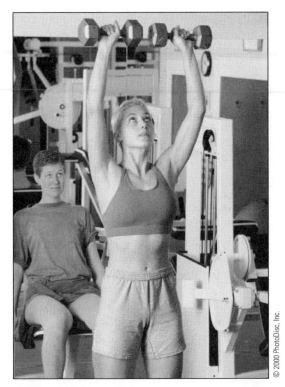

Physical education can help students develop strength and improve body image.

of physical activity and include behavioral skills such as decision-making, planning, and problem solving related to physical activity (Seefeldt, 1998). Physical educators can contribute to a healthy school environment by refusing to use physical activity as a disciplinary tool (CDC, 1997b). There is an obvious need to increase the number of children taking physical education daily. There also is a need to take a health-oriented approach to physical education. Both of these needs are more likely to be met when physical activity is enjoyable and increases students' feelings of competence for sustained participation. Teachers in both disciplines, as well as administrators, should be held accountable for maximizing vigorous physical activity during physical education classes.

## Component 5: Nutrition Services

Nutrition services should provide balanced, appealing, and varied meals and snacks to students. Reasons for offering a well-planned food service program include the following:

- Good nutrition promotes health and builds energy.

- Students are better able to learn and participate in school activities when they are well fed.

- Children have the opportunity to learn social aspects of dining as well as the sanitary aspects of foods and eating.

- If the nutrition service program is integrated into the instructional program, it can provide needed opportunities for teaching and learning about nutrition.

It is unrealistic to hold schools solely accountable for improving students' eating behaviors. Eating habits are shaped by a variety of powerful influences, including the family, sociocultural and economic factors, the food industry, peer pressure, and the mass media (Crockett & Sims, 1995; National Research Council, 1996). However, as part of the child's social environment, the school shapes children's behavior. The record shows that school-based programs can improve students' eating habits (Contento et al., 1995; Edmundson et al., 1996).

The essential functions of a school nutrition program are to provide (Caldwell, Nestle, & Rogers, 1998) the following:

- access to a variety of nutritious, culturally appropriate foods that promote growth and development, pleasure in healthy eating, and long-term health, as well as prevent school-day hunger and its consequent lack of attention to learning tasks

- nutrition education that empowers students to select and enjoy healthy food and physical activity

- screening, assessment, counseling, and referral for nutrition problems and the provision of modified meals for students with special needs

Food services have been a part of the school health program since President Harry Truman signed the National School Lunch Act in 1946. The Special Milk Program in 1954 and the School Breakfast Programs in 1966 and 1972 followed.

School nutrition programs are so entrenched that all states employ state-level food service directors (Pateman et al., 1995). Although poor children are assumed to be in greater need for nutrition services, youngsters from middle class and wealthy families also come to school unfed or poorly fed. Government supplementation of nutrition for children has been a benefit to all.

Although a great deal of federal funding is available for nutrition, only 43.1 percent of the states require that meals be offered during the school day. Still, 88.7 percent of districts participate in the National School Lunch Program, and 57.3 percent participate in the School Breakfast Program. More than 96 percent of the states recommend, and one state requires, that school meals be consistent with Dietary Goals for Americans. Although the National School Lunch Program is available to 92 percent of all students, more than 40 percent of students make other choices with no nutrition standards (Gleason, 1995). According to the School Health Policies and Programs Study (Pateman et al., 1995), more than half of all districts report responsibility for planning meals and for purchasing food, and about two of every five districts report some responsibility for preparing meals.

In addition to availability, other factors affect students' choice of foods, including history, culture, environment, and enjoyment. A comfortable and attractive social environment also contributes to establishing healthy eating patterns among students (Crockett & Sims, 1995). Federal recommendations include environmental factors such as adequate time and space for students to eat meals in a pleasant and safe environment (CDC, 1996b) and policies that will improve the cafeteria environment (Code of Federal Regulations, 1995).

Qualifications of those responsible for school nutrition currently are somewhat weak. Certification for district-level food service directors is offered by only 21.6 percent of all states, and required for employment by fewer than 1 in 10 states. At the school level, only 5.9 percent of the states require certification for food service directors. Only 2.8

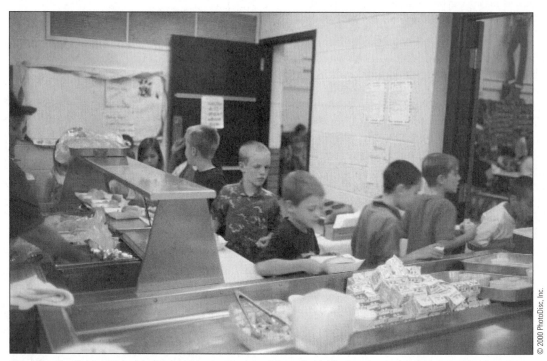

© 2000 PhotoDisc, Inc.

Opportunities for health instruction exist in many areas of the school. The lunch room and kitchen are areas that can be incorporated into health instruction.

percent of the persons most knowledgeable about the food service in the school were certified as Registered Dietitians by the American Dietetic Association (Pateman et al., 1995).

Recognizing that only 1 percent of schools offered lunches providing an average of 30 percent or less of calories from fat, Congress made improvements in several child nutrition programs in 1994. Under the Healthy Meals for Healthy Americans Act, amounts of fat, sodium, and cholesterol in school lunches and breakfasts were to be reduced to conform to the U.S. Department of Agriculture general dietary guidelines. The law required schools to meet the guidelines by the 1996–97 school year, with USDA assistance. The USDA mounted a comprehensive School Meals Initiative for Healthy Children in June 1994.

The unhealthy food choices of children and aggressive marketing that targets youngsters accentuates the need for solid nutrition education. Nutrition education is likely to be most effective when it is behaviorally oriented and emphasizes primarily skills needed to adopt and maintain specific healthy eating behaviors. Nutrition education that focuses narrowly on transmitting nutrition information typically produces gains in knowledge but has little effect on behavior (Contento et al., 1995; Lytle & Achterberg, 1995). Enlightened health educators coordinate classroom and cafeteria learning opportunities so that they afford skill practice and reinforce attitudes needed for behavior change. The Centers for Disease Control and Prevention (1996b) has identified the characteristics of nutrition instruction that are most likely to be effective:

- behaviorally focused content that is developmentally appropriate and culturally relevant

- active, participatory learning strategies

- fun activities

- repeated opportunities for students to taste foods that are low in fat, sodium, and added sugars and high in vitamins, minerals, and fiber

- positive, appealing aspects of healthy eating patterns

- presentation of the benefits of healthy eating behaviors in the context of what is already important to students

- "social learning" (Perry, Baranowski, & Parcel, 1990) techniques such as role modeling, providing incentives, enhancing students' self-confidence in their ability to make dietary changes, developing social resistance skills, working to overcome barriers to behavior change, and goal setting

The school nutrition service should look beyond the health instruction component to more fully integrate its objectives. Students are more likely to make healthy eating choices when they receive consistent, reinforcing messages from a number of credible sources who present positive role models of dietary habits.

Food service managers can reinforce classroom lessons by offering specific foods that coincide with lesson themes, displaying nutrition information about available foods, giving students a tour of the cafeteria kitchen, showing techniques for preparing low-fat meals, and involving students in planning menus (Caldwell, Nestle, & Rogers, 1998). Nutrition staff can collaborate with physical education and athletics staff to plan activities that teach students about the link between good nutrition and physical activity. There is also a natural link between food services and community health organizations, such as the National Dairy Council and American Heart Association, that provide services and educational programs in schools.

Beyond the obvious lessons in food selection, nutrition education provides other opportunities for development. Educators should implement strategies to allow students to gain etiquette and social skills associated with meals.

Finally, school district policy should contain guidelines for the sale of snack foods and foods sold at athletic, performance, and social events. It should also include foods donated for such events as school parties. Foods that fail to meet the USDA's "minimum nutritional value"—meaning that the food fails to provide at least 5 percent per serving of U.S. Recommended Dietary Allowance for each of eight specific nutrients—should be prohibited. This would bar the sale of hard candy, soda pop, and chewing gum and allow sale of candy bars made with milk or nuts and vitamin-fortified drinks, even though they have a high fat and sugar content (Naworski, 1994).

# Component 6: Psychological, Guidance/Counseling, and Social Services

A number of services are available in the school setting to help students overcome social and psychological obstacles to their performance. Although the classroom teacher may play a role in these services, they are best left to those with special preparation—the school psychologist, guidance counselor, and social worker. One of the more positive outgrowths of special education legislation has been the requirement for multidisciplinary teams to serve children. The general functions of the counseling, psychological, and social services component are to minimize barriers to student learning and promote students' healthy psychosocial development.

**Psychological Services**    Many schools employ school psychologists in roles that vary from school to school. Much of the psychologist's efforts are directed toward the following:

- psychoeducational evaluation
- educational programming for students with special needs
- individual and group appraisal of students
- coordination with child- and youth-serving community agencies and other pupil services
- counseling and psychotherapy
- crisis intervention and emergency assistance
- preventive mental health consultation
- inservice education
- data collection and research

Child study teams often are formed in school when a child is identified as needing psychological services. This team may include the school psychologist, special education teacher, social worker, school nurse, and others. Cooperation among the team members is imperative to maximize the team's productivity. Each member of the team brings a different perspective to the child's educational orientation. The school psychologist's contribution includes assessing behavior, personality, and educational achievement as it relates to the child's overall school functioning (Thomas, 1987) as well as

consultations and interventions to improve the child's adjustment to school. Specific duties of the school psychologist vary from state to state and even within a state.

Various procedures are available to test and evaluate certain aspects of personality, social acceptance, self-concept, intelligence, aptitude, achievement, and factors that might hinder optimum school performance. These should be administered by psychologists, psychometrists, and other specially trained mental health counselors, and only those with specific training should interpret the results. Results can be used to diagnose problems, prescribe therapy, place students in learning groups, provide education plans for students, and refer students for treatment. This function is reliant upon knowledge of learning theories, psychometric assessment, child development, and family systems, as well as a functional understanding

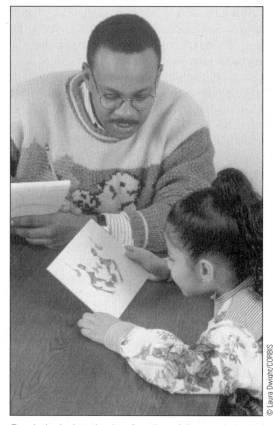

© Laura Dwight/CORBIS

Psychological testing is a function of the psychological services component of the CSHP.

of classroom analysis, school organization, and curriculum (Thomas, 1987). Written permission from parent or guardian must be obtained before administering these assessments. Results of these examinations should remain confidential.

The culmination of the child study is a conference with parents and teachers. The school's evaluations are reviewed; recommendations are made, explained, and discussed. Recommendations could include referral to outside professional mental health care, special classroom strategies, in-school counseling, special education, or a wide range of creative alternatives.

## Health Guidance

The aim of health guidance is to help pupils discover, understand, and resolve health matters through their own efforts. With guidance, pupils can uncover and use their own natural endowments to acquire the highest possible level of wellness. Teachers, especially at the elementary school level, work closely with children and have a unique opportunity to offer guidance.

Guidance can take many forms, including problem solving and helping children and parents see cause-and-effect relationships between behavior and outcomes. It also can serve as motivation to act.

Counseling is a significant part of guidance. Over the past several years, school counseling has shifted its emphasis from treatment and remediation to prevention. This change in emphasis brought about the development of a comprehensive model of school counseling, based on developmental principles (Perry, 1994). This model shifted the emphasis from reactive to more proactive and to establishing a comprehensive program to meet the needs of all students.

Counselors now are seen as an important part of the school health team. Cooperation and coordination of the school counseling and health education programs will strengthen and reinforce both approaches. Counseling programs approach student health from a social context viewpoint; they can offer valuable depth and support to health instruction. In addition, by consulting with school nurses about students' physical problems, with teachers about academic problems, with psychologists if educational or psychological testing seems

necessary, and with social workers if home visits or involvement of the courts are required, the counselor offers a range of services that benefit students. Counselors provide needs assessment and broad-based intervention programs to promote students' physical and emotional health. Interventions include assertiveness training, life skills training, peer-led discussions, problem-solving training, and programs to address esteem, loss of control, peer pressure, and adolescent rebellion (Klingman, 1984). Trained counselors can interpret a problem for students and parents and help them work out solutions so they can achieve high-level wellness through their own actions.

Counseling also frequently takes the form of one-on-one discussions with pupils or their parents, although it can involve both parents and children. This is often in response to a specific need. Counseling and follow-through can have tremendous value in promoting health.

The area of student health presents many opportunities for counselors to participate. Issues such as substance abuse, sexuality and pregnancy, depression, suicide, sexual and physical abuse, AIDS, and problems with family members or friends are all of interest to counselors. Counselors sometimes team-teach lessons concerned with these issues with health teachers. Classroom guidance can include sessions centering on discussions, media, or other activities appropriate to the student's developmental level. Individual, group, and family sessions can provide support, clarification of issues, information, identification of appropriate ways to express feelings and diffuse anger, coping skills, and referral to appropriate professionals.

## Social Workers

Social workers are part of the child study team. Many school districts employ social workers, and others utilize social workers employed by the local, state, or county office of social services. Social workers are primarily responsible for and interested in the relationships among the students, the school, and the community (Redican, Olsen, & Baffi, 1993). In this function, they may serve as "counselors," mediating differences between students, students and teachers, parents and teachers, and parents and children. Social workers also may serve in an advisory capacity to school administrators. Many times social workers serve as a referral service, assisting students and their families to locate needed services in the community. The social worker may be the only member of the school team who is allowed to conduct home visits to examine the family environment and living conditions.

## Component 7: Community and Family Involvement

Research indicates that teachers want parents and families involved with schools (Delgado-Gaitan, 1991; Chavkin & Williams, 1985) and parents want to help their children learn (Davies, 1991) and also support parental involvement in schools (Chavkin & Williams, 1985). Several researchers and experts have provided solid bases for a collaborative approach among the school, the community, and the family:

- Parent involvement is directly related to a significant increase in student achievement (Chavkin (1989).
- Parental involvement is related to increased student attendance, reduction in student dropouts, an improvement in student self-esteem, and more parent and community support for the school (Henderson, 1987).
- Schools do not exist in isolation from the community that sanctions and supports their existence through tax dollars (Gonder, 1981).
- Learning is not synonymous with schooling, because much of what is learned occurs outside the formal classroom setting (Silberman, 1976).
- The adoption of health-enhancing behaviors by students is increased if consistent messages are provided through multiple channels (home, school, community, media) and by multiple sources (such as parents, peers, health and education professionals, and media) (Pentz, 1986).
- School health education programs that incorporate parent involvement have been shown to effect positive changes in both children's diets and smoking behavior among parents, in addition to promoting child-parent discussion about health topics (Bernier, 1991; Perry, Crockett, & Pirie, 1987; Perry et al., 1988).

- The primary health status of students can be promoted through an aggressive school-based health services program that coordinates community personnel and resources to detect and remedy health problems that can adversely affect learning (Edwards, 1987; Kirby, 1986)

According to Hawkins, Catalano, and Miller (1992), students feel competent and do well in school when

- their communities have accessible resources and supportive networks and involve students in community services;
- their families seek preventive care, value and encourage education, spend time with their children, and have clear expectations;
- schools involve families and students and encourage the development of positive behaviors; and
- schools, families, and communities deliver clear, consistent messages.

When schools have good relationships with parents, parents are more likely to cooperate with school health efforts. Good school and family relationships also lay the groundwork in the home and community for an environment that models and reinforces classroom learning (NCPIE, 1995). The National PTA expressed similar sentiments in a statement shown in Box 7.4.

Successful parent involvement in schools is dependent upon several key factors (Redding, 1991). First, parents must be seen as full partners in the school community. Second, parental involvement should begin with parents most likely to respond and proceed in wider circles to reach other parents, using involved parents to recruit others. Third, parents must be involved in a meaningful activity. Finally, parent involvement must be measured by the quality of their involvement and not just their numbers.

The idea of cooperative planning among school and community leaders historically has been considered essential to advancement of an effective school health program. Involvement of families can take many forms. Most parents believe that they should be involved in school decision-making; this is an excellent opportunity to reach those who want

## Box 7.4  Comprehensive School Health Programs

National PTA believes that health is based on the quality of life of the whole child—emotional, intellectual, physical, social, and spiritual. All elements must be considered before optimum health can exist.

National PTA recognizes that:

- Social changes have produced major health problems among our children that have a direct impact on schools and their ability to educate;
- Academic achievement and student self-esteem and well-being are interrelated;
- While the well-being of children is primarily the responsibility of the home, responsibility for the emotional, intellectual, physical, and social health of children is shared by the whole community and all of its institutions;
- That, after the home, the school is often best positioned to serve as the community's center for meeting the needs of the whole child; and
- By encouraging creative integration of education, physical and mental health, housing, employment, and other social services, we can reach vulnerable families.

Source: National PTA. (1996). Position statement on comprehensive school health programs. Chicago. Reprinted by permission.

to become involved. School districts also benefit when parents are involved in curriculum development and selection. School health coordinating councils, which can operate at the building level, the district level, or both, have functioned as coordinating bodies for this cooperation and can be keys to promoting the school health program. They extend beyond the school to engage local business, media, political, religious, juvenile justice, and medical communities (Resnicow & Allensworth, 1996). Education programs for family members can be successful ways to get parents to reinforce what is taught in school and can be an overture to initiate family involvement. The programs can be offered at the same time or just before students study the health topics and skills in class.

Another approach is the interagency coalition, which involves schools and community agencies. This alliance can consist of voluntary health organizations, public health departments, professional associations, religious organizations, judicial bodies, and private foundations. The coalition can act as an advocate for school health programs and serve as a conduit to bring other community organizations and individuals into the school environment.

The school-based clinic is yet another approach to coordinating school and community health promotion efforts. The clinic may employ physicians, psychologists, social workers, and others who have links with many community agencies. Contact with these professionals can maximize the clinic's contribution to students' overall wellness.

Regardless of the model chosen to integrate school and community programs systematically, the structure of the individual school and the needs of its students should govern its implementation. In some cases, a combination of models may be useful. The appropriate vehicle to integrate school and community should do the following (Killup et al., 1987):

- provide primary health care for K–12 students in need
- deliver a comprehensive, integrated, sequential K–12 health education program
- coordinate a proactive health promotion program for faculty, staff, and students, utilizing an interdisciplinary team of administrators, teachers, nurses, counselors, psychologists, and health promotion and food service directors
- depend on a collaborative interagency network of health, educational, social, service, judicial, and recreational agencies to facilitate attainment of educational goals and improved health status for all K–12 students

Associations between schools and their communities can be structured in a number of ways. They may be short-term, such as enlisting a community dental hygienist to screen students for dental disease, or long-term, such as a police department's providing school resource officers. Multidimensional exchanges that occur with the formation of coalitions, consortiums, and health service networks tend to be formal, highly structured, long-term, proactive initiatives. They also have the most potential to mobilize and integrate all health and educational resources within the school and community (Killup et al., 1987).

The number and variety of contacts between school and community are almost limitless. Each practitioner associated with the school health program usually has contacts in the community. Examples are the food service director or nutritionist with the National Dairy Council; the physical education teacher with the President's Council on Fitness and Sport; the school nurse with hospitals, physicians, and the public health community; and the health educator with a plethora of voluntary health organizations. The responsibility for initiating these contacts was once limited to school personnel, but today community health agencies compete for instructional time and they often make the initial contact. They frequently bring with them professionally developed and produced instructional materials and curricula. Integrated school and community health programs truly benefit schools, community agencies, and students.

Parents and other family members can be strategic resources to the school and to the school health program. Student achievement improves (Chavkin, 1989), student self-esteem and parent support for schools increases (Henderson, 1987), and the quality of general education is enhanced (Solomon, 1991) when schools involve parents actively in the education process. Specific to health education, programs that include parent involvement have been shown to effect positive changes in children's diets (Perry et al., 1988), parents' smoking behavior (Bernier, 1991), parent eating and exercise habits (Hearn et al., 1992), and child-parent discussion about health topics (Perry, Crockett, & Pirie, 1987), including the presentation of a family perspective on values-laden topics (Birch, 1994). Family members and caregivers frequently have expertise in health-related areas that they can share with students and teachers. They can participate in program and curriculum development. In some limited ways, they can participate in school health services, such as vision screening. When parents participate in the activities of the school, they are more apt to take pride and feel ownership in the

school. Their participation as vital members of the community should be encouraged. A California task force (Solomon, 1991) outlined opportunities for parent involvement:

- Help parents develop parenting skills and foster communications at home that support learning.
- Provide parents with the knowledge of techniques designed to assist children in learning at home.
- Provide access to and coordinate community support services for children and families.
- Promote clear two-way communication between schools and families regarding school programs and children's progress.
- Involve parents in instructional and support roles in school.
- Support parents as decision-makers and develop their leadership in governance, advisory, and advocacy roles.

Students bring both their problems and their assets to school. Schools cannot carry all of the weight of the health and welfare of students. Schools, families, and communities must work together to create the climates that include support for children, high expectations for them, and a commitment to providing a safe, healthy environment.

## Component 8: Health Promotion for Faculty and Staff

Programs for educators are much less entrenched than worksite health promotion programs for employees in business and industry. Even though illness hampers teachers' effectiveness and puts children at risk, the health of school personnel is often ignored. However, given that new emphasis on school accountability and restructuring may place new pressures on school employees, new opportunities to assist faculty and staff are emerging.

A schoolsite health promotion program for faculty and staff may provide significant financial benefits. Most school districts provide medical care benefits; therefore, costs related to illness and premature death weigh heavily upon the districts.

Direct costs of health insurance are increased by indirect costs of absenteeism, disability, turnover, decreased productivity, and faculty and staff recruitment/replacement expenses. These costs can be reduced by implementing a schoolsite health promotion program (Committee on School Health Programs in Grades K–12, 1997; Blair, Tritsch, & Kutsch, 1987). In addition, studies show that these programs can result in fewer medical claims costs (Allegrante, 1998a) and reduced health care costs (Allensworth et al., 1994). Indeed, several studies have documented the cost-effectiveness of worksite health promotion programs (Lynch et al., 1990; Bellingham et al., 1987; Holzbach et al., 1990; Leutzinger & Blanke, 1991). Reduced school costs contribute to more positive, supportive attitudes in the community about school and open the opportunities for more creative programming.

A well-designed and implemented schoolsite health promotion program can help faculty and staff reduce weight, body fat, smoking, blood pressure, and depression; increase exercise; and improve diet. Fetro and Drolet (1991) reported that school staff from 25 states improved their safety, nutrition, and exercise behaviors through schoolsite health promotion programs. It has been demonstrated that schoolsite staff health promotion programs can improve health-related knowledge (Allegrante, 1998a) as well as improve attitudes and behaviors, including adopting healthful eating behaviors, stopping smoking, increasing physical activity, improving management of emotional stress (Williams & Kubik, 1990; Maysey, Gimarc, & Kronenfeld, 1988; Bishop, Myerson, & Herd, 1988), and improving instruction for students (Allensworth et al., 1994).

The ripple effect of these benefits can improve the school in many ways. Teachers are more energetic and are absent less (Jamison, 1993), school employees stay on staff longer, and school climate is more optimistic (Symons, Cummings, & Olds, 1994). Morale perceptions of the organizational climate are improved (Allegrante & Michela, 1990). These outcomes are bound to provide advantages to students.

Academic reasons also exist for instituting faculty-staff health promotion programs. Because schools have responsibility for the health of students during the day, the school environment and classroom teachers, as role models, should be primary links between students and their acquisition of health-enhancing knowledge and behaviors (Iverson, 1981; Stevens & Davis, 1974). As role models, when teachers or principals smoke or are obese, they are giving tacit approval for their pupils to follow suit. When teachers exercise regularly, maintain ideal weight, and demonstrate other health practices, their pupils also take note. Teachers who have participated in schoolsite health promotion programs report improved attitudes about their health (Health Insurance Association of America, 1985; Pine, 1985; Blair et al., 1984) and an improvement in quality of their instruction (Health Insurance Association of America, 1985; Passwater, Tritsch, & Slater, 1980).

The basic functions of a schoolsite health promotion program for staff are the promotion of physical, emotional, and mental health, as well as the prevention of disease and disability among employees. Programs typically involve health screening, education and supporting activities to reduce risk factors, an employee assistance program, organization policies that promote a healthful and psychologically supportive work environment, and employee health care through health insurance or managed care organization (Allegrante, 1998b).

A school health promotion program addresses changes in the entire employee population and promotes health-enhancing behaviors. Frequently, a health education program for school personnel can do wonders in changing adult behaviors. It should incorporate policies that prohibit smoking. It should utilize all of the school's resources, including the school nurse, health educators, wellness clinic, physical education program and facilities, and nutrition program. The program should utilize print and audiovisual materials, health assessment, counseling, classes conducted by experts, community resources, computer software, environmental alterations, and employee assistance programs. Program content should be chosen based upon the group's needs and interests and could include nutrition, weight control, stress management, and substance abuse prevention and treatment. The health promotion program should attempt to raise the target population's consciousness and increase interest in pursuing a healthy lifestyle, increase knowledge and understanding about health issues and behavioral options available to clients, and present opportunities for continued practice in the behavior.

School staff health promotion activities complement other components of the CSHP. Teachers who are interested in their own health are more likely to take interest in their students' health, thus benefiting the health instruction component. They understand the health needs of students and serve as role models. Because the gymnasium, pool, and other facilities are used, the physical education program becomes a partner in the program and gains prestige among the staff. School nurses, nutritionists, counselors, psychologists, and social workers can extend their expertise to the program. Finally, schoolsite health promotion programs provide an excellent medium for nurturing the bonds between a school and the community. With their expertise and facilities, schools serve as a focal point in the community for health promotion (Stokols, Pelletier, & Fielding, 1995, 1996).

# IMPLEMENTING CSHP

All schools have implemented some components of a coordinated school health program. It is a rare school that has implemented a fully functioning coordinated health program in which each of the eight components is completely developed and integrated with the others (Marx, 1998). Much work needs to be done in order to realize the promise of CSHP, but a local action plan should contain the following points:

- **Obtain a commitment from leadership.** Leaders at the state, local, and school levels must be committed to the notion that the school can be a place where students, families, and staff can adopt health-enhancing behaviors that can facilitate academic achievement and a lifetime of wellness. It is important to identify the key players and the people to whom they listen and gain their support.

- **Make a policy commitment.** Prepare a written policy supporting CSHP and share it with school staff and board. It is important that official policy makers, like local school boards and state departments of education, adopt policies supporting CSHP. You must consider state and federal requirements. You must also be willing to withstand controversies and opposition from businesses whose products damage health and community groups who oppose health education in any form.

- **Form a Healthy School Advisory Committee.** The committee should consist of community and religious leaders, school board members, administrators, teachers, school health education experts, representatives of higher education, businesspeople, parents, and students. The committee can provide information and feedback on needs and community reactions and can serve as a liaison to the community at large. It can also identify supports and challenges in the environment.

- **Assess needs, attitudes, and values.** Examine the reasons for opposition. Listen to people's statements, assess their attitudes and values. Determine if they reflect the community's philosophy of health and education. The advisory committee can be valuable in this function.

- **Appoint a school health coordinator.** The coordinator should be strong and knowledgeable about the goals and functions of the CSHP. He or she should be judicious and practical in working with community groups. The coordinator will oversee the program district-wide.

- **Set up a system that encourages integration of the components of CSHP.** It is crucial that strategies be developed to encourage communication among the various components and between the program and the district office. Communication helps to develop cooperation and ensures that individuals use the same language. Hold regular meetings so that ideas for sharing resources, plans, and needs can be aired and program activities can be coordinated. Encourage collaboration with community agencies and individuals with expertise.

- **Procure funding and commitment.** To succeed, the program must have a long-term commitment from administration. This requires budget development. Funding initially may come in the form of grants or from external sources such as medical societies, businesses, and service clubs. However, the state and the district must make a long-term financial commitment to the program to ensure its chances for success.

- **Select or develop a health education curriculum.** The coordinator and the advisory committee can fulfill this function. However, a separate committee could be appointed for this specific function. The process should be open and encourage comments from the community. The curriculum should emphasize skills development with objectives based upon the needs and interests of the students. The National Health Education Standards form an excellent framework for developing or assessing curricula. The curriculum should be sensitive to community values and ethnic and cultural diversity.

- **Develop an implementation plan.** Formulate a careful plan to implement the various components of the CSHP so that they are coordinated and integrated. Planning helps to reduce the chaos that often accompanies a new program.

- **Provide staff development.** Ongoing staff development allows teachers to assimilate new curricular methods and instructional strategies. Training helps teachers to be confident in their ability to implement the program.

- **Cultivate long-term community support and involvement.** In times of budget shortages, health education programs are often the first to be cut. Community support of the program may protect it.

- **Develop a health promotion program for staff.** The wellness program can build support from staff, good relationships among staff, and word-of-mouth publicity about the CSHP.

- **Provide for ongoing evaluation.** Based upon the goals and objectives of the CSHP, evaluation should take place often. It provides opportunities to upgrade programs, correct weaknesses, ensure accountability, and justify funding.

These steps can help a local school system reach the goal of an effective CSHP. However, on a broader scale, in order to make CSHP commonplace, government health, education, and social service agencies at the national, state, and local levels must work together as partners. National nongovernmental organizations must be involved and active while their affiliates work at the state and local levels. Universities must be engaged, conducting research, furnishing leadership and technical support to school districts, providing pre-service and inservice education and training. Philanthropic organizations should be integrally involved in efforts to improve schools. Some, such as the Carnegie Corporation of New York and the Robert Wood Johnson Foundation, have already provided support for educational reform and school health services.

# DEALING WITH CONTROVERSY

The underlying causes of controversy are the diversity in values found in a community (or the interpretation of those values) and the differences in ethnic and religious beliefs of various segments of a community (Ames et al., 1995). Controversy is to be expected in a democratic and pluralistic society such as that in North America. The skilled educator must manage controversy. The National School Boards Association (1993) highlighted this fact:

> Managing controversy is one of the most difficult and critical aspects of implementing a truly effective program; however, a health program that does not honestly address controversial issues in an age- and culturally-appropriate manner is, at best, ineffectual in helping children make appropriate choices and avoid risky behaviors.

Because of its nature and content, school health education naturally attracts controversy. Many of the most visible and controversial issues that school boards encounter—sexuality and family life education, mental health counseling, reproductive health counseling and services—are associated with school health programs (Marks & Marzke, 1993; Rienzo & Button, 1993). Other specific issues that may trigger controversy are anger management, sexual abuse,

**school health coordinator** the professional responsible for the management and coordination of all health education policies, activities, and resources within a school

child abuse, and death and dying. Those friendly to health education should be aware that opposition may come from individual concerned citizens, organized local groups, or well-orchestrated groups from outside the local community. Regardless of the source of the opposition, it should be taken seriously.

Many of the reasons for opposition deserve serious consideration by proponents of health education. For instance, differences in cultural mores, family values, and religious beliefs are often cited by opponents. Furthermore, curricula are sometimes implemented improperly or taught by persons who lack the academic preparation in health education. It is difficult to generate administrative support when this is the case. Of course, much opposition comes from conservative groups who simply oppose all open-ended decision-making processes and values-clarification activities.

Although policy may be mandated from state government, most curriculum decisions occur at the local level. It is important to seek out supporters for the CSHP on the local school board. Opposition groups often try to persuade school board members to oppose CSHP or even try to elect people to the board who share their view. Advocates must lay a firm foundation for support.

Advocates for school health education should do their homework. They should be aware of surveys indicating wide support, such as those mentioned earlier in this chapter. They should also be ready to cite studies showing parents' overwhelming support for such services as provision of all general health, counseling, parent education, and reproductive health services in school-based health centers (Glick et al., 1995). They should also know the facts about the local community and state, especially data relating to teen pregnancy, drug abuse, STD and HIV/AIDS incidence, violence, anorexia and bulimia, and fitness levels. An important part of the homework is to establish and maintain communication with all interested groups in the school and in the community.

A systematic curriculum planning process is essential. One effective strategy for deflecting controversy is to involve parents in program planning and advocacy (Committee on Comprehensive School Health Programs in Grades K–12, 1997). Build a broad-based planning group including any agency

or group that has legitimate interest in the health and safety of children (Sowers, 1990). Goals and objectives should be realistic and attainable; it does no good to set the program up for failure. Making sure that activities are age-appropriate is critical to gaining support. Once curricula are selected or developed, they should be available for review by parents and community leaders, including religious leaders.

Teachers should be qualified and committed to teaching health. They preferably have an academic degree in health education. Unfortunately, some foolish administrators invite controversy by assigning unqualified or reluctant teachers to health education. Teachers should use acceptable teaching methods and implement the district curriculum faithfully. Some useful guidelines for teaching controversial topics are presented in Box 7.5. Schools and teachers can reduce tension by having policies in effect that provide for handling parents' concerns quickly and thoughtfully. Teacher and administrator mistakes and failure to address parental concerns can undermine good health curricula.

Schools should be prepared to respond to disputes by developing policies and procedures for handling criticism. This is often done on the district level in public schools. Such policies should include, at a minimum, the following (Ames et al., 1995):

- Students have the right to study controversial issues that have political, economic, or social significance.

- Students have the right to free access of information.

- Students have the right to study under competent teachers in situations free from prejudice.

- Students have the right to form, hold, and express their own opinions without jeopardy of school reprimand.

- Teachers have the responsibility to guide discussions and class procedures with thoroughness and objectivity, to point out the possibility of alternative points of view, to show the importance of respecting conflicting opinions, and to carry out arguments with respect for the opinions of others.

**Box 7.5**  Teaching Controversial Topics

When teaching controversial topics, the teacher should

- refrain from forcing personal values on students
- maintain a scientific, unbiased approach
- take care not to ridicule or challenge the personal values of families and follow course and unit outlines recommended or approved by local school officials and allow parents to review them
- be sure the information being provided is scientifically accurate
- wherever possible, use materials that have been prepared by reputable groups and organizations
- use resources that are up to date and scientifically accurate
- keep school administrators informed of classroom activities
- inform parents of the intent of the program and the methods to be used (this might be a function of the school administrator)
- maintain adequate records of pupil activities, questions, interests, and problems

- never have "secret" lessons or admonish students not to discuss lessons at home
- be aware of school policy and do not violate that policy
- use accurate, nonsexist language and avoid stereotyping
- preview all audiovisual materials to be sure that they are scientifically accurate, age-appropriate, and germane to the objectives of the lesson, and allow parents to preview materials
- know all guest speakers, and have a preclassroom meeting with them to go over what will be presented in class
- invite parents to review materials that will be used
- never elicit confidential information from students that will be used in a classroom discussion
- be prepared for unexpected occurrences by having a good command of classroom management techniques

Source: *Health in elementary schools* (9th ed.), by H.J. Cornacchia, L.K. Olsen, & J.M. Ozias, 1996, St. Louis: Mosby. Reprinted by permission of the publisher.

- Students should understand the importance of and reasons for considering controversial issues.

Given that the school-based health center can be an easy target of opponents of the CSHP, the establishment of an advisory committee is often a successful approach. The advisory committee should include respected leaders in the medical and health professions, educators, parents, and other community leaders (Committee on Comprehensive School Health Programs in Grades K–12, 1997). Opposition can be diffused by allowing parents to choose services they wish to exclude for their children. Although this may be a case of missing children who need services most, compromises can help advance the larger program.

Advocates should be positive and present a professional demeanor. State mandates, popular support, and well-documented needs provide a basis for confidence. In addition, if advocates have built a strong coalition with broad-based planning and

clear goals, they should be ready for opposition. Being well-prepared can help deflect rumors, myths, and "dirty tricks" that may appear. It is important to respect differences of opinion and the rights of parents to participate in the process and even to exclude their children from particular lessons or services.

## KEY POINTS

1. Coordinated school health programs are strongly supported by students, parents, and administrators, as well as many national and federal organizations.

2. Evidence suggests that, by reducing children's health-risk behaviors and improving their level of health, school health education can contribute to improved overall academic performance.

3. School health education can be very cost-effective in reducing health care and related expenditures.

4. The National Health Education Standards provide an excellent framework for organizing health knowledge and skills into curricula at the state and local levels and for directing a move toward excellence in teaching health education.

5. The CSHP is made up of eight components: comprehensive school health instruction; healthy school environment; school health services; physical education; nutrition services; psychological, guidance/counseling, and social services; community and family involvement; and health promotion for faculty and staff.

6. The instructional component is the foundation of the CSHP. A major goal of health instruction is the advocacy of health as an instrumental value, focusing on beliefs of how people ought or ought not behave in order to maintain and enhance health.

7. Each of the other components of the CSHP can be linked with the comprehensive health education component.

8. School health services can be delivered through the traditional basic care model, the expanded school health services approach, or the comprehensive health services model.

9. A health-oriented approach to physical education would include emphasis on activities that can be enjoyed throughout life, are enjoyable, and will increase students' feelings of competency for sustained participation.

10. Although all schools implement some components of CSHP, few have a fully functioning program with all of the eight components well developed and implemented. Implementing a CSHP requires development and execution of a local action plan.

11. Opposition to health education often arises - because of diversity of values in a community. Proponents must be prepared to deal with controversy by understanding the opposition, building support, and involving parents and community members in curriculum development.

## REFERENCES

Allegrante, J.P. (1998a). School-site health promotion for faculty and staff: A key component of the coordinated school health program. *Journal of School Health, 68*(5), 190–195.

Allegrante, J.P. (1998b). School-site health promotion for staff. In E. Marx, S.F. Wooley, & D. Northrop (Eds.), *Health is academic: A guide to coordinated school health programs.* New York: Teachers College Press.

Allegrante, J.P. & Michela, J.L. (1990). Impact of a school-based workplace health promotion program on morale of inner-city teachers. *Journal of School Health, 60*(1), 25–28.

Allensworth, D. (1994). The research base for innovative practices in school health education at the secondary level. *Journal of School Health, 64*(5), 80–186.

Allensworth, D., & Kolbe, L. (1987). The comprehensive school health program: Exploring an expanded concept. *Journal of School Health, 57*(10), 409–412.

Allensworth, D.D., Simons, W.C., & Olds, R.S. (1994). *Healthy students 2000: An agenda for continuous improvement in America's schools.* Kent, OH: American School Health Association.

Allensworth, D., Wyche, J., Lawson, E., & Nicholson, L. (Eds.). (1995). *Defining comprehensive school health program: An interim statement.* Washington, DC: National Academy Press.

American Heart Association. (1995). *Strategic plan for promoting physical activity.* Dallas, TX.

American Medical Association. (1994). *Guidelines for adolescent prevention services (GAPS): Recommendations and rationale.* Baltimore: Williams & Wilkins.

American Nurses Association. (1991). *Nursing's agenda for healthcare reform.* Kansas City, MO.

Ames, E.E., Trucano, L.A., Wan, J.C., & Harris, M.H. (1995). *Designing school health curricula: Planning for good health.* Dubuque, IA: WCB Brown & Benchmark.

Arbeit, M.L., Johnson, C.C., Mott, D.S., Harsha, D.W., Nicklas, T.A., Webber, L.S., & Berenson, G.S. (1992). The heart smart cardiovascular school health promotion: Behavior correlates of risk factor change. *Preventive Medicine, 21*(1), 18–32.

Bellingham, R., Johnson, D., McCauley, M., & Mendes, T. (1987). Projected cost savings from AT&T communications total life concept (TLC) process. In J.P. Poatz (Ed.), *Health promotion evaluation: Measuring the organizational impact.* Stevens Point, WI: National Wellness Association.

Bernier, M.P. (1991). Parental involvement in health education. *The Eta Sigma Gamma Monograph Series 9*(1), 42–48.

Birch, D.A. (1994). Involving families in school health education. In P. Cortese & K. Middleton (Eds), *The comprehensive school health challenge, Vol. 2*. Santa Cruz, CA: ETR Associates.

Bishop, N., Myerson, W.A., & Herd, J.A. (1988). The school district for health promotion. *Health Values, 12*(2), 41–45.

Blair, S.N., Collingwood, T.R., Reynolds, R., Smith, M., Hagan, D., & Sterling, C.L. (1984). Health promotion for educators: Impact on health behaviors, satisfaction and general well-being. *American Journal of Public Health, 74*(2), 147–154.

Blair, S.N., Tritsch, L., & Kutsch, S. (1987). Worksite health promotion for school faculty and staff. *Journal of School Health, 57*(10), 469–473.

Botvin, G.J., Baker, E., Dusenbury, L., Botvin, E.M., & Diaz, T. (1995). Long-term follow-up results of a randomized drug abuse prevention trial in a white middle-class population. *JAMA, 273*(14), 1106–1112.

Boyer, E. (1983). *High school: A report on secondary education in America*. New York: Harper & Row.

Bremberg, S. (1991). Does school education affect the health of students? In D. Nutbeam (Ed.), *Youth health promotion: From theory to practice in school and community health*. London: Forbes Publications.

Briss, P.A., Sacks, J.J., Addiss, D.G., Kresnow, M., & O'Neil, J. (1994). A nationwide study of the risk of injury associated with day care centers attendance. *Pediatrics, 93*(3), 364–386.

Bryant, A.L. (1993). Hostile hallways: The AAUW survey on sexual harassment in America's schools. *Journal of School Health, 63*(8), 355–357.

Caldwell, D., Nestle, M., & Rogers, W. (1998). School nutrition services. In E. Marx, S.F. Wooley, & D. Northop (Eds.), *Health is academic: A guide to coordinated school health programs*. New York: Teachers College Press.

Carnegie Council on Adolescent Development. (1989). *Turning points: Preparing American youth for the 21st century. Report of the task force on education of young adolescents*. New York: Carnegie Corporation.

Carnegie Council on Adolescent Development. (1990). *Turning points: Preparing American youth for the 21st century: Recommendations for transforming middle schools*. Washington, DC.

Casamassimo, P. (Ed.). (1996). *Bright futures in practice: Oral health guide*. Arlington, VA: National Center for Education in Maternal and Child Health.

Centers for Disease Control and Prevention. (1996a, September 27). CDC Surveillance Summaries, 1995. *Morbidity and Mortality Weekly Report, 45* (SS-4).

Centers for Disease Control and Prevention. (1996b). Guidelines for school health programs to promote lifelong healthy eating. *Morbidity and Mortality Weekly Report, 45*(RR-9 Whole).

Centers for Disease Control and Prevention, Division of Adolescent and School Health. (1997a). *Is school health education effective? An exploratory analysis of selected exemplary components*. Unpublished manuscript.

Centers for Disease Control and Prevention. (1997b). Guidelines for school and community programs to promote lifelong physical activity among young people. *Morbidity and Mortality Weekly Report, 46*(RR-6), 1–36.

Centers for Disease Control and Prevention. (1999). Facts about violence among youth and violence in schools [On-line]. Available: http://cdc.gov/od/oc/media/fact/violence.htm

Centers for Disease Control and Prevention. (2000). *School health programs: An investment in our nation's future* [On-line]. Available: http://cdc.gov/nccdphp/dash/ataglanc.htm

Chavkin, N.F. (1989). A multicultural perspective on parent involvement: Implications for policy and practice. *Education, 109*(3), 276–285.

Chavkin, N.F., & Williams, D.L. (1985). *Executive summary of the final report: Parent involvement in education project*. Austin, TX: Southwest Educational Development Laboratory.

Children's Safety Network at Education Development Center, Inc. (1997). *Injuries in the school environment: A resource guide* (2nd ed.). Newton, MA: Education Development Center.

Code of Federal Regulations, Title 7. (1995). *School meals initiatives for healthy children rule* (Parts 210 and 220).

Collins, J.L., Small, M.L., Kann, L., Pateman, B.C., Gold, R.S., & Kolbe, L.J. (1995). School health education. *Journal of School Health, 65*(8), 302–311.

Commission on the Reorganization of Education. (1928). *Cardinal principles of secondary education* (Department of Interior, Bureau of Education, Bulletin No.35, 1918). Washington, DC: Government Printing Office.

Committee on Comprehensive School Health Programs in Grades K–12. (1997). *Schools & health: Our nation's investment*. Washington, DC: National Academy Press.

Committee on School Health, American Academy of Pediatrics. (1993). *School health: Policy and practice*. Elk Grove Village, IL: American Academy of Pediatrics.

Contento, I., Balch, G., Bronner, Y., Lytle, L., Maloney, S., Olson, C., Swadener, S., & Randell, J. (1995). The effectiveness of nutrition education and implications for nutrition education policy, programs, and research: A review of research. *Journal of Nutrition Education, 27*(6), 359.

Council of Chief State School Officers. (1991). *Beyond the health room*. Washington, DC.

Council of Chief State School Officers and State Collaborative on Assessment and Student Standards. (1999). *Achieving health literacy: A guide to portfolios* (2nd ed.). Soquel, CA: ToucanEd Publications.

Crockett, S., & Sims, L. (1995). Environmental influences on children's eating. *Journal of Nutrition Education, 27*(Suppl.), 235–249.

Davies, D. (1991). Schools reaching out. *Phi Delta Kappan, 72*(5), 376–382.

Davis, M., Fryer, G.E., White, S., & Igoe, J.B. (1995). *A closer look: A report of select findings from the National School Health Survey 1993–1994*. Denver: Office of School Health, University of Colorado Health Sciences Center.

Davis, T.M., & Allensworth, D.D. (1994). Program management: A necessary component for comprehensive school health program. *Journal of School Health, 64*(10), 400–404.

DeGraw, C. (1994). A community-based school health system: Parameters for developing a comprehensive student health promotion program. *Journal of School Health, 64*(5), 192–195.

Delgado-Gaitan, C. (1991). Involving parents in the schools: A process of empowerment. *American Journal of Education, 100*(1), 20–26.

Dhillon, H.S., & Tolsma, D. (1991). *Meeting global health challenges: A position paper on health education*. Geneva, Switzerland: World Health Organization.

Dryfoos, J.G. (1994). *Full service schools: a revolution in health and social services for children, youth, and families.* San Francisco: Jossey-Bass.

Dryfoos, J.G. (1998). School-based health centers in the context of education reform. *Journal of School Health, 68*(10), 404–408.

Dryfoos, J.G., Brindis, C., & Kaplan, D. (1996). Research and evaluation in school-based health care. In L. Juszczak & M. Fisher (Eds.), *Adolescent medicine: State of the art health care in schools.* Philadelphia: Hanley & Belfus.

Duncan, P. & Igoe, J.B. (1998). School health services. In E. Marx, S.F. Wooley, & D. Northrop (Eds.), *Health is academic: A guide to coordinated school health programs.* New York: Teachers College Press.

Dusenbury, L. & Falco, M. (1995). Eleven components of effective drug abuse prevention curricula. *Journal of School Health, 54*(6), 420–425.

Edmundson, E., Parcel, G., Feldman, H., Elder, J., Perry, C., Johnson, C., Williston, B., Stone, E., Yang, M., Lytle, L., & Webber, L. (1996). The effects of the child and adolescent trial for cardiovascular health upon psychosocial determinants of diet and physical activity behavior. *Preventive Medicine, 25*(4), 442–454.

Education Commission of the States. (1996). *Youth violence: A policymaker's guide.* Denver.

Edwards, L.H. (1987). The school nurse's role in school-based clinics. *Journal of School Health, 57*(4). 157–159.

Elam, S. & Lowell, C.R. (1995). The 27th annual Phi Delta Kappa/Gallup poll of the public's attitudes toward the public schools. *Phi Delta Kappan, 77*(1), 44.

English, J. (1994). Innovative practices in comprehensive health education programs for elementary schools. *Journal of School Health, 64*(5), 188–191.

Errecart, M.T., Walberg, H.J., Ross, J.G., Gold, R.S., Fielder, J.L., & Kolbe, L.J. (1991). Effectiveness of teenage health teaching modules. *Journal of School Health, 61*(special insert) (1), 26–30.

Fetro, J.V., & Drolet, J.C., (1991). State conferences for school worksite wellness: A content analysis of conference components. *Journal of Health Education, 22*(2), 80–84.

Fryer, G.E. & Igoe, J.B. (1996). Functions of school nurses and health assistants in U.S. school health programs. *Journal of School Health, 66*(2), 55–58.

The Gallup Organization. (1994). *Values and opinions of comprehensive school health education in U.S. public schools: Adolescents, parents, and school district administrators.* Atlanta: American Cancer Society.

The George Washington University. (1997). National survey of state SBHC initiatives, school year 1995–96 [On-line]. Available: http://gwu.edu/~mtg/sbhc/chart.html

Giordano, B.P. & Igoe, J.B. (1991). Health promotion: The new frontier. *Pediatric Nursing, 17*(5), 490–492.

Gleason, P. (1995). Participation in the national school lunch program and the school breakfast program. *American Journal of Clinical Nutrition, 61*(Suppl.), 213–220.

Glick, B., Doyle, L., Ni, H., Gao, D., & Pham, C. (1995, March 21). *School-based health center program evaluation: Perceptions, knowledge, and attitudes of parents/guardians of eleventh graders.* A limited dataset presented to the Multnomah County (Oregon) Commissioners.

Gold, R.S. (1994). The science base for comprehensive health education. In P. Cortese & K. Middleton (Eds.), *The comprehensive school health challenge, Vol. 2.* Santa Cruz, CA: ETR Associates.

Gonder, P.O. (1981). Exchanging school and community resources. In D. Davies (Ed.), *Communities and their schools.* New York: McGraw-Hill.

Hawkins, J.D., Catalano, R.F., & Miller, J.Y. (1992). Risk and protective factors in adolescence and early adulthood. *American Psychological Association Bulletin, 112*(1), 64–115.

Health Insurance Association of America. (1985). *Wellness at the worksite.* Washington, DC.

Hearn, M.D., Bigelow, C., Nader, P.R., Stone, E., Johnson, C., Parcel, G., Perry, C.L., & Luepker, R.V. (1992). Involving families in cardiovascular health promotion: The CATCH feasibility study. *Journal of Health Education, 23*(1). 22–31.

Henderson, A.C. (1994). The importance of a healthy school environment. In P. Cortese & K. Middleton (Eds.), *The comprehensive school health challenge, Vol. 1.* Santa Cruz, CA: ETR Associates.

Henderson, A.T. (1987). *The evidence continues to grow: Parent involvement improves student achievement.* Columbia, MD: National Committee for Citizens in Education.

Henderson, A., & Rowe, D.E. (1998). A healthy school environment. In E. Marx, S.F. Wooley, & D. Northrop (Eds.), *Health is academic: A guide to coordinated school health programs.* New York: Teachers College Press.

Hochbaum, G.M. (1982). Certain problems in evaluating health education. *Health Values: Achieving High Level Wellness, 6*(1), 14–20.

Holzbach, R.L., Piserchia, P.V., McFadden, D.W., Hartwell, T.D., Herrmann, A.A., & Fielding, J.E. (1990). Effect of a comprehensive health promotion program on employee attitudes. *Journal of Occupational Medicine, 32*, 973–978.

Iverson, D.C. (1981). Promoting health through the schools: A challenge for the eighties. *Health Education Quarterly, 8*(1), 6–14.

Jamison, J. (1993). Health education in schools: A survey of policy and implementation. *Health Education Journal, 52*(2), 59–62.

Johnson, D., & Johnson, R. (1982). Effects of cooperative, competitive, and individualistic learning experiences on cross-ethnic interactions and friendships. *Journal of Social Psychology, 118*(first half), 47–58.

Johnson, D., Johnson, R., Nelson, D., & Skon, L. (1981). Effects of cooperative, competitive, and individualistic goal structures on achievement: A meta-analysis. *Psychology Bulletin, 89*(1), 47–62.

Joint Committee on National Health Education Standards. (1995). *National health education standards: Achieving health literacy.* Atlanta: American Cancer Society.

Kann, L., Collins, J.L., Pateman, B.C., Small, M.L., Russ, J.G. & Kolbe, L.J. (1995). The school health policies and programs study (SHPPS): Rationale for a nationwide status report on school health programs. *Journal of School Health, 22*(2), 291–293.

Killup, D.C., Lovick, S.R., Goldman, L., & Allensworth, D.D. (1987). Integrated school and community programs. *Journal of School Health, 57*(10), 437–444.

Kime, R.E., Schlaadt, R.G., & Tritsch, L.E. (1977). *Health instruction: An action approach.* Englewood Cliffs, NJ: Prentice-Hall.

Kirby, D. (1986). A comprehensive school health clinic. A growing movement to improve adolescent health and reduce teen-age pregnancy. *Journal of School Health, 56*(7), 289–291.

Kirby, D., Short, L., Collins, J., Rugg, D., Kolbe, L., Howard, M., Miller, B., Sonenstein, F., & Zabin, L. (1994). School-based programs to reduce sexual risk behaviors: A review of effectiveness. *Public Health Reports, 109*(3), 339–360.

Klein, J.D., & Sadowski, L.S. (1990). Personal health services as a component of comprehensive health programs. *Journal of School Health, 60*(4), 164–169.

Klingman, A. (1984). Health-related school guidance: Practical applications in primary prevention. *Personnel & Guidance Journal, 62*(10), 576–579.

Knitzer, J., Steinberger, A., & Fleisch, B. (1990). *At the schoolhouse door: An examination of programs and policies for children with behavioral and emotional problems.* New York: Bank Street College of Education.

Kolbe, L.J. (1993). An essential strategy to improve the health and education of Americans. *Preventive Medicine, 22*(4), 544–560.

Kolbe, L.J., Iverson, D.C., Kreuter, M.W., Hochbaum, G., & Christensen, G. (1981). Propositions for an alternate and complementary health education paradigm. *Health Education, 12*(3), 24–30.

Kowalski, T. (1995). Chasing the wolves from the schoolhouse door. *Phi Delta Kappan, 76*(6), 486–489.

Lear, J.G. (1996). School-based services and adolescent health: Past, present and future. In L. Juszczak & H. Fisher (Eds.), *Adolescent medicine: State of the art reviews.* Philadelphia: Haneley and Belfus, Inc.

Leutzinger, J., & Blanke, D. (1991). The effect of a corporate fitness program on perceived worker productivity. *Health Values, 15*(5), 20–29.

Lohrmann, D.K., Gold, R.S., & Jubb, W.H. (1987). School health education: A foundation for school health programs. *Journal of School Health, 57*(10), 420–425.

Lohrmann, D.K., & Wooley, S.F. (1998). Comprehensive school health education. In E. Marx, S.F. Wooley, & D. Northrop (Eds.), *Health is academic: A guide to coordinated school health education.* New York: Teachers College Press.

Luepker, R.V., Perry, C.L., McKinlay, S.M., Nader, P.R., Parcel, G.S., Stone, E.J., Webber, L.S., Elder, J.P., Feldman, H.A., Johnson, C.C., Kelder, S.H., & Wu, M. (1996). Outcomes of a field trial to improve children's dietary patterns and physical activity: The Child and Adolescent Trial for Cardiovascular Health (CATCH). *JAMA, 275*(10), 768–776.

Lynch, W.D., Golaszewski, T.J., Clearie, A.F., Snow, D., & Vickery, D.M. (1990). Impact of a facility-based corporate fitness program on the number of absences from work due to illness. *Journal of Occupational Medicine, 32*(1), 9–12.

Lytle, L., & Achterberg, C. (1995). Changing the diet of America's children: What works and why? *Journal of Nutrition Education, 27*(5), 250–260.

Mack, M.G., Hudson, S.D., & Thompson, D. (2000). Playground safety: Using research to guide community policy. *Journal of Health Education, 30*(6), 352–357+.

Mack, M.G., Thompson, D., & Hudson, S. (1998). Playground injuries in the 90s. *Parks & Recreation, 33*(4), 88–95.

Making the Grade, George Washington University. (1996). School-based health centers continue to grow. *Access to Comprehensive School-Based Health Services for Children and Youth.* Washington, DC.

Making the Grade, George Washington University. (1997). *The picture of health: State and community leaders on school-based health care.* Washington, DC.

Marks, E.L., & Marzke, C.H. (1993). *Healthy caring: A process evaluation of the Robert Wood Johnson Foundation's school-based adolescent health care program.* Princeton, NJ: Mathtech.

Marx, E. (1998). Summary: Fulfilling the promise. In E. Marx, S.F. Wooley, & D. Northrop. (Eds.), *Health is academic: A guide to coordinated school health programs.* New York: Teachers College Press.

Maslow, A. (1986). Towards psychology of being. In V.F. Jones & L.S. Jones (Eds.), *Comprehensive classroom management* (2nd ed.). Boston: Allyn & Bacon.

Maysey, D., Gimarc, J.D., & Kronenfeld, J.J. (1988). School worksite wellness programs: A strategy for achieving the 1990 goals for a healthier America. *Health Education Quarterly, 15*(1), 53–62.

McKenzie, F.D., & Richmond, J.B. (1998). Linking health and learning: An overview of coordinated school health programs. In E. Marx, S.F. Wooley, & D. Northrop (Eds.), *Health is academic: A guide to coordinated school health programs.* New York: Teachers College Press.

Meeks, L., Heit, P., & Page, R. (1996). *Comprehensive school health education: Totally awesome teaching strategies* (2nd ed.). Blacklick: OH: Meeks Heit Publishing.

Meyers, A.F., Sampson, A.D., Weitzman, M., Rogers, B.L., & Kayne, H. (1989). School breakfast programs and school performance. *American Journal of Diseases and Children, 143*(8), 1234–1239.

National Association of State Boards of Education. (1996). *Someone at school has AIDS: A complete guide to education policies concerning HIV infection.* Alexandria, VA.

National Center for Education Statistics. (1998). Incidents of crime and violence in public schools [On-line]. Available: http://nces.ed.gov/pubs98/violence/98030003.html

National Coalition for Parent Involvement in Education. (1995). *Why a coalition for parent involvement?* Washington, DC.

National Commission on Children. (1991). *Beyond rhetoric: A new American agenda for children and families.* Washington, DC: Government Printing Office.

National Commission on the Role of the School and the Community in Improving Adolescent Health. (1990). *Code blue: United for healthier youth.* Alexandria, VA: National Association of State Boards of Education and American Medical Association.

National Education Goals Panel. (1994). *The National Education Goals Report: Building a nation of learners.* Washington, DC: U.S. Government Printing Office.

National Nursing Coalition for School Health. (1995). School health nursing services: Exploring national issues and priorities. *Journal of School Health, 65*(9), 370–385.

National PTA. (1992). *Position statement on comprehensive school health programs.* Chicago.

National Research Council. (1989). *Diet and health: Implications for reducing chronic disease risk.* Washington, DC: National Academy Press.

National Research Council. (1996). *National science education standards.* Washington, DC: National Academy Press.

National School Boards Association. (1993). *Issues brief no. 11: Controversy and pressure groups.* Arlington, VA: Author.

National School Boards Association, American Association of School Administrators, American Cancer Society, & National School Health Education Coalition. (1995). *Be a leader in academic achievement.* Alexandria, VA.

Naworski, P. (1994). The child nutrition program as a partner in comprehensive school health. In P. Cortese & K. Middleton (Eds.), *The comprehensive school health challenge, Vol. 1.* Santa Cruz, CA: ETR Associates.

1990 Joint Committee on Health Education Terminology. (1991). Report of the 1990 Joint Committee on Health Education Terminology. *Journal of School Health, 61*(6), 251–254.

Office of Technology Assessment. (1991). *Adolescent health: Volume I. Summary and policy options* (S/N 052–003–01234-1). Washington, DC: Government Printing Office.

Passwater, D., Tritsch, L., & Slater, S. (1980). *Seaside health education conference: Effects of three 5-day inservice conferences.* Salem, OR: Oregon Department of Education.

Pate, R.R., Corbin, C.B., Simons-Morton, B.G., & Ross, J.G. (1987). Physical education and its role in school health promotion. *Journal of School Health, 57*(10), 445–450.

Pate, R.R., Pratt, M., Blair, S.N., Haskell, W.L., Macera, C.A., Bouchard, C., Buchner, D., Ettinger, W., Heath, G.W., King, A., Kriska, A., Leon, A.S., Marcus, B.H., Morris, J., Paffenbarger, Jr., R.S., Patrick, K., Pollock, M.L., Rippe, J.M., Sallis, J., & Wilmore, J.H. (1995). Physical activity and public health: A recommendation from the Centers for Disease Control and Prevention and the American College of Sports Medicine. *JAMA, 273*(5), 402–407.

Pate, R.R., Small, M.L., Ross, J.G., Young, J.C., Flint, K.H., & Warren, C.W. (1995). School physical education. *Journal of School Health, 65*(8), 312–318.

Pateman, B.C., McKinney, P., Kann, L., Small, M.L., Warren, C.W., & Collins, J.L. (1995). School food service. *Journal of School Health, 65*(8), 327–332.

Pentz, M.A. (1986). Community organizations and school liaisons: How to get programs started. *Journal of School Health, 56*(9), 382–388.

Perry, C.L., Baranowski, T., & Parcel, G.S. (1990). How individuals, environments, and health behavior interact: Social learning theory. In K. Glantz, F.M. Lewis, & B.K. Rimer (Eds.), *Health behavior and health education: Theory, research, and practice.* San Francisco: Jossey-Bass.

Perry, C.L., Crockett, S.J., & Pirie, P. (1987). Influencing parental health behavior: Implications of community assessments. *Health Education, 18*(5), 68–77.

Perry, C.L., Luepker, R.V., Murray, D.M., Kurth, C., Mullis, R., Crockett, S., & Jacobs, D.R. (1988). Parent involvement in children's health promotion: The Minnesota home team. *American Journal of Public Health, 78*(9), 1156–1160.

Perry, N.S. (1994). Integrating school counseling and health education programs. In P. Cortese & K. Middleton (Eds.), *The comprehensive school health challenge, Vol. 1.* Santa Cruz, CA: ETR Associates.

Pine, P. (1985). *Promoting health education in schools: Problems and solutions.* Arlington, VA: American Association of School Administrators.

A point of view for health education. (1992). *Journal of Health Education, 23*(1), 4–6.

Policy Studies Associates. (1992). *Creating sound minds and bodies: Health and education working together.* Washington, DC: National Health/Education Consortium.

Pollock, M.B., & Middleton, K. (1994). *Health instruction: The elementary and middle school years* (3rd ed.). St. Louis: Mosby—YearBook.

Proctor, S.T., Lordi, S.L., & Zarger, D.S. (1993). *School nursing practice roles and standards.* Scarborough, ME: National Association of School Nurses.

Redican, K., Olsen, L., & Baffi, C. (1993). *Organization of school health programs* (2nd ed.). Dubuque, IA: Brown & Benchmark.

Redding, S. (1991). Creating a school community through parent involvement. *Education Digest, 57*(3), 6–9.

Resnicow, K., & Allensworth, D. (1996). Conducting a comprehensive school health program. *Journal of School Health, 66*(2), 59–63.

Rienzo, B.A., & Button, J.W. (1993). The politics of school-based clinics: A community-level analysis. *Journal of School Health, 63*(6), 266–272.

Robert Wood Johnson Foundation. (1995). *Special report: National school health services program.* Princeton, NJ.

Rothman, M.L., Ehreth, J.L., Palmer, C.S., Collins, J., Reblando, J.A., & Luce, B.P. (1993, October). *The potential benefits and costs of a comprehensive health education program.* Paper presented at the meeting of the American Public Health Association, San Francisco.

Rowe, D.E. (1987). Healthful school living: Environmental health in the school. *Journal of School Health, 57*(10), 426–431.

Santelli, J., Morreale, M., Wigton, A, & Grason, H. (1996). School health centers and primary care for adolescents: A review of the literature. *Journal of Adolescent Health, 18*(5), 357–366.

Schlitt, J.J. (1991). *Bring health to school: Policy implications for southern states.* Washington, DC: Southern Center on Adolescent Pregnancy Prevention.

Schultz, E.W., Glass, R.M., & Kamholtz, J.D. (1987). School climate: Psychological health and well-being in school. *Journal of School Health, 57*(10), 432–436.

Seefeldt, V.D. (1998). Physical education. In E. Marx, S.F. Wooley, & D. Northrop (Eds.), *Health is academic: A guide to coordinated school health programs.* New York: Teachers College Press.

Seffrin, J.R. (1990). The comprehensive school health curriculum: Closing the gap between state-of-the-art and state-of-the-practice. *Journal of School Health, 64*(4), 151–156.

Silberman, C. (1976). The Carnegie Study of Education of Educators: Preliminary statement of intent. In L.Cremin (Ed.), *Public education.* New York: Basic Books.

Sliepcevich, E.M. (1967). Health education: A conceptual approach to curriculum design. *School health education study.* St. Paul: 3M Education Press.

Small, M.L., Majer, L.S., Allensworth, D.D., Farquhar, B.K., Kann, L., & Pateman, B.C. (1995). School health services. *Journal of School Health, 65*(8), 319–325.

Solomon, L.P. (1991). California's policy on parent involvement: State leadership for local initiatives. *Phi Delta Kappan, 72*(5), 359–362.

Sowers, J.G. (1990). *Guidelines for dealing with resistance to comprehensive school health.* Hampton, NH: Sowers Associates.

Stevens, N.H., & Davis, L.G. (1974). *Something to get excited about: School health promotion in Oregon.* Salem: Oregon Department of Education.

Stokols, D., Pelletier, K.R., & Fielding, J.E. (1995). Integration of medical care and worksite health promotion. *JAMA, 273*(14), 1136–1142.

Stokols, D., Pelletier, K.R., & Fielding, J.E. (1996). The ecology of work and health: Research and policy directions for promotion of employee health. *Health Education Quarterly, 23*(2), 137–158.

Symons, C.W., Cummings, C.D., & Olds, R.S. (1994). Healthy people 2000: An agenda for schoolsite health promotion programming. In D.D. Allensworth, C.W. Symons, & R.S. Olds (Eds.), *Healthy students 2000: An agenda for continuous improvement in America's schools.* Kent, OH: American School Health Association.

Thomas, A. (1987). School psychologist: An integral member of the school health team. *Journal of School Health, 57*(10), 465–468.

Torabi, M.R., & Crowe, J.W. (1995). National opinion poll on school health education: Implications for the health care reform initiatives. *Journal of School Health, 26*(5), 260–266.

U.S. Census Bureau. (1997). Health insurance coverage: 1997 [On-line]. Available: http://census.gov/hhes/hlthin97/hi97e2.html

U.S. Congress, Office of Technology Assessment. (1995). *Risks to students in school.* Washington, DC: U.S. Government Printing Office.

U.S. Department of Education & U.S. Department of Health and Human Services. (1994). *Joint statement of school health by the Secretaries of Education and Health and Human Services.* Washington, DC: Office of Disease Prevention and Health Promotion.

U.S. Department of Health and Human Services. (1988). *The surgeon general's report on nutrition and health.* Washington, DC: U.S. Government Printing Office.

U.S. Department of Health and Human Services. (1996). *Physical activity and health: A report of the surgeon general.* Atlanta: U.S. Department of Health and Human Services, Centers for Disease Control and Prevention, National Center for Chronic Disease Prevention and Health Promotion.

U.S. Department of Health and Human Services (2000). *Healthy people 2010* (Conference ed. in two volumes). Washington, DC: U.S. Government Printing Office.

U.S. Department of Health and Human Services, Public Health Service. (1991). *Healthy people 2000: National health promotion and disease prevention objectives.* (DHHS Publication No. PHS 91-50213). Washington, DC: U.S. Government Printing Office.

U.S. House of Representatives, Select Committee on Children, Youth and Families. (1992). *A decade of denial: Teens and AIDS in America.* Washington, DC: Government Printing Office.

U.S. Senate, Subcommittee on Oversight of Government Management, Committee on Governmental Affairs. (1992). *Healthy schools, healthy children, healthy futures: The role of the federal government in promoting health through the schools.* Washington, DC: Government Printing Office.

VanDongen, R., Jenner, D.A., Thompson, C., Taggart, A.C., Spickett, E.E., Burke, V., Beilin, L.J., Milligan, R.A., & Dunbar, D.L. (1995). A controlled evaluation of a fitness and nutrition intervention program on cardiovascular health in 10- to 12-year-old children. *Preventive Medicine, 24*(1), 9–22.

Walter, H.J., Vaughan, R.D., & Wynder, E.L. (1989). Primary prevention of cancer among children: Changes in cigarette smoking and diet after six years of interventions. *Journal of the National Cancer Institute, 81*(13), 995–999.

Williams, P., & Kubik, J. (1990). The Battle Creek (Michigan) schools healthy lifestyles program. *Journal of School Health, 60*(4), 142–146.

Wooley, S.F. (1995). Behavior mapping: A tool for identifying priorities for health education curricula and instruction. *Journal of Health Education, 26*(4), 200–206.

World Health Organization. (1996). *Promoting health through schools.* Geneva, Switzerland: World Health Organization.

World Health Organization, United Nations Educational, Scientific, and Cultural Organization, and United Nations Children's Emergency Fund. (1992). Comprehensive school health education. *Hygiea, 11,* 8–15.

Zanga, J.R., & Oda, D.S. (1987). School health services. *Journal of School Health, 57*(10), 413–416.

# Governmental Initiatives

The federal government often sets priorities regarding education and health issues through presidential executive orders, laws enacted by Congress, or publications of cabinet-level departments, such as the Department of Health and Human Services. By setting priorities, the government sets in motion a huge and powerful bureaucracy whose actions can affect the everyday lives of all citizens. Federal priorities set the tone and direction of programs that deliver health education, health promotion, and health services. The impact reaches to the states, counties, towns, and private organizations.

The real work of educating youth and providing health services takes place at the state and local levels. The states have broad legal authority for a wide variety of programs. States' roles can take a number of forms, including

- assessing state and community needs and capacity for program development
- setting priorities for health promotion services
- authorizing or ordering that certain programs or content be included in (or excluded from) public education
- supporting the care and treatment of poor and chronically disabled people, including administration of federal and state Medicaid programs
- regulating insurance carriers
- authorizing local government health services

The states' own active policy agenda usually takes precedence in programming, although federal influences may sway priorities.

One aspect of federal government influence is its power to provide or withhold funds for states based on states' compliance with various federal requirements. The federal government also provides funding through a vast system of grants that may be awarded to, for instance, community agencies, departments of public health, and institutions of higher education.

The National Education Goals for the Year 2000 are one example of the federal government's attempt to improve the status of the American educational establishment. The goals, created by a federally convened panel of educators, served as a challenge to rebuild the education system to its former place as the best in the world. Two goals illustrate the importance of reducing risk factors so that students are better able to learn:

> Goal 1: ALL CHILDREN in America will start school ready to learn.
>
> Goal 2: EVERY SCHOOL in the United States will be free of drugs, violence, and the unauthorized presence of firearms and alcohol and will offer a disciplined environment conducive to learning.

Although the goals were set in 1991 (and signed into law in 1994) amid considerable acclaim and optimism, it quickly became obvious that they would not be met. However, the publication at least

191

announced the nation's acceptance of the decline in education and a commitment to improve. One positive effect of the National Education Goals was passage of the Safe Schools Act in 1994, which authorized grants to support a variety of activities, including identifying and assessing school violence and discipline problems, hiring security guards, training school personnel, and planning comprehensive violence prevention programs. It also authorized national activities, including research, program development and evaluation, data collection, and training and technical assistance.

Another example of federal involvement is in the area of school health education. One of the national health objectives for the year 2000 (U.S. DHHS, 1991) was the establishment of quality school health education for students in kindergarten through grade 12. This resulted in states mandating comprehensive health instruction in schools.

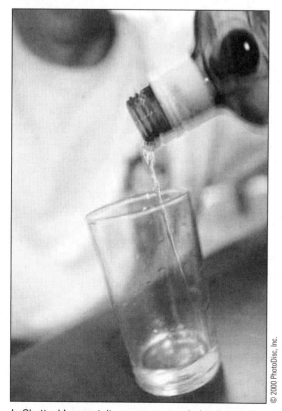

In Shattuck's report, it was recommended to "control" alcoholism. Today, we would try to treat it as a disease.

© 2000 PhotoDisc, Inc.

State and federal governments have historically addressed health concerns in response to crises. For instance, the boards of health in New York and Massachusetts were established in 1797 and the state health department of Louisiana was formed in 1855 to combat yellow fever outbreaks. Outbreaks of smallpox, tuberculosis, polio, and AIDS have prompted governmental action at many levels of government. Attempts to deal with health issues prior to the epidemics began only in the last half of the nineteenth century and escalated during the last half of the twentieth.

The *Report of the Sanitary Commission of Massachusetts: 1850* (Shattuck, 1850/1948) was a landmark in the history of American public health. Although it was a state, not a federal, report, it provided pioneering insights about and recommendations for public health and governmental action that are still not fully implemented. Among the commission's recommendations were the following:

— Establish state and local boards of health.

— Collect and analyze vital statistics.

— Develop sanitation programs for towns.

— Maintain a system of sanitary inspections.

— Study the health of children.

— Study and supervise health conditions of immigrants.

— "Supervise" mental disease.

— "Control" alcoholism.

— Control and reduce food adulteration.

— Control smoke nuisances.

— Preach health from the pulpit.

— Teach the science of sanitation in medical school.

— Include prevention as a part of medical practice.

— Support routine health examinations.

The *Nation's Health* (Federal Security Agency, 1948) is one of the most important documents in the history of health planning. It made recommendations and established goals related primarily to resources and financing of a health care system and a national health insurance program. It accentuated coordination of community action, programs of rehabilitation of people with disabilities, mental health services, and sufficient numbers of hospitals. Many of its proposals have become standard features of public health and the health care delivery system.

# AN OBJECTIVE APPROACH
## Health Objectives for the Year 1990

*Healthy People: The Surgeon General's Report on Health Promotion and Disease Prevention* (U.S. Department of Health, Education, and Welfare, 1979) set the stage for a different approach to dealing with health problems. The crisis management approach, although never abandoned, was augmented by long-term health objectives and development of programs and funding sources to reach those objectives. *Healthy People* proposed formulating objectives by building consensus among experts, professionals, and national advocacy organizations. The report identified five age-related population groups: infants, children, adolescents and young adults, adults, and older adults.

The report noted striking gains in the nation's health over the previous eighty years, but also verified that any further conspicuous improvement would require adoption of health promotion and disease prevention strategies and coordinated action to implement them.

*Healthy People* established quantifiable health goals for each of the five population groups and recommended actions necessary for attaining the goals in three categories: preventive health services, health protection, and health promotion. The goals were

**Infants** To reduce infant mortality by at least 35 percent, to fewer than nine deaths per 1,000 live births by 1990

**Children** To foster optimal childhood development; to reduce deaths among children ages 1 to 14 by at least 20 percent, to fewer than 34 per 100,000 by 1990

**Adolescents and Young Adults** To improve the health habits of adolescents and young adults; to reduce deaths among people ages 15 to 24 by at least 20 percent, to fewer than 93 per 100,000 by 1990

**Adults** To reduce deaths among people ages 25 to 64 by at least 25 percent, to fewer than 400 per 100,000 by 1990

**Older Adults** To improve the quality of life for older adults; by 1990, to reduce the average annual number of days of restricted activity because of acute and chronic conditions by 20 percent, to fewer than 30 days per year for people aged 65 years and older.

*Healthy People* placed great emphasis on decreasing deaths. However, with the exception of the older adult group, little mention is made of the quality of life, high level of wellness, or the ability to enjoy life. Although the government recognized the role that health promotion/education could play in attaining the goals, it seemed to overlook the very ideals that health educators hold dear.

The U.S. Department of Health and Human Services published *Promoting Health/Preventing Disease: Objectives for the Nation* in 1980. This document went beyond *Healthy People*, committing the United States to reaching 226 measurable and quantifiable objectives in fifteen priority areas by the year 1990. Box 8.1 displays the priority areas grouped by category. The publication also identified sources of national, state, and local data used to monitor progress toward the objectives, but stopped short of specifically identifying the governmental agencies that would have principal responsibility for attaining those objectives.

About 3,000 organizations were invited to review and comment on the document before its final publication. Many viewed it as a top-down, science-driven, professionally dominated set of objectives. They saw it as giving too little weight to social concerns and real quality-of-life issues and too much emphasis to bureaucratic and technocratic criteria such as morbidity, mortality, and cost containment.

Although the objectives for 1990 set in motion a ten-year plan for disease prevention and health promotion and contributed greatly to a new sense of purpose and focus for public health, school health, and preventive medicine, they had serious flaws. They were met with much skepticism by people representing the concerns of special populations, such as ethnic and racial minorities and the elderly. In setting objectives related to health and mortality of

| Box 8.1 | Priority Areas of the Year 1990 Health Objectives |
| --- | --- |

**Preventive Health Services**

Family planning

Pregnancy and infant care

Immunizations

High blood pressure control

Sexually transmissible diseases services

**Health Protection**

Toxic agent control

Occupational safety and health

Accidental injury control

Fluoridation of community water supplies

Infectious agent control

**Health Promotion**

Smoking cessation

Reducing misuse of alcohol and other drugs

Improved nutrition

Exercise and fitness

Stress control

*The 1990 Health Objectives for the Nation: A Midcourse Review* (U.S. DHHS, 1986) indicated a good deal of tangible evidence of progress toward meeting the objectives. It suggested that a lack of data to measure the status of many objectives indicated that they were unlikely to be achieved. Specific priority areas showing the greatest progress included high blood pressure control, immunization, control of infectious disease, and smoking. It was revealed later that the priority areas showing the least progress included pregnancy and infant health, family planning, and physical fitness and exercise (McGinnis & DeGraw, 1991).

By the end of the 1980s, most states had accepted the necessity to establish and pursue health objectives. In 1989, 90 percent of the states and territories had established objectives for at least some of the priority areas in the 1990 national objectives. About forty states had established centralized units within the state health agency to promote and coordinate health promotion/disease prevention operations.

By 1990, three of the original goals from *Healthy People* had been accomplished. Targets for reduction in mortality of infants, children, and adults were met. Adolescent mortality did not decline. Data systems were not able to track the goal of improving quality of life for older adults.

## Health Objectives for the Year 2000

As a result of *Healthy People*, the national efforts to improve the health of the populace became oriented toward the accomplishment of ambitious objectives established through the Department of Health and Human Services. This approach was continued with the publication of *Healthy People 2000: National Health Promotion and Disease Prevention Objectives* (U.S. DHHS, 1991). The Office of Disease Prevention and Health Promotion (ODPHP) of the U.S. Public Health Service (PHS) coordinated the development of the Year 2000 Objectives.

The Year 2000 Objectives bore some resemblance to the 1990 objectives, breaking down the population by age group: infants, children, adolescents and young adults, and older adults. It proposed three overarching public health goals that permeate the structure and content of the document:

1. To increase the span of healthy life for Americans

the whole American population, the objectives ignored and hid the wide variations among distinctive populations such as white and non-white, old and young, and rich and poor.

Consistency of funding for programs to address the objectives and priority areas was also lacking. The Reagan administration's philosophy was to reduce large-scale public sector spending on domestic activities and return power and responsibilities to the states. Many viewed this ideology as a mechanism to reduce federal expenditures for domestic activities and to abandon the national commitments to certain costly social programs, including some of those that served to guard people's health. The resulting transfer of responsibility to the states and their political subdivisions without adequate funding forced a struggle at state and local levels to provide for human services in the face of diminishing financial resources.

2. To reduce health disparities among Americans

3. To achieve access to preventive services for all Americans

The Year 2000 Objectives listed 22 priority areas under three broad categories: health promotion, health protection, and preventive services. An additional category, surveillance and data systems, stands alone. These systems were developed to monitor progress toward the objectives. Box 8.2 lists the categories and their respective priority

---

### Box 8.2   Priority Areas of the Year 2000 Health Objectives

**Health Promotion**

Physical activity and fitness
Nutrition
Tobacco
Alcohol and other drugs
Family planning
Mental health and mental disorders
Violent and abusive behavior
Educational and community-based programs

**Health Protection**

Unintentional injuries
Occupational safety and health
Environmental health
Food and drug safety
Oral health

**Protective Services**

Maternal and infant health
Heart disease and stroke
Cancer
Diabetes and chronic disabling conditions
HIV infection
Sexually transmitted diseases
Immunization and infectious diseases
Clinical preventive services

**Surveillance and Data Systems**

Surveillance

---

areas. When *Healthy People 2000* was published, it contained 298 specific objectives. Through the decade of the 1990s, objectives were revised and added, bringing the total to 376—of which 319 were unduplicated (U.S. DHHS, 1999a).

McGinnis and DeGraw (1991) provided an excellent explanation of the three broad categories:

1. **Health promotion strategies** are related to individual lifestyle—personal choices made in a social context—that can have a powerful influence over one's health prospects. Educational and community-based programs can address lifestyle in a cross-cutting fashion.

2. **Health protection strategies** are related to environmental or regulatory measures that confer protection on large population groups. Interventions addressing these issues are not exclusively protective in nature and must have a substantial health promotion element as well.

3. **Preventive services strategies** include counseling, screening, immunization, and chemoprophylactic interventions for individuals in the clinical setting.

Obviously overlap exists among these three broad categories.

To ensure participation of groups with specific expertise and to increase the likelihood of achieving the objectives, the ODPHP provided funding and cooperated with various organizations that work with certain high-risk groups in specific settings. In cooperation with the PHS, the American School Health Association published a compilation of the *Healthy People 2000* objectives related to school health. The PHS, under a cooperative agreement with the American Association of School Administrators, worked with school administrators nationwide to increase awareness of the Year 2000 Objectives as they relate to schools and to promote adoption of school health programs. ODPHP worked through the Maternal and Child Health Bureau of the Health Resources and Services Administration to publish *Healthy Children 2000*, a compilation of the Year 2000 objectives that relates to mothers, infants, children, adolescents, and youth. The American Medical Association was identified to receive funding to focus on the adolescent population through the Healthier Youth by the Year 2000 Project. *Healthier Youth 2000* (AMA, 1991) included objectives from *Healthy People 2000* that relate to the 10- to 24-year age group. Together, *Healthy Children 2000* and *Healthier Youth 2000* illustrated the enormous health problems facing the youth of America and highlighted the significant role of health educators in the health of the nation's young people. They stimulated development and revision of programs.

Many of the Year 2000 Objectives are related directly to the performance of schools. We should never lose sight of the link between children's health and their academic performance. The risks of adolescence and childhood can be reduced by a comprehensive, planned, and sequential health instructional program within a coordinated school health program (discussed in Chapter 7). More than one-third of the Year 2000 Objectives had the potential to be achieved directly by schools, or the schools could affect their attainment significantly. Objective 8.4 accentuated the fact that schools offer the most efficient means available to improve the health of young people and to enable them to avoid risks to their health:

> Increase to at least 75 percent the proportion of the nation's elementary and secondary schools that provide planned and sequential, quality school health education kindergarten through 12th grade.

Sadly, this objective is far from being met.

Progress toward accomplishing the Year 2000 Objectives was evaluated several times, including near the end of the decade (National Center for Health Statistics, 1999). Data indicated that 14 percent of the objectives were met by 1999, movement toward the targets had been made for 45 percent of the objectives, and 18 percent showed movement away from the targets. Data for 6 percent of the objectives showed mixed results, and 3 percent showed no change from the baseline. There were insufficient data to evaluate progress on the remainder (about 14 percent) of objectives. Movement toward or away from target is determined by the direction of the change between the baseline and the most recent data point. Table 8.1 shows progress (or lack of it) toward the 376 objectives in all 22 priority areas.

## Health Objectives for the Year 2010

*Healthy People 2010* (U.S. DHHS, 2000), a continuation of the national prevention initiative that identifies opportunities to improve the health of all Americans, specifies national health objectives to be reached by the year 2010. With 467 objectives in 28 focus areas, it is an agenda for the nation and a tremendously valuable asset to health planners, medical practitioners, educators, and elected officials. Nearly all states, the District of Columbia, and Guam have developed their own Healthy People plans. Most have built on national objectives, but virtually all have tailored them to their own specific needs. Local health departments also use the objectives in their planning. Healthy People objectives have been specified by Congress as the measure for assessing the progress of the Indian Health Care Improvement Act, the Maternal and Child Health Block Grant, and the Preventive Health and Health Services Block Grant.

Individuals, groups, and organizations are encouraged to integrate *Healthy People 2010* into current programs, special events, publications, and meetings. Businesses can use the framework, for example, to guide worksite health promotion activities as well as community-based initiatives. Schools, colleges, and civic and faith-based organizations can undertake activities to further the health of all members of their community. Health care providers can encourage their patients to pursue healthier lifestyles and to participate in community-based programs. By selecting from among the national objectives, individuals and organizations can build an agenda for community health improvement and can monitor results over time (Office of Disease Prevention and Health Promotion, 2000).

The context of *Healthy People 2010* differs from that of the previous two sets of objectives and will continue to evolve throughout the decade. Advances in preventive therapies and strategies, vaccines and pharmaceuticals, assistive technologies, and computerized systems will change the face of how health care and health promotion will be practiced. Demographic changes in the United States, reflecting an older and more racially diverse population, will create new demands on public health and the overall health care system. Global forces,

**Table 8.1**   Healthy People 2000 Objectives: Summary of Progress by Priority Area

| Priority area | Met goal | Moved toward target | Moved away from target | Insufficient data, mixed results, or no change | Total |
|---|---|---|---|---|---|
| 1. Physical activity and fitness | 1 | 6 | 5 | 1 | 13 |
| 2. Nutrition | 5 | 13 | 6 | 3 | 27 |
| 3. Tobacco | 4 | 15 | 3 | 4 | 26 |
| 4. Substance abuse: Alcohol and other drugs | 1 | 8 | 4 | 7 | 20 |
| 5. Family planning | 0 | 8 | 1 | 3 | 12 |
| 6. Mental health and mental disorders | 4 | 3 | 6 | 2 | 15 |
| 7. Violent and abusive behaviors | 3 | 6 | 5 | 5 | 19 |
| 8. Educational and community-based programs | 3 | 3 | 2 | 6 | 14 |
| 9. Unintentional injuries | 6 | 9 | 2 | 9 | 26 |
| 10. Occupational safety and health | 3 | 10 | 5 | 2 | 20 |
| 11. Environmental health | 2 | 11 | 1 | 3 | 17 |
| 12. Food and drug safety | 2 | 5 | 1 | 0 | 8 |
| 13. Oral health | 1 | 8 | 2 | 6 | 17 |
| 14. Maternal and infant health | 1 | 8 | 5 | 3 | 17 |
| 15. Heart disease and stroke | 2 | 12 | 3 | 0 | 17 |
| 16. Cancer | 6 | 10 | 0 | 1 | 17 |
| 17. Diabetes | 1 | 5 | 11 | 6 | 23 |
| 18. HIV infections | 2 | 7 | 3 | 5 | 17 |
| 19. Sexually transmitted diseases | 4 | 6 | 1 | 6 | 17 |
| 20. Immunization and infectious diseases | 1 | 9 | 2 | 7 | 19 |
| 21. Clinical preventive services | 0 | 2 | 1 | 5 | 8 |
| 22. Surveillance and data services | 0 | 6 | 1 | 0 | 7 |

Source: National Center for Health Statistics. (1999). *Healthy People 2000 Review, 1998–99*. Hyattsville, MD: Public Health Service.

including food supplies, emerging infectious diseases, and environmental interdependence, will present new public health challenges and require new relationships among public and community health organizations, the health care system, and health promoters/educators.

**Important Revisions**   The Year 2010 Objectives are distinguished from the Year 2000 Objectives by a broadened prevention science base; improved surveillance and data systems; a heightened awareness and demand for preventive health services and quality health care; and changes in demographics, science, technology, and disease spread that will affect the public's health in the twenty-first century.

These developments will provide both challenges and essential tools for health promotion.

*Healthy People 2010* identified two broad types of objectives: **Measurable objectives** provide direction for action. They have baselines that use valid and reliable data from currently established, nationally representative data systems. These baseline data provide the point from which a 2010 target can be set. For example, based on baseline data

**measurable objectives**   in the context of *Healthy People 2010*, objectives for which there are valid and reliable data from currently established, nationally representative data systems indicating that 77 percent of the population had a usual primary care provider in 1996, Objective 1-5 reads, "Increase the proportion of persons with a usual primary care provider," with a target of 85 percent. **Developmental objectives** provide a vision for a desired outcome or health status. Current surveillance systems do not provide data on these objectives, so there are no baseline data. Developmental objectives identify areas that are important and drive the development of data systems to measure them. Objective 1-2 is an example of a developmental objective: "Increase the proportion of insured persons with coverage for clinical preventive services." *Healthy People 2010* objectives are constructed around two major goals.

## Goal 1. Increase Quality and Years of Healthy Life

This goal emphasizes the health status and nature of life, not just longevity. Health status includes preventing disability, improving functioning, and relieving pain and distress caused by physical and emotional symptoms. It encompasses the full range of functional capacity at each stage of life, allowing one the ability to enter into satisfying relationships with others, to work, and to play. Many individuals and organizations have begun developing new measures that reflect life duration, morbidity and health-related life quality (Field & Gold, 1998). A range of measures will be used to evaluate progress toward accomplishing this goal.

## Goal 2. Eliminate Health Disparities

The Year 2000 Objectives contained the goal of reducing disparities in health status, health risks, and use of preventive interventions among population groups. However, most progress toward the objectives appears to primarily reflect the achievement among the higher socioeconomic groups. In a bold step, *Healthy People 2010* added the goal of eliminating these disparities entirely, regardless of race, ethnicity, gender, disability status, income, or educational level.

Eliminating disparities will require new knowledge about the determinants of disease and effective interventions for prevention and treatment. It will also require improved access for all to the resources that influence health. Reaching this goal will necessitate improved collection and use of

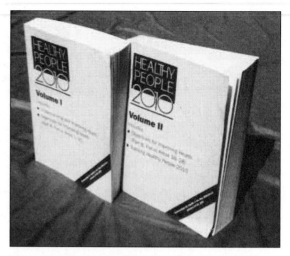

The national health objectives for both 2000 and 2010 addressed health disparities as a major goal. Many of the disparities can be traced to poverty.

standardized data to correctly identify all high-risk populations and monitor the effectiveness of health interventions targeting these groups. Research dedicated to a better understanding of the relationships between health status and income, education, race and ethnicity, cultural influences, environment, and access to quality medical services will help us acquire new insights into eliminating the disparities and developing new ways to apply our existing knowledge toward this goal (U.S. DHHS, 1999b).

**Monitoring Progress**    Figure 8.1 is useful in appreciating the vision required for development of the *Healthy People 2010* objectives from the two goals and, in broad terms, the variables to be observed in monitoring progress toward the objectives. It also indicates how the depth of the topics covered by the objectives reflect the wide array of critical influences that determine the health of individuals or communities. These **determinants of health**, borrowed from the Health Field Concept, are biology and behaviors, social and physical environments, and access to quality health care. An additional determinant, policies and interventions, was added because they have such a powerful influence on the health of individuals and communities. The figure also underscores the importance of understanding the health status of a population though monitoring

**Figure 8.1** Healthy People in Healthy Communities

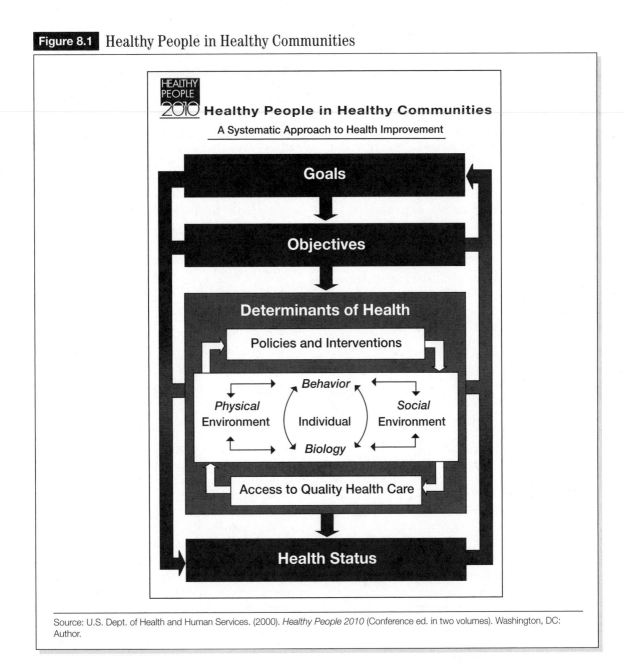

Source: U.S. Dept. of Health and Human Services. (2000). *Healthy People 2010* (Conference ed. in two volumes). Washington, DC: Author.

and evaluating the consequences of the determinants of health. Health status is measured by birth and death rates, life expectancy, quality of life, morbidity from specific diseases, risk factors, use of ambulatory care and inpatient care, accessibility of health personnel and facilities, financing of health care, health insurance coverage, and many other factors.

**developmental objectives**    in the context of *Healthy People 2010*, objectives for which current surveillance systems do not provide sufficiently valid and reliable data to establish a baseline

**determinants of health**    critical influences that determine the health of individuals and communities

The nation's progress in achieving the two goals of *Healthy People 2010* will be monitored in all 467 objectives, which are arranged in the 28 focus areas shown in Box 8.3. Many objectives focus on interventions designed to reduce or eliminate illness, disability, and premature death among individuals and communities. Others focus on broader issues, such as improving access to quality health care, strengthening public health services, and improving the availability and dissemination of health-related information. Each objective has a target for specific improvements to be achieved by the year 2010.

---

**Box 8.3**  Healthy People 2010 Focus Areas

Access to quality health services
Arthritis, osteoporosis, and chronic back conditions
Cancer
Chronic kidney disease
Diabetes
Disability and secondary conditions
Educational and community-based programs
Environmental health
Family planning
Food safety
Health communication
Heart disease and stroke
HIV
Immunization and infectious diseases
Injury and violence prevention
Maternal, infant, and child health
Medical product safety
Mental health and mental disorders
Nutrition and overweight
Occupational safety and health
Oral health
Physical activity and fitness
Public health infrastructure
Respiratory diseases
Sexually transmitted diseases
Substance abuse
Tobacco use
Vision and hearing

---

*Healthy People 2010* also identified leading health indicators—areas of major public health concern in the United States. These were chosen based on their ability to motivate action, the availability of data to measure their progress, and their relevance as broad public health issues. The indicators illuminate individual behaviors, physical and social environmental factors, and important health system issues that greatly affect the health of individuals and communities. Underlying each of these indicators is the significant influence of income and education. The leading health indicators are:

— Physical activity
— Overweight and obesity
— Tobacco use
— Substance abuse
— Responsible sexual behavior
— Mental health
— Injury and violence
— Environmental quality
— Immunization
— Access to health care

The indicators will be used to track progress and provide a snapshot of the health of the nation. For each leading health indicator, specific objectives will be used to measure progress among children, adolescents, and adults. These objectives are presented in Appendix D. The leading health indicators can become the basic building blocks for community health initiatives. Developing strategies and action plans to address one or more of these indicators can increase the quality of life and the years of healthy life and help eliminate health disparities, thus creating healthy people in healthy communities.

# SPECIFIC FEDERAL INTERVENTIONS

Although the federal government has historically approached health issues with many overlapping departments, agencies, and bureaus, the health objectives for the nation have helped to produce some very positive initiatives. For instance, at least seven cabinet departments play important roles in adolescent health, but *Healthy People 2000* and *Healthy People 2010* made it possible to assign major responsibility for reaching specific objectives to particular departments within government. As a result, many health promotion programs have emerged from the morass of governmental offices. The following discussion, though not meant to be complete, describes some important federal health and health promotion/education programs.

## Department of Health and Human Services

The Department of Health and Human Services (HHS) is the department

> most concerned with the Nation's human concerns. In one way or another HHS touches the lives of more Americans than any other federal agency. It is literally a department of people serving people, from newborn infants to persons requiring health services to our most elderly citizens (National Archives and Records Administration, 1996).

In terms of budget, HHS is the second largest department in the federal government. The department comprises twelve operating divisions, eight of which constitute the Public Health Service (PHS):

**Operating Divisions of the Department of Health and Human Services**

Administration on Aging

Administration for Children and Families

Agency for Healthcare Research and Quality*

Agency for Toxic Substances and Disease Registry*

Centers for Disease Control and Prevention*

Food and Drug Administration*

Health Care Financing Administration

Health Resources and Services Administration*

Indian Health Service*

National Institutes of Health*

Program Support Center

Substance Abuse and Mental Health Services Administration*

*Part of the U.S. Public Health Service

The mission of the PHS is to protect and advance the health of the American people by

- conducting and supporting biomedical, behavioral, and health services research and communicating research results to health professionals and the public;

- preventing and controlling disease, identifying health hazards, and promoting healthful behaviors for the nation's citizens;

- monitoring the adequacy of health personnel and facilities available to serve the nation's needs;

- improving the organization and delivery of health services and bringing good health care within the reach of all Americans;

- ensuring that drugs and medical devices are safe and effective and protecting the public from unsafe foods and unnecessary exposure to radiation;

- administering block grants to the states for preventive health and health services; alcohol, drug abuse, and mental health services; maternal and child health services; and

- working with other nations and international agencies on global health problems and their solutions.

Within this mission, the divisions of the PHS conduct and support health promotion in many ways. Following are some highlights of the divisions' activities.

### Administration on Aging

The Older Americans Act of 1965 established the AoA and called for a range of programs that offer services and opportunities for older Americans. AoA is the federal focal point and advocate agency for older Americans, tracking the characteristics, circumstances, and needs of older people. It works to heighten awareness among other federal agencies, organizations, groups, and the public about the valuable contributions that older Americans make to the nation and alerts them to the needs of vulnerable older people.

AoA administers key programs at the federal level mandated under the Older Americans Act.

Programs offer opportunities for older people to enhance their health and to be active contributors through employment and volunteer programs. Services include nutrition, transportation, health promotion, and homemaker services. Emphasis is also placed on elder rights, including nursing home ombudsman programs, legal services, insurance counseling, and elder abuse prevention.

The Elderly Nutrition Program provides grants to support nutrition services to older people. It is intended to improve the participants' dietary intakes and to offer opportunities to form new friendships and to create informal support networks. The program provides meals in a variety of settings, such as senior centers, schools, and individual homes. It also provides a range of related services, including nutrition screening, assessment, education, and counseling. Services help older participants learn to shop for, plan, and prepare meals that are economical and that may help manage specific health problems as well as enhance health and well-being. Positive byproducts of the nutrition program are the social contacts provided for participants and opportunities for practitioners to check on the welfare of homebound clients (AoA, 1999).

AoA awards funds to state agencies on aging and to 216 tribes and organizations to meet the needs of older Native Americans, including Aleuts, Eskimos, and Hawaiians. Funds are also awarded to support research, demonstration, and training programs. Some successful demonstration projects have laid the groundwork for ongoing nationwide programs, such as the Nutrition Program for the Elderly and the elder abuse prevention program (AoA, 1997).

## Administration for Children and Families

ACF provides direction and leadership for all federal programs that affect children and families. Two of the most noteworthy federal programs are Head Start and Early Head Start, which provide comprehensive child development programs for children from birth to age 5, pregnant women, and their families (ACF, 1999a). The overall goal of the programs is to increase the school readiness of young children in low-income families. Grants are awarded to local public agencies, private organizations, Native American tribes, and school systems to operate Head Start programs in the local community. Programs include a wide range of individualized services in the areas of education and early childhood development; medical, dental, and mental health; nutrition; and parent involvement. The entire range of Head Start services is responsive and appropriate to each child's and family's developmental, ethnic, cultural, and linguistic heritage and experience.

The Early Head Start program provides services for low-income families with infants and toddlers and for pregnant women. Early Head Start provides resources to community programs to address the needs for children's physical, social, emotional, and cognitive development; to enable parents to be better caregivers and teachers of children; and to help parents meet their own goals, including economic independence. Services are provided through an appropriate mix of home visits, experiences at the Early Head Start Center, and in other settings, such as center-based child care. Connections are developed with other service providers to ensure that a comprehensive array of health, nutrition, and other services is provided (ACF, 1999b).

## Agency for Healthcare Research and Quality

This agency, established in 1989 as the Agency for Health Care Policy and Research and renamed in 1999, is the lead federal agency on quality research. It is charged with supporting research designed to improve the quality of health care, reduce its cost, and broaden access to essential services. AHRQ's broad programs of research bring practical, science-based information to medical practitioners, consumers, and other health care purchasers. AHRQ carries out its mission by (AHRQ, 1999)

- supporting and conducting research that creates the science base for improvements in clinical care and in the organization and financing of health care;

- promoting the incorporation of science into practice through the development of databases and research tools for public and private decision-makers at all levels of the health care system; and

- establishing public-private partnerships and practice networks to identify and develop research priorities, design and conduct studies, translate research and implement findings into clinical practice, and disseminate information from health care research for public use.

## Agency for Toxic Substances and Disease Registry
ATSDR was created by the Comprehensive Environmental Response, Compensation, and Liability Act (Superfund legislation) of 1980. The legislation was enacted to ensure the cleanup of hazardous substances in the environment. The mission of ATSDR is "to prevent exposure and adverse human health effects and diminished quality of life associated with exposure to hazardous substances from waste sites, unplanned releases, and other sources of pollution present in the environment" (National Archives and Records Administration, 1996). Its specific goals are to identify people who are at health risk because of their exposure to hazardous substances in the environment; evaluate relationships between hazardous substances in the environment and adverse human health outcomes; and intervene to eliminate exposures of health concern and prevent or mitigate adverse human health outcomes related to hazardous substances in the environment (ATSDR, 1999).

In furtherance of these goals, the agency conducts assessments of waste sites, keeps registries of exposures to hazardous substances, and maintains a list of areas closed to the public or restricted in use because of contamination. ATSDR supports health promotion by providing consultation and education concerning specific hazardous substances and training to ensure adequate response to public health emergencies.

## Centers for Disease Control and Prevention
The mission of CDC is to promote health and quality of life by preventing and controlling disease, injury, and disability (CDC, 1999a). In 1996, in celebrating its fiftieth anniversary, CDC identified five priority areas in public health for the next century: strengthen essential public health services, expand capacity to respond to urgent health threats, develop nationwide prevention strategies, promote women's health, and invest in the health of youth. Much of this work is carried out in the National Center for Chronic Disease Prevention and Health Promotion (NCCDPHP).

CDC works with state and local health departments to develop, operate, and evaluate disease control programs. Examples include fluoridation of water, childhood immunization, diabetes control, and HIV prevention and surveillance. CDC assists state and local governments in case of disease outbreaks by providing laboratory services, rare vaccines, therapeutic drugs, and by supporting quarantine of ports of entry. It is the lead agency for working with the states and communities to track and implement the health objectives for the nation.

Health education activities have always been in the forefront of CDC activities. The mission of the Division of Adolescent and School Health (DASH), located in the NCCDPHP, is to identify the highest priority health risks among youth, monitor the incidence and prevalence of those risks, implement national programs to prevent risks, and evaluate and improve those programs (CDC, 1999b). DASH monitors incidence and prevalence of critical behaviors among youth with the Youth Risk Behavior Survey. In 1994, CDC implemented the School Health Policies and Programs Study to monitor critical state policies and programs, critical district policies and programs, and critical local school policies and programs. Based on monitoring activities, DASH has supported and conducted efforts to develop improved health education through schools, health care providers, community organizations, and other routes. DASH supports national, state, and local agencies and organizations that have the capacity to improve child and adolescent health, including 57 state and territorial education agencies, 18 local education agencies, 31 national organizations that are leaders in promoting school health education, three demonstration centers that train policy makers and program managers, and a national network of training centers that help over 180,000 teachers in every state administer HIV education programs within comprehensive school health instruction. It has developed a number of education programs covering HIV/AIDS, family planning, violence prevention, smoking cessation, and physical activity.

CDC is heavily involved in promoting comprehensive school health instruction. It has assisted several state education agencies to plan, implement, and evaluate effective school health programs to prevent tobacco use, dietary patterns that contribute to disease, and physical inactivity. It also supports training of teachers to provide education to prevent sexual behavior that results in HIV infection and other sexually transmissible diseases. CDC also coordinates the state education agencies and state health agency programs, policies, and personnel related to the school health program. CDC has helped improve the school health education curricula and teacher training programs in many states, particularly with emphasis on nutrition, tobacco use, physical activity, and prevention of HIV and other STDs. To facilitate state and district implementation of school health programs, CDC has developed guidelines for HIV/AIDS education, tobacco prevention education, nutrition education, promotion of physical activity, and school health education. CDC evaluates and identifies effective programs and curricula for HIV prevention and tobacco use prevention. More than $9.6 million in funding for fiscal year 1999 was devoted to strengthening national efforts for coordinated school health education and providing direct support for fifteen states.

CDC established a national framework to support coordinated health education programs in schools. More than forty professional and voluntary organizations work with CDC to develop model policies, guidelines, and training to help states implement high-quality school health education. As part of this effort, CDC collaborates with scientists and education experts to identify curricula that have successfully reduced health risk behaviors among young people. CDC provides resources to ensure that these curricula, including training for teachers, are available nationwide for state and local education agencies. Schools themselves decide which curricula best meet their students' needs (CDC, 1999d).

CDC/DASH provides information, training, and technical assistance to help federally qualified health centers and state and regional primary care associations establish and strengthen health center partnerships in schools. CDC/DASH maintains a database on health center school-based and school-linked programs so that information about effective programs can be showcased and disseminated (Allensworth et al., 1997).

CDC conducts a wide range of health promotion activities, including administering the National Immunization Program, which promotes immunizations for children and adults. NIP also provides research and surveillance to obtain and publish information about vaccine safety. It maintains the Immunization Registry Clearinghouse, which provides expert recommendations for the handling and storing of vaccines. NIP provides consultation, training, promotional, educational, epidemiological, and technical services to help health departments plan, develop, and implement immunization programs (CDC, 1999e).

The Health Promotion and Disease Prevention Research Centers Program, administered by CDC, integrates the experience, expertise, and resources of academic institutions committed to research that benefits the public's health. CDC supports a national network of 23 centers focusing on reducing and preventing death and disability from the nation's leading causes of death. University-based research centers work closely with state and local health departments, community-based organizations, and national nonprofit organizations to ensure that promising research findings result in practical, cost-effective, and innovative prevention programs that can be applied at the community level (CDC, 1999c). Prevention research is an indispensable part of the process of developing effective prevention programs.

**Food and Drug Administration**    FDA "activities are directed toward protecting the health of the Nation against impure and unsafe foods, drugs and cosmetics, and other potential hazards" (National Archives and Records Administration, 1996). The agency is charged with ensuring the safety and effectiveness of foods, drugs, cosmetics, and medical devices. This includes vaccines, diagnostic tests, ionizing and nonionizing radiation-emitting electronic products, and veterinary products. Regulation and setting of health and safety standards are a part of its mandate. However, much of the enforcement of FDA regulations is left to other agencies and other departments.

**Health Care Financing Administration**
Created in 1977, the HCFA unites under one administration an agency responsible for overseeing

the Medicare program, the federal portion of the Medicaid program, the Children's Health Insurance Program (CHIP), and ensuring that those programs are properly run by contractors and state agencies. HCFA establishes policies for paying health care providers who care for the 75 million Americans who receive health coverage through Medicare, Medicaid, and CHIP (HCFA, 2000). It also performs a number of quality-focused activities, including regulation of laboratory testing; surveys and certification of health care agencies such as nursing homes, intermediate care facilities for the mentally retarded, and hospitals; development of coverage policies; and quality-of-care improvement.

HCFA initiatives include reducing health care fraud and abuse. It also has authority to enter into contracts with entities to promote the integrity of the Medicare program and is involved in insurance reform.

The Early and Periodic Screening, Diagnosis, and Treatment (EPSDT) program provides Medicaid-eligible children with these services for health deficiencies. If a district or school provides these services, it is eligible for reimbursement for these services. Reimbursement is also available for case management and administrative expenses.

## Indian Health Service

The IHS provides a comprehensive health services delivery system for Native Americans and Alaska Natives that allows maximum tribal involvement in developing and managing programs. The mission of the IHS is to raise the physical, mental, social, and spiritual health of Native Americans, including Alaska Natives, to the highest level. To carry out its mission, the IHS (1) assists tribes in developing their health programs through activities such as health management training, technical assistance, and human resource development; (2) helps tribes coordinate health planning; obtain and use health resources available through federal, state, and local programs; operate comprehensive health care services, and evaluate health programs; (3) provides comprehensive health care services, including hospital and ambulatory medical care, preventive and rehabilitative services, and development of community sanitation facilities; and (4) serves as the principal federal advocate for Native Americans in the health field to ensure that they receive comprehensive health services (IHS, 1999a).

IHS constructs sanitation facilities, develops community-oriented care programs, and operates 43 hospitals. It has also implemented a variety of preventive programs, including prenatal, postnatal, and well-baby care; family planning; dental health; nutrition; immunizations; and health education. Because the current age-adjusted alcoholism death rate is 440 percent higher for Native Americans than for the general U.S. population (IHS, 1999b), extensive alcoholism and substance abuse treatment and prevention programs have been developed by IHS.

## National Institutes of Health

NIH is the principal biomedical research agency of the federal government. The mission of NIH is to uncover new knowledge that will lead to better health for everyone with the goal of helping prevent, detect, diagnose, and treat disease and disability (NIH, 1999). It comprises 25 separate institutes and centers.

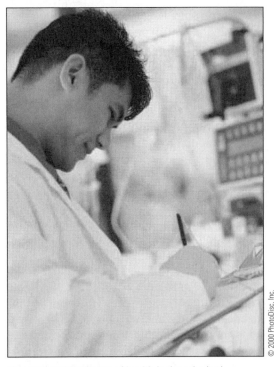

The National Institutes of health is the principal biomedicine research agency of the federal government.

About 82 percent of the NIH budget supports research and training in more than 2,000 institutions in the U.S. and abroad. This is in addition to the research conducted in its own laboratories. Patients come from all over the world to the Warren Grant Magnuson Clinical Center (NIH's research hospital in Bethesda, Maryland) to participate in clinical research studies. The Mark O. Hatfield Clinical Research Center (also in Bethesda) is expected to be open in 2002, allowing a link between rapidly moving biomedical findings in the laboratory and the mainstream of medical practices.

In addition to clinical research, NIH also operates two components of the National Library of Medicine: the Lister Hill National Center for Biomedical Communications and the National Center for Biotechnology Information.

NIH has played a major role in making possible many achievements in health improvement. These include a drop of 36 percent in mortality from heart disease between 1977 and 1999; 50 percent decrease in death from stroke in the same period; increase of the relative 5-year survival rate for people with cancer to 60 percent; development of vaccines against infectious diseases that once killed and disabled millions of people; and development of dental sealants that have proved 100 percent effective in protecting the chewing surfaces of children's molars and premolars where most cavities occur.

**Program Support Center**   The center is a relatively new addition to the Department of HHS. Its mission is to provide qualitative and responsive administrative support services on a cost-effective, competitive, fee-for-service basis to HHS components and other federal agencies. Services and products are available in the areas of human resources, financial and property management, and information technology (PSC, 1999).

**Substance Abuse and Mental Health Services Administration**   SAMHSA's mission is to provide substance abuse and mental health services and to ensure that up-to-date information and state-of-the-art practice is effectively used for treatment and prevention of addictive and mental disorders. It works to improve access to quality, effective programs and services for individuals suffering from or at risk for these disorders, as well as their families and communities. SAMHSA is composed of three centers:

- The Center for Mental Health Services heads efforts to speed the application of mental health treatments for patients with mental illness.

- The Center for Substance Abuse Treatment has programs designed to improve treatment services and make them more available to those in need.

- The Center for Substance Abuse Prevention leads federal efforts to prevent alcohol and other drug abuse and often works with other federal offices such as the Department of Education and the Food and Drug Administration.

Here, as in many government functions, the challenge is often to prevent duplication among federal agencies.

In addition, six special offices focus and coordinate the agency's work in certain areas. The Office of Applied Studies is the focal point for the agency's activities in gathering, analyzing, and disseminating substance abuse data. The Office on AIDS coordinates and monitors SAMHSA activities that address the critical health problems posed by HIV among substance abusers and persons with mental illness. The Associate Administrator for Alcohol Prevention and Treatment Policy promotes and monitors SAMHSA's efforts to address national alcohol-abuse issues and coordinates them with other public and private organizations. The other special offices are the Office of Managed Care, the Office for Women's Services, and the Associate Administrator for Minority Concerns (SAMHSA, 1999).

## Department of Agriculture

The USDA is heavily involved in provision of services and programming centered on nutrition and food safety. The Food and Nutrition Service of the USDA provides food and dietary guidance for children and adults. In addition, the National School Lunch Program and the School Breakfast Program, both administered by the Food and Nutrition Service, provide a nutritious breakfast for over 7 million and lunch for more than 25 million children each day (USDA, 1999a,b). Meals are provided free or at a reduced cost. USDA also provides support for the Special Milk and Snack Programs. The Nutrition Education and Training Program places a coordinator in each state. It provides some funding for nutrition education for food service directors and classroom health educators.

In 1995, the USDA created the School Meals Initiative for Healthy Children, which requires that school meals meet the Dietary Guidelines for Americans, supply certain proportions of recommended daily allowances of particular nutrients, include foods from different cultures, and appeal to the consumer. Regulations later allowed increased flexibility in meeting the Dietary Guidelines. USDA developed tools to institute and monitor menu planning, established technical assistance for training food preparation staff, created new recipes, and created the Team Nutrition Schools program. Over 15,000 schools participate in the Team Nutrition Schools effort, which includes training food service managers to be effective team members and helping them meet the regulations.

The department has provided support for a number of education programs. Working through USDA, the Partnership for Food Safety Education, a public/private alliance, provides education about safe food handling. "Fight BAC" is a program to teach young children about the importance of safe food practices. Teacher training is included. The USDA also operates the Conflict Prevention and Resolution Center to help the department better handle conflict that arises in the conduct of department duties—workplace conflict, conflict with farmers and ranchers, even conflict with other agencies. The center focuses on developing employee skills for managing conflict effectively and using alternative dispute resolution methods to resolve disputes (USDA, 1999c).

## Department of Education

Soon after the Goals 2000: Educate America Act became law in 1994, the secretaries of the Department of Education and the Department of Health

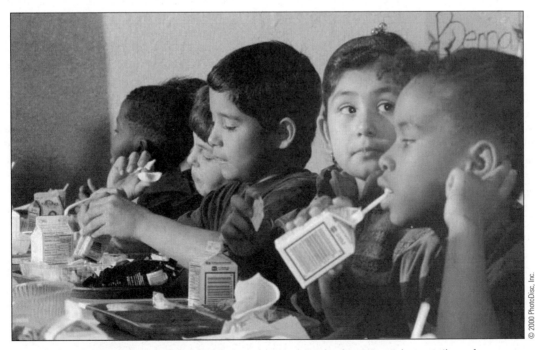

© 2000 PhotoDisc, Inc.

The U.S. Department of Agriculture requires that meals served at schools meet certain proportions of recommended daily allowances for nutrients.

and Human Services released a joint statement announcing a new level of interagency cooperation and affirming the importance of school health programs in accomplishing education goals. Both departments have been intimately involved in achieving both the education goals and health objectives for the nation. As the focal point for the nation's educational efforts, the DoEd is especially important in program development in many school health education areas. Two examples of this involvement are the Safe and Drug-Free Schools Program (discussed in Chapter 4) and programs related to the Individuals with Disabilities Education Act.

### The Safe and Drug-Free Schools and Communities Program
Created under Title IV of the Improving America's Schools Act, this is the federal government's primary vehicle for reducing violence and curbing alcohol, tobacco, and other drug use through education and prevention activities in our nation's schools. Initiatives are designed to prevent violence in and around schools, strengthen prevention programs, and involve parents. There are two major programs: (1) State Grants for Drug and Violence Prevention Programs is a formula grant program that provides funds to state and local education agencies and governors for a wide range of school- and community-based education and prevention activities. The funding allows the work to be developed based on needs within a state so that agencies can establish, operate, and improve local programs of drug and violence prevention, early intervention, rehabilitation referral, and education in schools. State education agencies can use funding for training and technical assistance. Public agencies, private nonprofit organizations, and institutions of higher education often utilize these funds to conduct training, demonstrations, evaluation and supplementary services. (2) National Programs carries out a variety of discretionary initiatives that respond to emerging needs. Among these are direct grants to school districts and communities with severe drug and violence problems, program evaluation, and information development and dissemination (U.S. DoEd, 1998).

The DoEd requires that local school districts use Safe and Drug-Free Schools and Communities funds based on the following four principles of effectiveness:

- Conducting a needs assessment
- Setting measurable goals and objectives
- Using effective research-based programs
- Evaluating program impacts and outcomes

### The Individuals with Disabilities Education Act
IDEA was first implemented in 1975. Over the years, research has provided practical answers about how to best educate infants, toddlers, children, and youth with disabilities. The DOEd has responsibility to make sure that the provisions of IDEA and the findings of the research are implemented. This includes increasing parental involvement in the education of their children and ensuring that regular classroom teachers are involved in planning and assessing children's progress. Another important strategy is to include children with disabilities in assessments, performance goals, and reports to the public. Meeting the goals of the act requires supporting quality professional development for all personnel who are involved in educating children with disabilities (U.S. DOEd, 1999). IDEA has profound implications for school health services and for the environment of the school. For example, funding is available to schools to provide health, counseling, and related services to students with disabilities. DOEd provides assistance to local curriculum developers by reviewing and disseminating exemplary health education curricula through its National Diffusion Network.

The DOEd funds and promotes many other programs under the Improving America's Schools Act. Title I of the act makes available funding for schools to provide additional health and social services to selected students and their families. The 1995 version of the act specifically provided for funds to state education agencies to help disadvantaged students meet high educational standards. Title II supports staff training and assists school reform efforts. Under Title III, schools receive funding to support activities directed toward neglected or delinquent youth or students at risk for dropping out of school, such as counseling, social work, and psychological services; drop-out prevention programs; and before- and after-school programs. Title XI allows school districts to use a portion of the funds received under the act to develop, implement, or expand a coordinated services project.

It should be obvious that the bulk of federal program support for health education has been categorical, i.e., applied to a specific topic or health problem. During the 1980s, Congress provided funding to the Department of Education to support a more comprehensive approach to health education in schools. This approach is now referred to as coordinated school health programs (discussed in Chapter 7).

## Interagency Cooperation

### Interagency Committee on School Health

This committee is composed of representatives from all federal agencies and offices that provide funding and other resources for programs related to school health. With leadership from the DOEd, the ICSH is concerned with all federal policies and programs related to school health. Its mission is to increase the overall effectiveness of federal involvement in school health. The charter of ICSH (U.S. DOEd, 1994) indicated that it would

- improve communication, planning, coordination, and collaboration among federal agencies engaged in ongoing activities of relevance to school health or planning such activities;

- identify needs and facilitate the planning and updating of strategies to improve federal leadership for school health;

- identify opportunities for federal policies to facilitate the development and implementation of school health programs and identify and address policies and practices that may be acting as barriers to effective school health programs;

- facilitate the identification, coordination, and dissemination of promising programs, information, or materials relevant to school health generated by federally conducted or supported programs or activities;

- provide a focal point for identification of, and interaction and coordination with, efforts in the private and voluntary sectors to promote the implementation of school health programs;

- help private and voluntary sectors identify federal policies, programs, initiatives, and materials that support the implementation of school health programs; and

- prepare reports and make policy recommendation to the relevant officials on special topics identified by the committee.

Although the committee has not yet lived up to expectations and has been rather dormant, it holds great potential for promoting school health education. Its formation—a product of the efforts of two federal departments—is significant in itself.

### National Coordinating Committee on School Health

The purpose of the NCCSH is to bring together representatives of major national education and health organizations to support coordinated school health programs. The committee's mission statement (Allensworth et al., 1997) declares its responsibilities to be

- providing national leadership for the promotion of quality comprehensive (coordinated) school health programs;

- improving communication, collaboration, and sharing of information among national organizations;

- developing a clear vision of the role of school health programs in improving the health and educational achievement of children;

- identifying local, state, and federal barriers to the development and implementation of effective school health programs;

- collecting and disseminating information on effective school health programs; and

- establishing and monitoring national goals for strengthening school health programs.

NCCSH has made the marketing of school health programs to communities one of its primary activities. This includes use of community focus groups, involvement of youth, business sector participation, and research demonstrating the effectiveness of school health programs.

## KEY POINTS

1. The real work of educating youth and providing health services takes place at the state and local levels.

2. The government of the United States has historically addressed its health concerns primarily in response to crises.

3. Beginning with the 1979 publication of *Healthy People: The Surgeon General's Report on Health Promotion and Disease Prevention*, the federal government took a different approach to dealing with health problems—a long-term approach that developed programs to achieve national health objectives. Objectives have been developed for the years 1990, 2000, and 2010.

4. Various departments within the federal government—including the Departments of Education, Health and Human Services, and Agriculture—develop and support health promotion programs.

5. The Congress mandates the development of many health promotion programs.

## REFERENCES

Administration for Children and Families. (1999a). *Head Start: General information* [On-line]. Available: http://www2.acf.dhhs.gov/programs/hsb/about/mission.htm

Administration for Children and Families. (1999b). Early Head Start [On-line]. Available: http://www2.acf.dhhs.gov/programs/hsb/about/programs/ehs.htm

Administration on Aging. (1997). *The Administration on Aging and the Older Americans Act* [On-line]. Available: http://www.aoa.dhhs.gov/aoa/pages/aoafact.html

Administration on Aging. (1999). *The Elderly Nutrition Program* [On-line]. Available: http://www.aoa.gov/factsheets/enp.html

Agency for Healthcare Research and Quality. (1999). *AHRQ* [On-line]. Available: http://www.ahcpr.gov

Agency for Toxic Substances and Disease Registry. (1999). *The goals of ATSDR* [On-line]. Available: http://www.atsdr.cdc.gov/goals.html

Allensworth, D., Lawson, E., Nicholson, L., & Wyche, J. (1997). *Schools & health: Our nation's investment.* Washington, DC: National Academy Press.

American Medical Association Healthier Youth by the Year 2000 Project. (1991). *Healthier youth 2000: National health promotion and disease prevention objectives for adolescents.* Chicago: AMA.

Centers for Disease Control and Prevention. (1999a). *About CDC* [On-line]. Available: http://www.cdc.gov/aboutcdc.htm

Centers for Disease Control and Prevention. (1999b). *What is DASH?* [On-line]. Available: http://www.cdc.gov/nccdphp/dash/what.htm

Centers for Disease Control and Prevention. (1999c). *Prevention research centers: Investing in the nation's health* [On-line]. Available: http://www.cdc.gov/nccdphp/prcaag.htm

Centers for Disease Control and Prevention. (1999d). *School health programs: An investment in our nation's future* [On-line]. Available: http://cdc.gov/nccdphp/dash/ataglanc.htm

Centers for Disease Control and Prevention. (1999e). *About NIP* [On-line]. Available: http://cdc.gov/nip/aboutnip.htm

Federal Security Agency, U.S. Office of Education. (1948). *The nation's health.* Washington, DC: Government Printing Office.

Field, M.J., & Gold, M.R. (Eds.). (1998). *Summarizing population health: Directions for the development and application of population metrics.* Washington, DC: Institute of Medicine.

Health Care Financing Administration. (2000). *About HCFA* [On-line]. Available: http://www.hcfa.gov/about.htm

Indian Health Service. (1999a). *Comprehensive health care program for American Indians and Alaska Natives: Mission statement* [On-line]. Available: http://www.ihs.gov/NonMedicalPrograms/Profiles/profileMission.asp

Indian Health Service. (1999b). *Comprehensive health care program for American Indians and Alaska Natives: IHS accomplishments* [On-line]. Available: wysiwyg://74/http://ihs.gov/NonMedicalPrograms/Profiles/profileAccomp.asp

McGinnis, J.M., and DeGraw, C. (1991, September). Healthy schools 2000: Creating partnerships for the decade. *Journal of School Health, 61*: 292–297.

McKenzie, J.F., Pinger, R.R., & Kotecki, J.E. (1999). *An introduction to community health* (3rd ed.). Boston: Jones and Bartlett.

Moore, J.R., Daily, L., Collins, J., Kann, L., Dalmat, M., Truman, B.I., & Kolbe, L.J. (1991). Progress in efforts to prevent the spread of HIV infection among youth. *Public Health Reports, 106*(6), 678–686.

National Archives and Records Administration. (1996). *The United States government manual 1996/1997.* Washington, DC: U.S. Government Printing Office.

National Center for Health Statistics. (1999). *Healthy people 2000 review, 1988–99.* Hyattsville, MD: Public Health Service.

National Institutes of Health. (1999). *National Institutes of Health* [On-line]. Available: http://www.nih.gov

Office of Disease Prevention and Health Promotion. (2000). *Healthy people 2010: Healthy people in healthy communities.* Washington, DC: U.S. Dept. of Health & Human Services.

Program Support Center. (1999). *About the program support center* [On-line]. Available: http://www.psc.gov

Shattuck, L. (1948). *Report of the Sanitary Commission of Massachusetts: 1850.* New York: Cambridge University Press. (Originally published in 1850)

Substance Abuse and Mental Health Service Administration. (1999). *SAMHSA's programs and services* [On-line]. Available: http://www.samhsa.gov/programs/index.htm

U.S. Department of Agriculture. (1999a). *School breakfast program history* [On-line]. Available: http://www.fns.usda.gov/cnd/Breakfast/AboutBFast/ProgHistory.htm

U.S. Department of Agriculture. (1999b). *National School Lunch Program* [On-line]. Available: http://edweek.org/context/orgs/nslp.htm

U.S. Department of Agriculture. (1999c). *Conflict prevention and resolution* [On-line]. Available: http://www.usda.gov/cprc/

U.S. Department of Education. (1994). *Interagency committee on school health charter.* Washington, DC: U.S. Department of Health and Human Services.

U.S. Department of Education. (1998). *About Safe & Drug-Free Schools Program* [On-line]. Available: http://www.ed.gov/offices/OESE/SDFS/aboutsdf.html

U.S. Department of Education. (1999). *IDEA '97: Overview* [On-line]. Available: http://www.ed.gov/offices/OSERS/IDEA/overview.html

U.S. Department of Health, Education and Welfare. (1979). *Healthy people: The surgeon general's report on health promotion and disease prevention* (PHS Publication No. 79-55071). Washington, DC: Government Printing Office.

U.S. Department of Health and Human Services. (1986). *The 1990 health objectives for the nation: A midcourse review* (PHS Publication No. 191-691/70228). Washington, DC: Government Printing Office.

U.S. Department of Health and Human Services. (1991). *Healthy people 2000: National health promotion and disease prevention objectives* (PHS Publication No. 91-50212). Washington, DC: Government Printing Office.

U.S. Department of Health and Human Services. (1999a). *Healthy people 2000 review (1998–99).* DHHS Publication No. 99-1256). Hyattsville, MD: DHHS.

U.S. Department of Health and Human Services. (1999b). *Healthy people 2010 objectives: Draft for public comment.* Washington, DC: U.S. Government Printing Office.

U.S. Department of Health and Human Services. (2000). *Healthy people 2010* (Conference Edition in Two Volumes). Washington, DC: U.S. Government Printing Office.

# Effective Programs

The following descriptions of actual health promotion and health education programs demonstrate the kinds of efforts that have been successful. Many, but not all, of the programs described here are currently in use in the setting and location in which they are presented. Many of the programs were developed to assist in reaching Healthy People objectives.

## HEALTH EDUCATION CENTERS

A relatively recent phenomenon in the field is the health education center. Over 25 centers throughout the United States currently offer education services to their communities in many formats. These centers are different from the traditional community health agency in which education is only one of the services. In a health education center, education is the primary and sometimes only service.

## Weller Health Education Center

The Lehigh Valley in Pennsylvania is home to the Weller Health Education Center, which provides health education to more than 50,000 children and adults in 205 school districts within an eighty-mile radius of the city of Easton (Weller Health Education Center, 1999). The center offers over 25 programs, but the premiere exhibit is the "talking"

transparent anatomical model. The model fascinates visitors by describing its body systems and their functions, how to keep healthy, and the effects of health-risky behavior. School children are bused regularly to the center.

The Anatomy Academy is a 6,000 square foot interactive children's museum. It offers hands-on exhibits that absorb entire families in learning about the human body. Exhibits include "World of the Brain," featuring a walk-through brain with ears as the entrance and exit and interactive video and sound to teach children about functions of the brain; "Impaired Driving Simulator," which provides a perilous ride from the perspective of an intoxicated driver and a sober passenger; "AIDS Exhibit," featuring a telephone connection to the U.S. Centers for Disease Control and Prevention, where representatives answer questions; and "To Market We Go," a mini-grocery store, which contains computerized scanners, check-out stations, and kid-sized shopping carts to help educate children to make healthy food choices.

The Weller Center also offers a mobile van equipped to take its programs to people who cannot visit the center. Both mobile and center programs can be tailored to meet the particular needs of the audience. Programs are facilitated by highly skilled instructors using the latest technologies and teaching exhibits. Programs focus on general health, nutrition, family life, and drug abuse

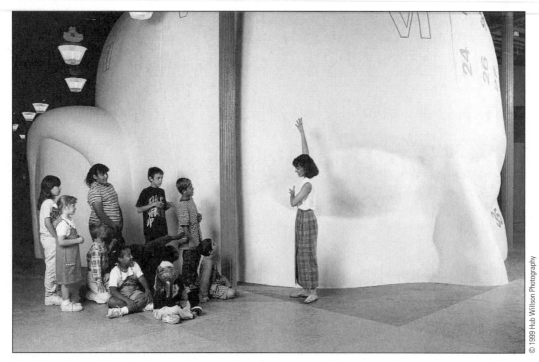

© 1999 Hub Willson Photography

The Weller Health Education Center offers a number of hands-on exhibits designed to pique young people's interest in health.

prevention and carry catchy titles like "The Food You Chews," "AIDS: Blood, Sweat, and Fears," "Where Did I Come From?" and "All-American Drugs."

## Hult Health Education Center

The Hult Health Education Center is located in Peoria, Illinois. The purpose of the center is to promote healthy lifestyles through preventive education and rational decision making, and its mission is "to teach people of all ages to respect and take better care of themselves in order to live longer, healthier lives" (Hult Center, 1999). Programs are designed to complement existing health education offered by schools, families, civic groups, social agencies, and health care institutions. The center houses five learning theaters, which provide a stimulating learning environment. It utilizes state-of-the-art visual displays, interactive models, electronic displays, and

audio-visual presentations are used during presentations by health educators.

The Hult Center offers programs in general health, nutrition, substance abuse prevention, and family life education. Specific classes in each program area are age- and developmentally appropriate. More than 40,000 students enjoy the center each year.

Through a grant from the Illinois Board of Education, the center works directly with 24 K–12 classrooms throughout the state via the Internet. A unique "Engaged Learning" project will be developed by each school as they visit the center. The center's exhibits and interactive teaching theaters can be explored and manipulated by each student. Several partners have collaborated on the project, including Bradley University, University of Illinois College of Medicine at Peoria, and Dynamic Graphics, Inc.

The center also offers employee health programs on corporate sites. Programs include lifestyle screening, exercise and fitness, stress management, sexuality education, and cholesterol and blood pressure education.

# PROGRAMS IN CLINICAL SETTINGS

## The Lifestyle Heart Trial

The Lifestyle Heart Trial was a program in which patients with documented coronary heart disease were randomly assigned to treatment and control groups. The usual-care (control) group received traditional medication, surgery options, cardiac rehabilitation, and standard dietary exercise recommendations. The treatment group received a low-fat vegetarian diet, stress management training, and moderate exercise. A diet analyzer and self-report questionnaires were used to monitor compliance with dietary, stress management, and exercise regimens. The interventions were presented as a model for enhancing spiritual health (Hawks et al., 1995) and based upon the rationale and methods depicted in Figure 9.1. The major premise behind this approach was that the earlier the intervention in the

multicausal chain of illness, the more beneficial the effects (Ornish, 1992). The trial emphasized treating the earliest links in the chain of heart disease, thereby hoping to eliminate the need for the biomedical approach of treating the later causal factors with surgery, aggressive drug therapy, or both. This philosophy of treatment reflects the view that a lack of emotional and spiritual health, with its resultant stress, is the most elemental cause of heart disease.

After one year, angiography showed that the treatment group had significant regression in the extent of occluded arteries, whereas the usual-care group experienced an increase in level of blockage. The treatment group's reductions in blood cholesterol levels, blood pressure, body weight, and angina pain were similar to those obtained with aggressive drug therapy, but with no side effects (Ornish et al., 1990; Ornish, 1991; Ornish et al., 1983). There appeared to be a causal relationship between adherence to the program and improved outcomes (Hawks et al., 1995). Disease reversal was seen in 82

---

**Figure 9.1**  Intervention Options Within the Causal Chain of Coronary Heart Disease

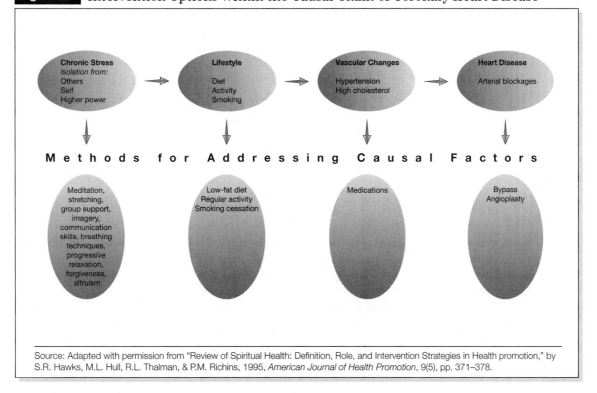

Source: Adapted with permission from "Review of Spiritual Health: Definition, Role, and Intervention Strategies in Health promotion," by S.R. Hawks, M.L. Hull, R.L. Thalman, & P.M. Richins, 1995, *American Journal of Health Promotion*, 9(5), pp. 371–378.

percent of the treatment group after one year with no side effects, whereas patients in the usual-care group continued to worsen. Participation in the treatment program is cost-effective, costing one-tenth the cost of a single bypass surgery (Mental Medicine Update, 1993).

## Stress Reduction Clinic

The University of Massachusetts Medical Center is home to the Stress Reduction Clinic, which provides services to patients experiencing chronic pain, insomnia, cancer, hypertension, stress, and other disorders that have not responded fully to traditional treatment. Group-based meditation—including formal "sitting" meditation and yoga, walking meditation and daily mindfulness—form the basis of the clinic's practice. Participants are taught to live in the moment and become more aware of feelings, sensations, and thoughts. They become better able to control pain, insomnia, fear, or stress. They also learn to respond to their feelings and sensations in more meaningful ways. Spiritual health is enhanced by emphasizing connectedness with self and others.

Several published studies indicate the usefulness of the stress reduction clinic in reducing physical symptoms (Kabat-Zinn, Lipworth, & Burney, 1985; Kabat-Zinn et al., 1986) and psychological problems such as anxiety, stress, and depression (Kabat-Zinn et al., 1992; Tate, 1994). Hawks et al. (1995) reported that results from other studies show strong support for the efficacy of this clinic's intervention.

## Asthma Intervention Program

The Great Brook Valley Health Center (GBVHC) in Worcester, Massachusetts, is part of a community health center–owned health maintenance organization. Its Asthma Intervention Program (Gallivan et al., 1998) was based on the principles of the Health Resources and Services Administration, U.S. Department of Health and Human Services (1998). The goal of the program was to improve the health status and quality of life of the asthmatic clients served by GBVHC. Target audiences were clients with asthma and their families and medical providers at the health center.

Keys to the program's success were (1) identifying an "opinion leader" among medical providers who was knowledgeable about guidelines and committed to improvement in care and (2) employment of a bilingual asthma nurse to implement case management and patient education. The asthma nurse is immediately notified of any emergency room visit or admission of a patient with asthma, so that the patient can be followed up at the health center. The nurse also provides education to asthmatic clients who come to the center for urgent care.

A six-session asthma education model features understanding asthma; identifying and reducing the asthma triggers in the environment; instruction on use and care of a peak flow-meter, a spacer, and a nebulizer; describing asthma medications and how they should be used; and explaining the signs and precursors of an asthma exacerbation and what to do. Creative arrangement with pharmaceutical companies helped obtain medications and equipment for asthma control. Patients never leave the center without the necessary equipment and medication, regardless of their ability to pay. Other important services include nutrition, smoking cessation, and asthma camp for children. Group education is also offered as a supplement to individual education.

In the Asthma Outreach Program, an adjunct to the intervention program, educational techniques for the health center patients are taught at schools and day care centers, at open houses and health fairs, and in residents' homes.

Evaluations have been favorable. Quality of life questionnaires administered pre- and post-intervention indicate significant improvement in functional status. Peak flow measurements also showed significant improvement. The Asthma Intervention Program has become highly visible in the Worcester community and has attracted patients to the health center.

# COMMUNITY SETTINGS

## Healthy Smiles

Baby bottle tooth decay (BBTD)—a specific form of severe and rampant decay of the primary teeth of infants (Barnes et al., 1992)—is preventable. The decay, which is caused by allowing babies to fall asleep with their bottle of milk, formula, or sugary drink remaining in their mouths (King, 1998), is associated with increased infections, impaired nutrition, sleeplessness, low self-esteem, lethargy, and poor concentration (Ohio Department of Health, 1995; Ripa, 1988).

Healthy Smiles is a multidisciplinary BBTD prevention campaign implemented in northwest Ohio. The program was established with the leadership of the Dental Center of Northwest Ohio, a nonprofit dental agency, with the goals of decreasing incidence of BBTD and increasing the number of children between 2 and 5 years old who are regularly examined by dentists. Based on incidence data, low-income day care centers were targeted.

The first step in the program was to have day care staff distribute fact sheets and other educational materials and articles to parents of children in the centers. Follow-up phone calls were made to day care center directors to encourage the distributions. Inservice programs on BBTD were offered to staff and parents associated with the centers. Alternatives to putting infants to bed with a bottle were emphasized. Later, discussions with the Ohio Department of Health and Human Services produced recommendations to distribute the most current BBTD information to area prenatal clinics and hospital maternity wards. Many clinics inserted the BBTD information into their educational classes. Pediatricians were urged to check each child for signs of BBTD and provide educational information to patient parents. Healthy Smiles is an excellent example of professionals working together in multiple community settings to reduce a health problem.

## Project Freedom

Recognizing that minors' access to alcohol is a major public health concern and that many stores sold alcohol to underage customers in Wichita, Kansas, a substance abuse community coalition implemented Project Freedom. The project was an attempt to educate merchants and influence them to refuse to sell alcohol to minors.

To achieve a baseline, the project started with a pretest in which adolescents attempted to purchase alcohol illegally. The result of each attempt was recorded. Approximately six weeks after the pretest, a press conference was held to alert citizens and store clerks of the ease with which adolescents could purchase alcohol. If the store was willing to sell to minors, coalition members issued a citation to the clerk; if not, a commendation was awarded. One week after the press conference, minors again attempted to purchase alcohol.

Although no formal education took place, results were impressive. The overall percentage of store clerks willing to sell alcohol to minors decreased markedly from a pretest level of 55 percent to 41 percent at post-test. Among merchants who received the intervention (citations or commendations), the level of willingness to sell dropped from 83 percent to 33 percent. Those who did not receive the intervention showed a decrease from 45 percent to 36 percent, possibly as a result of the press conference or word-of-mouth information about Project Freedom.

Concurrently to the alcohol sales, coalition members duplicated the procedures with tobacco sales. No positive differences were observed from pretest to post-test. One possible explanation of this was that, whereas merchants who sell alcohol in Kansas must obtain a license and may lose it for selling to minors, no license was required to sell tobacco products. Therefore, merchants ran less risk in selling tobacco to minors (Lewis et al., 1996).

## SEARCH Program

The Southeast Louisiana Area Health Education Center developed the SEARCH program to improve the health status of migrant farmworkers and their families in rural Louisiana. Recognizing that preventive medicine is cost-effective, the community outreach program was designed to reach the approximately 3,000 migrant farmworkers and their 300 children in the area.

SEARCH employed a Hispanic man who had been a migrant farmworker, because his ethnicity and familiarity with the clients' lifestyle and culture helped gain trust. A curriculum was developed in Spanish to be taught in the homes of migrant farmworkers during the summer. The classes were informal, fun, and flexible, because the age range of children could be from 3 to 14 years. The lessons covered topics such as personal hygiene, nutrition, car safety, and smoking. The lessons were reinforced by repeat visits. Each class started with a review of previous material.

Because the classes were conducted at the clients' homes, which were located in clusters, it was convenient for children to attend. It was also possible to identify problems in the home environment, take corrective action, and measure improvement in subsequent visits. Parents' awareness was also increased, because they often observed the classes.

The program was successful at expanding contacts between the health education center and the community. There was also observational evidence of positive changes in children's behavior (Marier, 1996).

## Obesity Prevention Among Inner-City Females

African-American women and their daughters were the target of this program, because obesity rates among African-American women are significantly higher than rates for white women (Kumanyika, 1994), and African Americans have higher-than-average cardiovascular disease mortality (Kumanyika, 1990; Otten et al., 1990). Specifically, girls and their mothers who live in Chicago's inner city and attend a local tutoring program were targeted. Participants were within walking distance of the program.

Parental participation was considered to be imperative because of the mothers' limited access to dietary and physical activity information and because of all participants' needs for nutrition and health knowledge and for support in making dietary changes. It was also recognized that mothers usually prepare meals for their daughters, and eating patterns are usually influenced by the home.

The twelve-week culture-specific curriculum (Stolley & Fitzgibbon, 1997) addressed the particular needs of the target population. All activities in the curriculum involved tasting foods, comparing high-fat to low-fat foods, changing recipes, and planning meals. Participants were asked to bring their favorite recipes or foods to be analyzed for fat and caloric content. The group visited local grocery stores to better understand product selection, practice using food labels to shop more healthfully, and assess availability of certain products. Culturally relevant music and dance were used for a number of exercise and diet-related activities. Appropriate materials gathered from magazines geared toward African Americans were distributed and reviewed for information on diet and exercise. Risks of high-fat and benefits of low-fat foods were presented, with emphasis on selection of fast foods. Discussion of how to make exercise a part of daily life and of low-impact aerobics classes were included; mothers and daughters met separately for these sessions.

Participants were assessed before and after taking part in the program for body weight, height, percentage overweight, daily caloric intake, total fat gram intake, percentage calories in fat, saturated fat intake, and dietary cholesterol. Results were compared with a control group. The study demonstrated the efficacy of a culturally specific obesity prevention program (Stolley & Fitzgibbon, 1997). However, most of the measurable benefit from the program was detected in the mothers. They reported receiving less than 32 percent of their calories from fat compared to 40 percent before the program. They also reported an average intake of 11.5 grams of saturated fat as compared to nearly 14 grams pretreatment. The results confirm the importance of parental involvement in dietary interventions with children.

## SCHOOL-BASED PROGRAMS

### Growing Healthy

*Growing Healthy* is a widely respected and used school-based health education curriculum. Although billed as "America's first comprehensive school health education curriculum," (National Center for Health Education, 1997), it is actually a program for grades K–6. Various training models are offered to teachers, and training is required. It is one of few school health education curricula to be cited by the U.S. Department of Education as exemplary. The content is laid out as shown in Table 9.1.

The largest study ever done on comprehensive school health education was initiated in 1983; it is considered the definitive study of the effectiveness

**Table 9.1** *Growing Healthy* Content Overview

| Grade | Title | Content Summary |
|---|---|---|
| Kindergarten | Happiness Is a Healthy Me | Overview of the five senses. Differences make life interesting. Discover special features that make each student unique. Make self-portraits and sign them with fingerprints, reinforcing uniqueness. Dental professional visits class to teach about tooth care and function and development of teeth. |
| Grade 1 | Super Me | Focuses on taste, touch, and smell. Bodies are precious "machines" that enable us to have healthy and active lives. Students compare new self-portraits with others' to see differences and similarities. Discussions to build assertiveness skills and self-esteem. |
| Grade 2 | Sights and Sounds | Focuses on sight and hearing. Students look at optical illusions to illustrate that we need to look carefully to be sure we are seeing what is really there. Exercises include writing in Braille and navigating their way while blindfolded. Hand puppets aid in discussing feelings, body language, and how the tone of their voice indicates feelings. Study includes noise pollution concentration and solutions. |
| Grade 3 | Movement and the Human Body | Focuses on muscular and skeletal systems. Students make a mannequin to illustrate muscles and bones and movement. Interactive video assists in daily exercises and movement activities while applying muscles to activity. Chicken leg dissection teaches about muscles and joints and movement. Study includes safety at home. |
| Grade 4 | Our Digestion, Our Nutrition, Our Health | Energy transfer is demonstrated by popping popcorn. Food Guide Pyramid is used to study energy in the diet, snacks, and nutritious, balanced meals. "Web of Life" game reinforces ecosystem relationships. Digestive process is studied daily. |
| Grade 5 | Our Lungs & Our Health | Appreciation of the respiratory system is the focus. Students conduct air experiments to determine the levels of pollution and create solutions. Smoking machine illustrates passive smoke. Students practice ways to say "No" to peer pressure to use cigarettes and other drugs. Lung dissections aid in understanding lung diseases. First aid skills are taught. |
| Grade 6 | Our Heart & Our Health | Students build time capsule collage to reinforce "how we've changed" and identify health and other goals for age 18. Demonstrations include how bleeding is controlled, listening to the heart with a stethoscope, calculating pulse rate, and heart dissection to explore the structure and function of the heart. Causes of stress are explored and refusal skills are reinforced. |

Source: Adapted with permission from *Growing Healthy: Content Overview* [On-line], 1997, National Center for Health Education. Available: http://www.nche.org/ghfinalpg/ghctover.htm

of school health education. *Growing Healthy*, then called the School Health Curriculum Project, was evaluated with three other school health education programs. A sample of 30,000 students in twenty states was included in the study. Four measures of program effectiveness were used: overall knowledge, attitudes, practices, and program-specific knowledge. The study found that, of all programs studied, SHCP showed the strongest statistically significant effects on overall knowledge, attitudes, and behavior. Importantly, teacher training, full implementation, and fidelity of program design were found to be important factors in the program's success (Connell, Turner, & Mason, 1985).

In a second study (Andrews & Moore, 1987), students in this program were tracked from kindergarten through seventh grade and followed up at grades 9–12. This study also revealed that, when compared to a traditional health curriculum, *Growing Healthy* students had significantly higher levels of knowledge about health and how to maintain health and more positive attitudes and behaviors. They also had significantly lower levels of experimentation with smoking or illegal drugs, which persisted for years after the class. Other evidence suggested that *Growing Healthy* students showed improved mathematics and reading scores (Schoener, 1988), a positive link between health education and general academic performance.

## Teenage Health Teaching Modules

The *Teenage Health Teaching Modules* (*THTM*), a grade 7–12 health education curriculum, was developed to be compatible with the *Growing Healthy* K–6 program. It contains 21 instructional modules organized by developmentally-based health tasks of concern to adolescents. Modules range from 6 to 15 class sessions and address issues such as violence prevention, tobacco, alcohol and other drug use, and HIV/AIDS. *THTM* is intended to address five skill areas: self-assessment, communication, decision making, health advocacy, and health self-management.

Comprehensive evaluation has confirmed *THTM*'s effectiveness, including strong positive net gain in health knowledge and, compared to control groups, a net gain in health-related attitudes and total health practices. (Gold et al., 1991; U.S. Department of Education, 1995).

## The Healthy Lifestyles Program

The Greater Battle Creek (Michigan) schools, with a grant from the W.K. Kellogg Foundation, developed a project to improve the knowledge, attitudes, and behaviors of students in kindergarten through grade 12 in four target areas: substance use, fitness, nutrition, and stress management. In order to increase the likelihood of success and to obtain their commitment, parents and staff were also targeted for wellness programs. By taking this approach, parents, families, and school staff served as role models to encourage and reinforce healthy habits among pupils. The key to the overall success of the program was the belief in the benefits of the program by the board of education, superintendent, and teacher union representatives. Community agencies—such as hospitals, health departments, American Red Cross, American Cancer Society, American Heart Association, parks and recreation departments, Y-centers, and employee assistance groups—became involved. This helped to develop ownership and personal and community pride in the program.

Staff participation was crucial to success with students. Recognizing that students watch staff and are influenced by them was one of the key points in the recruitment of staff. Needs assessment and inquiring about staff interest provided data useful in planning programs and recruiting. Communication flowed freely in both top-down and bottom-up directions. A monthly newsletter included special topics on health, a profile of a "wellness person of the month," and a schedule of events. Classes were offered in stress management, weight loss, fitness, healthy cooking, and other areas. Smoking cessation groups were put in place. Special activities such as cross-country skiing were implemented. A Staff Shape-Up program encouraged friendly competition among buildings.

Staff members' efforts to improve their health carried over into their interactions with students. School staff petitioned the administration to offer salad bars in elementary schools, and students eagerly joined in. Teachers interested in walking found students following them. Walking maps began to appear in and out of buildings, and walking groups formed in cooperation with parents in after-school programs. High school physical education began to place greater emphasis on aerobic classes.

Appreciating the importance of the health of their children, parents became more involved, leading the way to health initiatives in their schools. Schools began to implement extensive sexuality education courses with little or no conflict from outside interests. Perhaps the most significant outcome was the development of a comprehensive health education curriculum for all kindergarten through grade six students.

## Know Your Body

*Know Your Body* (*KYB*) is a skills-based K–6 curriculum that seeks to provide students with knowledge, attitudes, skills, and experience they need to practice positive health behaviors. The lessons in *KYB* address the six health-risk behaviors identified by the Centers for Disease Control and Prevention and the ten content areas of comprehensive health instruction (see page 148). The program consists of five components—two core components and three optional—and recommended enhancements. The core components are the curriculum and the teacher training; the enhancements are extracurricular activities, biomedical screening, and program evaluation. *KYB* has been revised and updated several times.

*KYB* covers a wide range of health topics using ten modules at each level. It contains a "skill builders" unit in which five life skills—self-esteem, decision making, assertive communication, goal setting, and stress management—are practiced and reinforced. The skills are woven throughout the curriculum in all grades. A range of 36 to 72 sessions per year is necessary to implement the core lessons.

The theoretical framework that forms the foundation for *KYB* includes social cognitive theory, the Health Belief Model, and the PRECEDE-PROCEED Model (discussed in Chapter 11). Developmental appropriateness is based on the intellectual development theories of Piaget and Bloom.

*KYB* has been evaluated extensively. Longitudinal studies indicate that the curriculum has a significant positive impact on children's health behaviors. Health knowledge of students and parents regarding nutrition and early detection of disease is significantly improved (Marx, 1995).

## HeartReach

The Heart and Vascular Network of Butterworth Hospital in Grand Rapids, Michigan, provided HeartReach, a school-based heart health education program. HeartReach focuses on four major areas: **H**eart-health Education, **A**dvocacy, **R**esearch, and **T**eam-building (Walton, Heine, & DeLaFuente, 1998).

The Heart-health Education facet acts as a resource for teachers. The program offers free classroom cardiovascular health screenings for grades 5–12. Results are examined by trained health educators in the classroom in a format of lecture and question and answers. Parents are notified and follow-up actions are recommended if their child has abnormal measures. Classroom education includes beef and pig heart/lung dissection in upper grades to teach anatomy and heart function. Elementary children receive dissection demonstrations using a beef heart. Schools conduct health fairs and family nights. The staff dietician offers nutrition education to teachers, food service personnel, and students. Food service personnel are trained to prepare heart-healthy foods at workshops.

Staff members attempt to affect community and school programs, policies, and curricula that deal with cardiovascular health in youth. They also advocate for the reinstitution of daily physical and health education. They are engaged in community playground projects, school health curriculum committees, and a tobacco education consortium.

The HeartReach research component tracks data points in an attempt to define the cardiovascular health profiles of area children. Low HDL levels, high body fat and body mass index levels, and high and borderline blood pressure and total cholesterol levels are tracked. Educational outcomes are measured by pre- and post-test surveys.

The program attempts to forge partnerships between HeartReach, school districts, individual schools, local colleges and universities, other hospitals, the health department, and other health service programs. Many partnerships are mutually beneficial and thriving.

## Project ALERT

*Project ALERT* is a substance use prevention curriculum for middle grades, designed by RAND Corporation and marketed nationwide. It consists of a two-year curriculum containing eleven lessons in the core year followed by three lessons in the booster year. Teacher training is required. An optional Teen Leader component is available to trained teachers.

*Project ALERT* is based on the social influence model, which emphasizes teaching students how to recognize pressures to use drugs and how to use strategies and skills to resist those pressures. The interactive curriculum provides much opportunity to practice those skills, with several lessons centered on videos with accompanying activities. Student-centered activities include role-plays, instructional games, reasons lists, advertisement analysis and rewrites, and homework to be done with parents or guardians.

The curriculum was tested in thirty middle schools in longitudinal studies (Bell, Ellickson, & Harrison, 1993; Ellickson & Bell, 1990; Ellickson,

Bell, & McGuigan, 1993). When compared with children who did not get *Project ALERT*, students initiated marijuana and tobacco use one-third less and initiated alcohol use by 28 percent less; experimenters reduced current marijuana and cigarette use by 50–60 percent; smokers showed moderate increase in quitting smoking; and experimenters with alcohol showed a 44 percent reduction in monthly use. *Project ALERT* students felt more able to resist offers of a drug. The results were consistent across ethnic groups and urban, rural, and suburban populations.

## Safer Choices

*Safer Choices* uses a multicomponent approach designed to reduce risk behaviors or increase protective behaviors to prevent HIV infection, other STDs, and pregnancy in students ages 14–18 (Coyle et al., 1996). The program, which seeks to shape both individual and environmental influences, is based upon social cognitive theory, social influence theories, and school change/improvement models. Although curriculum and instruction were included, the school environment is the central focus of *Safer Choices*.

The program recommends that a School Health Promotion Council be established at the school to

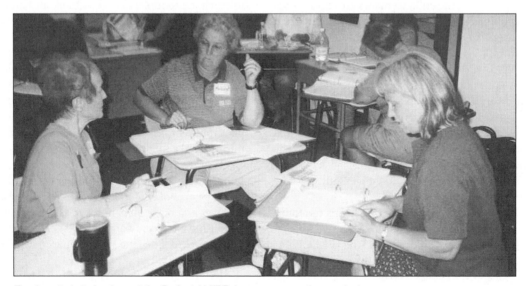

Teachers train to implement the Project ALERT drug use prevention curriculum.

make sure that the interventions become an integral part of the school environment and culture. The council includes parents, teachers, administrators, other staff, students, and community agencies. The council works with staff to plan, conduct, and/or monitor activities of the four components: curriculum and staff development, peer resources and school environment, parent education, and community-school links.

The curriculum, based on *Reducing the Risk: Building Skills to Prevent Pregnancy* (Barth, Middleton, & Wagman, 1989), consists of separate ten-lesson series for grades 9 and 10. The lessons address attitudes and beliefs, social skills, functional knowledge, social and media influences, peer norms, and parent-child communication. They consistently stress that it is not healthful to engage in unprotected intercourse and that unprotected sex is against the norm. Students are given structured opportunities to practice skills so that they develop self-efficacy. Peer facilitators are used in some activities.

*Safer Choices* saturates the school environment with activities, information, events, and services to reinforce key messages of classroom instruction. It also fosters an environment that supports prevention of HIV, STD, and pregnancy. This approach, using peer education, provides positive role models, reinforces norms against unprotected sex, provides opportunity for youth to help one another, and empowers students by establishing meaningful involvement and personal responsibility.

The parent education component is important as a means to help parents provide accurate information to their children and reinforce norms against unprotected intercourse. Parents receive project newsletters providing background information on *Safer Choices* and information regarding HIV/AIDS, STDs, and pregnancy as well as tips on talking with teens. Student/parent homework activities are included.

The program provides links with community resources. Students are encouraged to access these services. The Health Promotion Council develops links and a resource guide for youth services agencies.

Research (Coyle et al., 1999) indicates that *Safer Choices* enhanced 9 of 13 psychosocial variables including knowledge, self efficacy for condom use, normative beliefs and attitudes regarding condom use, perceived barriers to condom use, risk perceptions, and parent-child communication. It also reduced the frequency of intercourse without a condom in the previous three months, increased use of condoms at last intercourse, and increased use of selected contraceptives at last intercourse.

## Gimme 5

The National Cancer Institute initiated the national *5-A-Day for Better Health Program* in 1991 to achieve a per capita intake of five servings of fruits and vegetables a day. *Gimme 5: A Fresh Nutrition Concept for Students* was one of nine NCI-funded research studies. *Gimme 5* focused on increasing fruit and vegetable consumption of students in nineteen high schools in the archdiocese of New Orleans, Louisiana. The population of the schools under study were heavily weighted with Caucasians from a middle-to-upper socioeconomic background (Nicklas et al., 1998).

*Gimme 5* contained multiple interventions. The media campaign provided appealing messages and

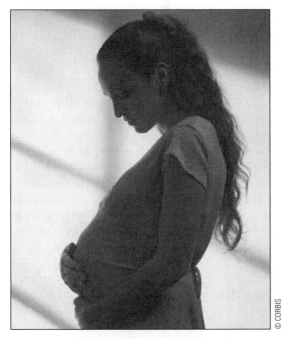

Reducing teen pregnancy is one of the goals of Safer Choices.

© CORBIS

activities that would increase awareness, reinforce concepts, and promote positive attitudes toward consumption of fruits and vegetables. Monthly activities included marketing stations, taste tests, public service announcements, student contests, and fruit and vegetable baskets. Five 55-minute workshops, which contained unique themes, a variety of learning strategies, and a student focus, were Fresh Start, Body Works: Eating for Athletic Performance and Appearance, Fresh Snax to the Max, Fast Food—Go for the Greens, and Microwave Magic and Other Quick Fixes. Supplementary activities were included in required academic courses using fruit and vegetables in the lesson design to increase and maintain awareness. Fresh Choices was a meal modification component designed to increase the availability, variety, and taste of fruits and vegetables that met the *5-A-Day* serving size and nutrient criteria (Havas et al., 1995). The program included training of food service staff. A parent component provided education, stimulated awareness, and elicited parental support for *Gimme 5* with the objective of encouraging increased availability of fruits and vegetables in the home (Nicklas et al., 1998).

When compared with the control group, the *Gimme 5* intervention students had significantly higher group knowledge scores. Both groups were evaluated to determine which of the stages of change (precontemplation, contemplation, preparation, action, or maintenance) (Prochaska & DiClemente, 1992) they occupied. The intervention group showed a progressive shift from precontemplation and contemplation to preparation—an encouraging outcome—and an increased awareness of the *5-A-Day for Better Health Program*. The reported daily servings of fruit and vegetables usually consumed increased by 14 percent over two years in the intervention group, whereas no significant increase occurred in the control group.

# WORKSITE HEALTH PROMOTION

## Lifestyle Improvements for Everyone (L.I.F.E.) at Physicians Health Plan

The L.I.F.E. program (Brey, Tyler, & Brooks, 1998), a voluntary health promotion program built on the power of incentives, is the worksite program at Physicians Health Plan, a health maintenance organization in Fort Wayne, Indiana. Employees who are considering participation receive an instruction manual that describes the program, health promotion activities, and an activity guide. Those who enroll report their participation in the activity guide and turn the guide in to employees (known as LIFESAVERs) who review the guides and forward them to the Health Education Department. Eventually, the results of the self-report activity guides are translated into money added to the employee's paycheck four times per year.

Other incentives are used as well. Monthly drawings are held for a gift certificate related to the L.I.F.E. program. Employees are paid small sums to have their blood pressure checked, their teeth cleaned, and their body composition measured.

Evaluation sought to determine participation among employees and in different facets of the program. In 1997, 67 percent of employees participated in L.I.F.E. In order of most rewards given, the nutrition program was highest, followed by aerobic exercise, stress management, not smoking, strength training, and wearing seatbelts. The average expenditure per year was $80 per participating employee.

## City of Birmingham's Good Health Program

The city of Birmingham, Alabama, developed the Good Health Program, a comprehensive worksite health promotion program that has paid handsome dividends (Pelletier, 1993). Smoking among street and sanitation workers decreased from 53 percent to 32 percent. The fraction of participants having cholesterol above 200 ml/dl dropped from 56 percent to 45 percent. Medical costs per employee dropped over a five-year period. The program received the prestigious C. Everett Koop National Worksite Health Award in 1993 (Brown et al., 1995).

The program is configured to reach employees at multiple sites throughout the city of Birmingham. Initially, the program was designed to reduce risk factors for cardiovascular disease and promote the practice of good health habits at the worksite. To meet the needs of a diverse population in multiple locations, it was placed under the city's "Working Well" initiative, which includes worksite-hazard identification, safety training for injury prevention, health insurance, medical management of on-the-job injuries, FitCheck health and fitness program for public-safety workers, and employee assistance services.

The Good Health Program is multi-faceted. One major component is the use of health-risk appraisals (HRAs) and screening to help employees recognize age-related and lifestyle threats to health. HRAs and screenings are a condition for enrollment in city-sponsored health insurance benefits. At their option, employees may go to their private physicians for screening, although few choose to do so. Employees are measured for several health indicators and receive immediate health counseling, referrals to physicians if necessary, and health education materials. Follow-up procedures are important to the screening: Medical appointments and referrals to the employee assistance service are made, and data are stored on a confidential computer database. Health awareness, smoking cessation, hypertension control, nutrition and cholesterol education, exercise, and back-care education interventions are offered.

The program keeps employees informed about a variety of health issues. Tip sheets attached to paychecks, posters, bulletin boards, health booths, pamphlets, and articles and updates on health are provided regularly.

Smoking cessation is another dominant component of the Good Health Program. Recruitment booths and incentives are utilized. Self-help kits are given to each smoker. Contests are held to encourage cessation. Participants are telephoned weekly with encouragement.

Hypertension control has taken a variety of forms, including weekly group sessions and one-on-one appointments with a registered nurse. These have been shown to be effective: At the most recent screening, about one-third of city employees were found to have controlled their blood pressures.

Various interventions have been used to affect nutrition and cholesterol. Open classes, nutrition booths, taste tests, displays, and cash incentives have been used. Cash incentives and groceries have been awarded in contests. Nutritionists have taught nutrition and cholesterol modification at fire stations.

Exercise is one of the most popular interventions. The city owns a fitness center. Physical fitness, job task performance, nutrient intake, and selected lifestyle behaviors are assessed annually in the FitCheck program. This has led to required fitness training for the city's firefighters.

A rehabilitation program for employees with back injuries was initiated. Back-care education, lifestyle instruction, daily flexibility, strengthening, and aerobic exercises are offered to employees who had previously incurred medical costs for back injuries.

## Hoechst Marion Roussel Employee Wellness Program

Hoechst Marion Roussel has been offering programs and services to associates, retirees, and their families since 1986 (WellTech International, 1999). The medically based program, under the management of Bethesda Preventative Health Systems, is designed to provide education and opportunity to improve fitness, nutrition, and other health practices through behavior modification.

Services include a bimonthly newsletter, an annual health fair, quarterly incentive programs for all associates, biannual programs for fitness center members, quarterly health screenings, bimonthly brown-bag presentations and awareness programs, and safety meeting presentations. There is an outdoor walking trail, onsite fitness center, aerobics program, and a resource library.

Given that participation is one measure of success, this program succeeds. Approximately 25 percent of associates are fitness center members, 94 percent of all associates participate in at least one health promotion or fitness program each year, and 67 percent participate in two or more. About 50 percent of all associates received a blood pressure screen, and 10 percent received a skin cancer screen in a recent year. Fitness center members are charged a nominal fee, and most exercise incentive and awareness programs are free. Screenings are subsidized in varying amounts.

## Chevron's Health Quest

The worksite wellness programs of Chevron's Preventive Health Services, collectively known as

Health Quest (Kashima, 1999), include eight corporate owned and operated fitness centers around the United States. Health Quest's primary goals include increasing productivity, reducing health risks, reducing absenteeism, and improving safety incident rates.

During 1997, employees in the marketing division voluntarily took a health risk appraisal, which was processed by StayWell Health Management Systems. Safety specialists coordinated the HRA program at the company's many locations. A total of 1,045 marketing employees participated, over 50 percent of the marketing population. The HRA was used to assess needs and establish baseline information on the health risks of the marketing staff.

Marketing employees were asked to select the health area that they were interested in changing in the next six months. Five areas were identified: eating habits, exercise, stress, weight control, and cholesterol. Health Quest programs were planned to target poor nutrition and exercise, the areas most often identified. Health Quest staff planned programs addressing these problems and used its local existing safety committees to implement the program. Safety specialists and committees proved to be effective assets by integrating Health Quest programs into their existing efforts.

"Focused Intervention" is an example of one of the programs developed at Health Quest. The program works with high-risk employees to improve their health status in one of six areas: exercise, back care, eating habits, smoking or tobacco use, stress, and weight control. Focused one-on-one counseling is conducted by StayWell. Employees work with one of StayWell's health educators to reduce one risk at a time. Follow-up calls come at six and twelve months after completing the program.

"Maintain Don't Gain" is an awareness program given during the holiday season that targets poor nutrition and lack of exercise. Goals are to help employees maintain their pre-holiday weight and increase awareness about nutrition and exercise. During the eight-week program, employees can choose to participate as individuals or in groups of three. Although this is not a weight-loss program, during one year employees lost over 300 pounds during the eight weeks. In addition, 94 percent of participants felt the program was worth their time,

74 percent learned something about nutrition, 71 percent improved their knowledge about fitness, and 74 percent felt the program had helped them maintain their weight during the holidays.

The "Leadership in Health and Safety Coaching" program was to teach managers how their leadership in health and safety can affect employees and help managers become more personally responsible for health and safety. Instruction was given on use of ergonomically correct equipment, inclusion of a health topic during meetings, and permission for time away from work to exercise or stretch. Managers were encouraged to actively participate in health promotion programs. As a result of the program, 82 percent of managers enhanced their communication with employees relative to health and safety, 53 percent integrated health and safety initiatives into their business plans, 76 percent implemented and continued to endorse ergonomic training for employees, and 64 percent committed to a personal exercise program.

# UNIVERSITY/COLLEGE CAMPUS SETTINGS

## WellnessWorks

The University of South Carolina's WellnessWorks program is available, not only for faculty and staff, but also for the university community. It receives counsel from the Employee Wellness Program Advisory Committee. The Health Ambassador Committee is a team of USC faculty members who serve as liaisons between WellnessWorks and their academic departments.

WellnessWorks provides clients with a Personal Wellness Profile, including comprehensive screening followed by advice on identifying health strengths and areas of improvement and planning actions to increase wellness. Nutrition and exercise consultations are available. Smoking cessation programs, stress management, and weight management classes are popular. Self-paced programs, including a walking program, cholesterol reduction, managing stress, and back pain and injury prevention are also offered. First aid and CPR courses are available. Some services require a fee.

Special events include the Health Expo, which showcases campus and community resources for health and fitness. Walking Works is a five-week walking challenge for teams. The Great Weight Maintenance Marathon is a five-week program during the holiday season to encourage healthy eating.

WellnessWorks functions in cooperation with other university services. For instance, the Counseling and Human Development Center is fully accredited and offers psychotherapy. Fitplace provides structured exercise programs for individuals interested in monitored exercise. The Employee Assistance Program provides comprehensive services for faculty and staff.

# Health Education and Lifestyle Promotion (H.E.L.P.)

Missouri University is home to the H.E.L.P. program, whose goal is to improve levels of physical, intellectual, emotional, social, spiritual, and vocational health experienced by participants as a result of health-related knowledge acquired, attitudes changed, and behaviors modified (Watts et al., 1992). The overarching expected outcome is health promotion habit formation.

The fundamental interventions are physical activity, nutrition education, and stress awareness and management. Additional expected outcomes are assumption of personal health "response-ability" and enhancement of positive self-image. Within each fundamental intervention are various components that enable maximal, measurable effects. As part of the physical activity intervention, extensive blood chemistry analyses are performed before and after a fifteen-week regimen is begun. A thorough assessment of physical fitness is also done before and after exercise intervention. An individualized exercise prescription is prepared for each participant, tailored to his or her personal needs, interests, and capabilities.

The H.E.L.P. nutrition intervention has three components. First, dietary modification prescriptions are prepared for each participant based on blood lipid profile and dietary analysis. Second, body fat reduction and management plans are developed for each participant, based on body composition data and recommended dietary changes that are acceptable to the individual. Participants are taken on a supermarket tour that emphasizes how to shop for groceries more healthfully and cost effectively. Third, stress awareness and management techniques are taught and practiced. Information on time management, stressor identification, and relaxation exercises are included. Emphasis on a strong, positive self-image is an integral part of this intervention.

The noontime wellness lifestyle course is an important part of H.E.L.P. Participants bring and eat their lunches while undergoing a comprehensive health education experience. The class meets at noon twice each week for a total of thirty sessions.

Evaluation of H.E.L.P. indicated that a statistically significant health-positive change occurred in seven physiological variables measured in program participants. These included dry body weight, body fat, total cholesterol, systolic blood pressure, diastolic blood pressure, resting heart rate, and exercise heart rate.

# Pure Energy Wellness Program

Chattanooga State Technical Community College is home to the Pure Energy Wellness Program, the fundamental purpose of which is to provide all staff members and students with quality programs from each dimension of wellness to enhance health status and quality of life. When implemented, Pure Energy set very challenging objectives, including (1) to reduce the incidence of smoking among employees by 50 percent within three years; (2) to have "heart healthy" food choices with appropriate nutritional information at each meal served in the college cafeteria within one year; and (3) to include the college's wellness initiative as an integral piece of the institutional goals in the college's strategic plan.

The program includes classes of varying lengths, including Fitness for Living, Concepts of Wellness, Bicycling, Step Aerobics, Hiking and Backpacking, and WaistWatchers Plus. Pure Energy offers seminars such as Roadblocks to a Healthy Lifestyle and What to Do When Life is Making You Crazy. Special outings including rafting, canoeing, and bicycling trips, some of which offer extensive travel. There are also special interest classes, such as Photography for the Beginner and Writing Popular Fiction. The program and its members participate in fund-raising activities for nonprofit organizations such as the Alzheimer's Memory Walk and the Multiple Sclerosis 150 Bicycle Ride. It sponsors a health fair that features a variety of health screenings.

Employees may participate in the Lifestyle Assessment Questionnaire, a computerized assessment of nutrition, weight management, and personality type. Pure Energy also works with the campus employee assistance program to provide services, including support groups. Employees, retirees, and immediate family members have free access and exclusive usage hours in the Fitness Center.

The program uses both intrinsic and extrinsic incentives for employee participation. To promote intrinsic motivation, program directors provide information in promotional materials about the practical health benefits of the programs. They also use small extrinsic incentives, such as refrigerator magnets, free healthy snacks, and participation buttons. At the conclusion of each program, they present special recognition certificates to each individual who completes the program. They also use door prizes, recognition articles in the monthly newsletter, and point systems.

Wellness staff have conducted numerous evaluations of Pure Energy. Results have shown consistent increases in the proportion of employees who have regular blood pressure and cholesterol checks and who do regular self-examination for cancer. There has been much improvement in the percentage of employees who participate in formal exercise regularly. Since inception of the program, indicators of attitudes about the work setting have improved. Many positive benefits have also been demonstrated among students.

# FAITH COMMUNITY SETTINGS

## Jackson County (FL) Alcohol and Other Drug Prevention Partnerships

A group of six African-American churches spurred the development of the Jackson County Alcohol and Other Drug Prevention Partnership in Florida (Sutherland et al., 1997). They expanded the initiative to include the school board, law enforcement, the health department, local businesses, a sorority, and a service organization. A primary objective of the partnership was to reduce drug use risk by increasing resiliency among African-American youth in the county. According to Bernard (1991), resilient children are those with (1) social competence, (2) problem-solving skills, (3) autonomy, (4) a sense of purpose, and (5) a sense of some degree of environmental control. The focus was increasing youth anti-drug resiliency and supporting the family unit as an institution.

The coalition of six churches formed in the mid-1980s to provide prevention services to older church and community members (Cowart, Sutherland, & Harris, 1995). The church appears to be particularly suited to provide entree into the community because it possesses many desirable features, including a history of volunteerism, influence on families, members who live close to the church, social networks, serving as a source of community identity, and established communication networks. These characteristics make the church a viable and useful partner in primary prevention initiatives (Sutherland et al., 1997).

All of the coalition churches formed Health Advisory Councils (HAC) to plan and implement prevention programs. HAC members receive training by professional staff and receive monthly continuing education. Training includes alcohol and other drug content; basic community organizational skills; and structured program planning, budgeting, implementation, assessment, evaluation, and reporting procedures. Training includes how to develop a church drug prevention program and how to integrate prevention strategies into other church activities.

Programming options were varied. Church health committees, assisted by HAC, selected their own options. Choices included competitions and cooperative activities between and among churches, excellence recognition for youth programs, youth mentoring, parent skills training, keeping youth successful in school, providing viable alternatives to drugs, peer-resistance training, public education, intergenerational activities, health/drug awareness Sundays, interchurch prevention activities, and summer and after-school programs.

Over a three-year period, there was a 123 percent increase in youth participation, an indication of the program's attractiveness. Several significant changes in drug-related attitudes resulted, most in a positive direction. More youth reported counting on friends when faced with a serious problem and more were less likely to imitate a friend's negative behavior, suggesting less vulnerability to peer pressure. Self-concept indicators, including family life quality, were significantly improved. Few youths reported problems at school and feeling lonely. Sutherland et al. (1997) concluded that the church is almost indispensable in prevention activities because, of all social institutions, it is among the closest to the family.

## Health Enhancement Ministries

Health Enhancement Ministries is housed at Hickory Grove Baptist Church in Charlotte, North Carolina. H.E.M. provides programming for the optimal wellness of body, mind, and spirit through a Biblical perspective. It offers counseling from both professionals and "lay counselors"; share groups (wherein people talk about and share experiences),

whose topics include "divorce care," panic disorders, and diabetes; and health fairs. There are recreation and exercise facilities and programs. H.E.M. provides seminars in a variety of health-related subjects and renewal retreats that feature meditation, spiritual development, and inner healing. There are also recovery groups, including a twelve-step program for alcoholics and programs for children of alcoholics and co-dependents. Project H.O.P.E. (Healing of Painful Experiences) is a multidimensional offering that includes the physical and the spiritual. There is also a pain management program by accredited therapists. H.E.M. is a multifaceted program to link religious and spiritual services with overall wellness programs.

## KEY POINTS

1. Health promotion programs take place in a variety of settings.

2. Health promotion programs can succeed in diverse settings with a variety of objectives and various offerings to reach the objectives.

## REFERENCES

Andrews, R.L., & Moore, D.D. (1987). Growing Healthy: A longitudinal study—kindergarten through grade nine. Monograph, The College of Education, University of Washington, Seattle.

Barnes, G.P., Parker, W.A., Lyon, Jr., T.C., Drun, M.A., & Coleman, G.C. (1992). Ethnicity, location, age, and fluoridation factors in baby bottle tooth decay and caries prevalence of Head Start children. *Public Health Reports, 107*(2), 167–173.

Barth, R.P., Middleton, K., and Wagnan, E. (1989). A social and cognitive skill-building approach to preventing teenage pregnancy. *Theory Into Practice, 28*(3), 183–189.

Bell, R.M., Ellickson, P.L., & Harrison, E.R. (1993). Do drug prevention effects persist into high school? How Project ALERT did with ninth graders. *Preventive Medicine, 22*(4), 463–483.

Bernard, B. (1991). *Fostering resiliency in kids: Protective factors in the family, school, and community.* Portland, OR: Northwest Regional Laboratory.

Brey, R.A., Tyler, H.A., & Brooks, B.L. (1998). Lifestyle improvements for everyone (L.I.F.E.): A worksite health promotion incentive program. *Journal of Health Education, 29*(6), 376–380.

Brown, K.C., Hilyer, J.C., Artz, L., Glasscock, L., & Weaver, M. (1995). The Birmingham good health program: Meeting healthy people 2000 objectives. *Health Values, 19*(6), 45–53.

Connell, D.B., Turner, R.R., & Mason, E.F. (1985). Summary of findings of the school health education evaluation: Health promotion effectiveness, implementation, and costs. *Journal of School Health, 55*(8), 316–321.

Cowart, M.E., Sutherland, M., & Harris, G.J. (1995). Health promotion for older rural African Americans: Implications for social and public policy. *The Journal of Applied Gerontology, 14*(1), 33–46.

Coyle, K., Basen-Engquist, K., Kirby, D., Parcel, G., Banspach, S., Harrist, R., Baumler, E., & Weil, M. (1999). Short-term impact of Safer Choices: A multicomponent, school-based HIV, other STD, and pregnancy prevention program. *Journal of School Health, 69*(5), 181–188.

Coyle, K., Kirby, D., Parcel, G., Basen-Engquist, K., Banspach, S., Rugg, D., & Weil, M. (1996). Safer Choices: A multicomponent school-based HIV/STD and pregnancy prevention program for adolescents. *Journal of School Health, 66*(3), 89–94.

Ellickson, P.L., & Bell, R.M. (1990). Drug prevention in junior high: A multi-site longitudinal test. *Science, 247*(4948), 1299–1305.

Ellickson, P.L., Bell, R.M., & McGuigan, K. (1993). Preventing adolescent drug use: Long-term results of a junior high program. *American Journal of Public Health, 83*(6), 856–861.

Gallivan, L.P., Lundberg, M.E., Fiedelholltz, J.B., Andringa, K., Stableford, S., & Visser, L. (1998). *Journal of Health Education, 29*(5-supplement), S28–S33.

Gold, R.S., Parcel, G.S., Walberg, H.J., Leupker, R.V., Portnoy, B., & Stone, E.J. (1991). Summary and conclusions of the THTM evaluation: The expert work group perspective. *Journal of School Health, 61*(1), 39–42.

Havas, S., Heimendinger, J., Damron, D., Nicklas, S.A., Cowan, A., Beresford, S.A.A., Sorensen, G., Buller, D., Bishop, D., Baranowski, T., & Reynolds, K. (1995). 5-a-day for better health: Nine community research projects to increase fruit and vegetable consumption. *Public Health Reports, 110*(1), 68–79.

Hawks, S.R., Hull, M.L., Thalman, R.L., & Richins, P.M. (1995). Review of spiritual health: Definition, role, and intervention strategies in health promotion. *American Journal of Health Promotion, 9*(5), 371–378.

Health Resources and Services Administration. (1998). *Grants and contracts* [On-line]. Available: http://www.hrsa.dhhs.gov

Hult Center. (1999). *All things Hult* [On-line]. Available: http://www.hult-health.org

Kabat-Zinn, J., Lipworth, L., & Burney, R. (1985). The clinical use of mindfulness meditation for the self-regulation of chronic pain. *Journal of Behavioral Medicine, 8*(2), 163–190.

Kabat-Zinn, J., Lipworth, L., Burney, R., & Sellers, W. (1986). Four year follow-up of a meditation-based program for the self-regulation of chronic pain: Treatment outcomes and compliance. *Clinical Journal of Pain, 2*, 159–173.

Kabat-Zinn, J., Massion, A., Kristeller, J., Peterson, L., Fletcher, K.E., Pbert, L., Lenderkins, W.R., & Santorelli, S.F. (1992). Effectiveness of meditation-based stress reduction program in the treatment of anxiety disorders. *American Journal of Psychiatry, 149*(7), 936–943.

Kashima, S. (1999). Using three CHES responsibilities in a comprehensive worksite health promotion program. *The CHES Bulletin, 10*(2), 41–50.

King, K.A. (1998). Healthy smiles: A multidisciplinary baby bottle tooth decay prevention program. *Journal of Health Education, 29*(1), 4–7.

Kumanyika, S.K. (1990). Diet and chronic disease issues for minority populations. *Journal of Nutrition Education, 22*(2), 89–96.

Kumanyika, S.K. (1994). Obesity in minority populations: An epidemiologic assessment. *Obesity Research, 2,* 166–182.

Lewis, R.K., Paine-Andrews, A., Fawcett, S.B., Francisco, V.T., Richter, K.P., Copple, B., & Copple, J.E. (1996). Evaluating the effects of a community coalition's efforts to reduce illegal sales of alcohol and tobacco products to minors. *Journal of Community Health, 21*(6), 429–436.

Marier, A.E. (1996). A health education program for migrant children. *American Journal of Public Health, 86*(4), 590–591.

Marx, E. (1995). *Choosing the tools: A review of selected K–12 health education curricula.* Newton, MA: Education Development Center, Inc.

Mental Medicine Update. (1993). Insuring behavioral medicine. *The Mind/Body Newsletter, 2,* 1.

National Center for Health Education. (1997). *Growing healthy* [On-line]. Available: http://www.nche.org/ghfinalpg/ghhome.html

Nicklas, T.A., Johnson, C.C., Myers, L., Farris, R.P., & Cunningham, A. (1998). Outcomes of a high school program to increase fruit and vegetable consumption: Gimme 5—A fresh nutrition concept for students. *Journal of School Health, 68*(6), 248–253.

Ohio Department of Health. Bureau of Dental Health. (1995). *The oral health of Ohioans, 1993. The Ohio health monograph series.* Columbus, OH.

Ornish, D. (1991, May). Can life-style changes reverse coronary atherosclerosis? *Hospital Practice, 26*, 123–132.

Ornish, D. (1992). *Dr. Dean Ornish's program for reversing heart disease.* New York: Ballantine Books.

Ornish, D., Brown, S., Scherwitz, L., Billing, J.H., Armstrong, W.T., Ports, T.A., McLanahan, S.M., Kirkeeido, R.L., Brand, R.J., & Gould, K.L. (1990). Can lifestyle changes reverse coronary heart disease? *Lancet, 336*(8708), 129–133.

Ornish, D., Scherwitz, L., Doody, R., Keston, D., McLanahan, S.M., Brown, S.E., DePuey, E.G., Sonnemaker, R., Haynes, C., Lester, J., McAllister, G.K., Hall, R.J., Burdine, J.A., & Gotto, Jr., A.M. (1983). Effects of stress management training and dietary changes in treating ischemic heart disease. *JAMA, 249*(1), 54–59.

Otten, Jr., W., Tuetsch, S.M., Williamson, D.F., & Marks, J.S. (1990). The effect of known risk factors on the excess mortality of black adults in the United States. *JAMA, 263*(6), 845–850.

Pelletier, K.R. (1993). A review and analysis of the health and cost-effective outcome studies of comprehensive health promotion and disease prevention programs at the worksite: 1991–1993 update. *American Journal of Health Promotion, 8*(1), 50–62.

Prochaska, J.O., & DiClemente, C.C. (1992). Stages of change in the modification of problem behaviors. In M. Hersen, R.M. Eisler, & P.M. Miller (Eds.), *Progress in behavior modification.* Sycamore, IL: Sycamore Press.

Ripa, L.W. (1988). Nursing caries: A comprehensive review. *Pediatric Dentistry, 10*(2), 268–282.

Schoener, J.E. (1988). The effects of the growing healthy program upon children's academic performance and attendance in New York City, 1987–1988. New York: New York City Board of Education.

Stolley, M.R., & Fitzgibbon, M.L. (1997). Effects of an obesity prevention program on the eating behavior of African American mothers and daughters. *Health Education & Behavior, 24*(2), 152–164.

Sutherland, M.S., Hale, C.D., Harris, G.J., Stalls, P., & Foulk, D. (1997). Strengthening rural youth resiliency through the church. *Journal of Health Education, 28*(4), 205–214.

Tate, D. (1994). *Mindfulness meditation group training: Effects on medical and psychological symptoms and positive psychological characteristics.* Unpublished doctoral dissertation, Brigham Young University, Provo, UT.

U.S. Department of Education. (1995). *Educational programs that work—1995* [On-line]. Available: http://www.ed.gov.pubs/EPTW/eptw9/eptw9h.html

Walton, J.A., Heine, L.D., & DeLaFuente, K.A. (1998). Heartreach: Reaching the hearts of youth before disease does. *Journal of Health Education, 29*(1), 51–53.

Watts, P.R., Waigandt, A., Londeree, B.R., & Sappington, M. (1992). A university worksite health promotion and wellness education program model. *Journal of Health Education, 23*(2), 87–94.

Weller Health Education Center. (1999). *Weller Health Education Center* [On-line]. Available: http://www.wellercenter.org

WellTech International. (1999). *Hoechst Marion Roussel, Inc., employee wellness program* [On-line]. Available: http://www.welltech.com/programs/hoechst.html

# Learning and Behavior Change: Theories and Models

At the most basic level, the goals of health education involve either changing human behavior or establishing preferred behavior. Principles of learning, theories of human behavior, and models provide frameworks for understanding how people learn and how and why people behave as they do, as well as bases for interventions to effect behavior change.

No single theory or model dominates research or practice in health education and health promotion. The health educator/promoter is best advised to apply the one most relevant to the situation and setting. The principles of learning, the domains of learning, and several theories of human behavior presented in this chapter are easily applied to health education and promotion. In addition, the discussion includes several theories of human behavior developed specifically to explain health-related action.

Traditionally, learning has been categorized into three domains:

1. The **cognitive domain** involves acquiring knowledge and information on an intellectual level.

2. The **affective domain** involves acquiring and changing emotions, feelings, and attitudes.

3. The **psychomotor** (sometimes called action or behavioral) **domain** involves acquiring physical skills and the aspects of learning in which the individual applies accumulated knowledge and attitudes to behavior or action.

## DOMAINS OF LEARNING

### Cognitive Domain

Learning within the cognitive domain principally involves the acquisition of **knowledge**, the intellectual acquaintance with facts, truth, and principles. In recent years, acquisition of knowledge has lost some of its emphasis among health educators, supplanted first by more emphasis on attitudes and values and, later, by acquisition of skills. In truth, the acquisition of knowledge is only one key to behavior. Rudd and Glanz (1991) wrote, "Knowledge is considered necessary but not sufficient . . . to guide . . . health actions and to stimulate health-enhancing behavior." Certainly, minimizing the significance of cognitive learning would be a mistake.

**cognitive domain**   learning, consisting of acquiring knowledge and information on an intellectual level

**affective domain**   emotions, feelings, and attitudes

**psychomotor domain**   physical skills and the aspects of learning in which the individual applies accumulated knowledge and attitudes to behavior or action

**knowledge**   the intellectual acquaintance with facts, truth, or principles

The cognitive domain traditionally has been depicted in terms of Bloom's (1956) Taxonomy of Educational Objectives. The taxonomy is arranged from simple to complex and implies intellectual abilities. Some educational objectives are listed below (in Bloom's order of simplest first), followed by examples of cognitive abilities required for each:

1. **Knowledge**—naming, defining, listing, identifying
2. **Comprehension**—explaining, describing, interpreting
3. **Application**—illustrating, predicting, applying
4. **Analysis**—analyzing, categorizing, classifying, differentiating
5. **Synthesis**—concluding, proposing, synthesizing
6. **Evaluating**—contrasting, comparing, evaluating

Teacher preparation programs and, therefore, public and private schools have leaned heavily upon Bloom's taxonomy. Although it still forms the basis of much of cognitive teaching-learning strategy, it is challenged by a number of theories. Regardless of one's view of Bloom's taxonomy, its vast following and its historical significance demand that educators be familiar with it.

Closely related to knowledge and existing on the edge of cognition are **beliefs**, acceptance of or confidence in an alleged fact or body of facts as true or right without positive knowledge or truth (Simons-Morton, Greene, & Gottlieb, 1995). As we shall see later in this chapter, although one's beliefs may be considered true or false by others, they have a powerful influence on behavior.

## Affective Domain

The affective domain consists of emotions, personal interests, values, and attitudes. Knowledge is necessary to guide behavior choices, but knowledge is not enough. Knowledge coupled with affective associations can be highly effective in shaping health-related behavior.

**Attitudes** can be described as perceptions that people have about their environment and the things in it. They can be a reason to act. Attitudes about health, however, are influenced by (1) the acquisition of health concepts that result from knowledge, (2) comprehension, (3) application of health knowledge and (4) one's beliefs. The development of positive health attitudes is a fundamental factor in improving health behaviors and, therefore, health status. Values are more complex and more deeply internalized than attitudes. They are also more difficult to change. Values exert a powerful force on behavior by assigning rightness or wrongness, goodness or badness.

Krathwohl, Bloom, and Masia (1964) suggested several processes, from simple to complex, that constitute affective learning:

1. **Receiving**—being aware of or attending to something in the environment
2. **Responding**—showing some new behaviors as a result of experience
3. **Valuing**—showing some definite involvement or commitment
4. **Organization**—integrating a new value into one's general set of values; giving it some ranking among one's general priorities
5. **Characterization** by a value or value complex—acting consistently with the new value

Affective development can be influenced in a number of ways. The long-term goal of health education, however, is *voluntary* behavior that is conducive to health. Inflicting health attitudes upon learners is unethical. Choices should remain personal and individual and not the result of indoctrination or brainwashing. The development of attitudes and feelings conducive to health should be the result of rational reflection, not authoritarian strategy. This rational reflection, coupled with knowledge, produces attitudes, beliefs, and values.

## Psychomotor Domain

The psychomotor domain is concerned with human movement, including motor skills and coordination, and the development of behavioral patterns. The latter, of course, is the essence of health education. The acquisition of skills is often necessary to perform actions and establish patterns of behavior.

Behavioral patterns are made by choice. Thus, certain variables contribute to making the choice from different alternatives. These variables include knowledge, attitudes, beliefs, and feelings. Therefore, the cognitive and affective domains affect the psychomotor domain. Health education can foster the variables that encourage people to behave in ways that enhance their health. Indeed, this is its purpose.

# CONCEPTS AND PRINCIPLES OF LEARNING

Educators, especially health educators, are devoted to promoting change. Change can occur in three ways: maturation, learning, or a combination of maturation and learning. **Maturation** is a developmental process within which a person manifests traits, the blueprint of which is carried on the genes. **Learning** is change of behavior brought about by experience, insight, perception—or a combination of the three—that causes the individual to approach future situations differently.

Learning is a dynamic process that begins with some motivation (desire, urge, drive) and leads the learner to be receptive to outside stimuli. **Mediators** (e.g., social norms, social supports, values, knowledge, attitudes) facilitate the change. If the learner trusts and is satisfied with his or her present facts, perceptions, values, and assumptions, he or she will have no need to seek new knowledge, skills, or attitudes (Knutson, 1965). A learning environment and activity must be present. Learning also requires a process of some kind. Finally, the learner must be able to use the new knowledge or skills in future applications.

According to Coleman (1969), the learning process consists of four critical factors: the learner, the task, the procedure, and the learning situation.

1. The **learner** brings all of his or her experience to the situation, including successes and failures. The learner also brings his or her resources, skills, motivations, and tendencies. Moreover, the learner's own personal frame of reference may greatly affect his or her ability to comprehend and apply what is to be learned. A certain level of maturity and adjustment fosters factors such as patience, concentration, and objectivity.

2. The **task** itself is defined by its size, complexity, and clarity. The task also is affected by the conditions and procedures applied to the learning experience. Familiarity with the task makes for a more suitable beginning. A small, simple body of knowledge is easier to assimilate, especially if it is built upon existing skills and knowledge.

3. The **procedure**, consisting of learning opportunities, is critical to the learning experience. College-level "methods and materials" courses emphasize the selection and implementation of procedures that best suit the learner, based on a multitude of factors such as age and maturity, proficiency in the language, reading level, gender, and other indicators of readiness.

4. The **learning situation**—the time and place of the experience—is expedited by using the best and most appropriate resources and facilities available for the individual learner.

Simons-Morton and associates (1995) suggested some basic conditions for learning that, for best results, should be present in any teaching situation: (1) The learner understands the objectives of the educational sessions, (2) instruction proceeds from the known to the unknown and from the simple to the complex, and (3) information and skills are supported with meaningful methods, including examples, practice, and feedback. Variables in teaching-learning methods are thus dependent upon

**beliefs** acceptance of or confidence in an alleged fact or body of facts as true or right without positive knowledge or proof; perceived truth

**attitudes** people's perceptions of or feelings about their environment and the things in it

**maturation** a developmental process during which a person manifests traits, the blueprint of which is carried on the genes

**learning** change of behavior brought about by experience, insight, perception, or a combination of the three, that causes the individual to approach future situations differently

**mediators** factors that facilitate or help bring about a change in personal behavior

the goals of the program, the nature of the behavior, the characteristics and abilities of the learner, the setting, the time allotment, and the frequency of the activities.

The following **principles**, or general guidelines for action (Green & Lewis, 1986), are applicable to health education:

1. Learning is continuous; it is not a single event.

2. Learning is facilitated if several of the senses are used.

3. People learn by doing, by being actively engaged.

4. Without sufficient readiness on the learner's part, learning is inefficient and possibly harmful.

5. Motivation is necessary for learning.

6. Learning is facilitated if the learning encounter is pleasant and if learning is recognizable to the learner.

7. Immediate responses, or reinforcement, enhance effective learning.

8. Transfer and generalization are not automatic; the learning situation must provide for them by presenting responses in the way they are going to be used and in ways applicable to several settings.

9. Learning is enhanced if material to be learned starts with what is known and simple and proceeds to the unknown and more complex.

10. People vary in how they perceive a stimulus, and their responses vary according to their perceptions.

11. Responses vary according to the learning environment; distractions and discomfort can interfere.

12. We cannot teach another person, only facilitate his or her learning.

13. The learner learns only what he or she perceives as relevant.

14. Experiences that involve a change in the self tend to be resisted, and experiences that are perceived as inconsistent with the self can be assimilated only if the organization of the self is relaxed.

The final three principles, attributed to Carl Rogers (1967), are particularly interesting to health educators. Lest we de-emphasize the learner's role in his or her own learning, we have to recognize our role as facilitator (in item 12 of list) and accept the learner's role as more important. As a kindly professor always announced to her students on the first day of class, "You have two teachers: you and me. By far, you are the more important." The final principle implies that the most effective learning situations are those that reduce to a minimum the threat to the learner. If the student is relaxed and comfortable, he or she will be more able to learn.

# THEORIES AND MODELS: WHAT'S THE BIG DEAL?

Theory and its value to education sometimes are underappreciated. Failure to hold the relationship of theory and real-world practice in high regard has damaged academic endeavors and research for years. Yet, as Shirreffs (1984) wrote, "One of the fundamental characteristics of a true profession is that it has a theoretical base underlying its practice." Two definitions of "theory" help to clarify its nature:

> A set of interrelated concepts, definitions, and propositions that present a systematic view of events or situations by specifying relations among variables in order to explain and predict the events or the situations. (Glanz, Lewis, & Rimer, 1997)

> A systematic arrangement of fundamental principles that provide a basis for explaining certain happenings of life. (McKenzie & Smeltzer, 1997)

Theories are testable and, when tested, can be applied to practice with confidence.

**Concepts** are major components of a theory. When theoretical concepts are developed or adopted for specific use in a theory, they are called **constructs** (Kerlinger, 1986). The **variables** of concepts are the operational definitions (Green & Lewis, 1986). They are the practical-use form of concepts.

Hochbaum, Sorenson, and Lorig (1992) described the value of theory to health educators:

> Theories aim at identifying and helping us understand elements that affect seemingly diverse classes of behaviors and tell us how these elements function. They may also suggest or actually offer ideas of how we can influence

such elements under a variety of circumstances and thereby furnish us with valuable tools for solving a wide variety of problems in our work. In the context of our professional practice, our theories can be regarded as being essentially statements identifying factors that are likely to produce particular results under specified conditions. To put it in other words, good and proven theories, if well chosen and skillfully adapted, can help us predict what consequences various interventions are likely to have even in situations we have never before encountered.

Theory can be applied in the real world of health promotion/education in a number of ways. It can

— *explain* relationships—the whats, hows, whens, and whys—allowing the practitioner to focus on a limited number of variables and providing a comprehensive grasp of the problem

— be used as a *basis for research* and a *basis for formulating hypotheses*

— be used as a *basis for needs assessment and intervention approaches*, thus for *planning*

— be used to *predict outcomes* of interventions and research procedures

— aid in *measuring the impact* of interventions and in *reformulation* and *generalization*

The quality of generalizability allows health promoters to adapt theory-based programs to a wide variety of settings.

A completely developed theory contains the major explanatory factors that influence the phenomena of interest, the relationship among these factors, and the conditions under which these relationships do and do not occur (Kerlinger, 1986). **Models,** a subclass of a theory, are less complete and detailed than theories and usually only specify explanatory factors and the relationships among them. They may draw on a number of theories to help people understand a specific problem and organize information. They are often used to represent processes, sometimes to explain them. Models can provide health educators with a framework on which to create plans for programs (Cottrell, Girvan, & McKenzie, 1999), including the implementation and evaluation of programs.

Health education/promotion has evolved without a theoretical base, indicating that its evolution still may be in its early stages. Although the theories and models discussed in this chapter have their foundations in different disciplines, they help the aspiring health educator/promoter comprehend some of the processes that affect health-related behavior. If health educators are to be successful in changing or establishing health behavior, they must be cognizant of the factors affecting behavior and how people learn. Theory helps with this process. In order for health educators/promoters to utilize theory to its fullest advantage, they must possess the requisite skills and information necessary for applying theory to health problems, feel confident that they will be able to use theory appropriately, and believe that developing theory-based interventions will produce good results (van Ryn & Heaney, 1992).

# THE STAGES OF CHANGE OR TRANSTHEORETICAL MODEL

The stages of change or transtheoretical model (Prochaska & DiClemente, 1983, 1984; Prochaska & Velicer, 1997; Velicer & Prochaska, 1997) draws on diverse theories of behavior change. It provides a description of a logical series of decision stages of change. These stages, closely related to individual motivation, are the following:

1. The **precontemplation** stage is characterized by the individual's neither considering nor being interested in change. He or she is, in fact, unaware of risk associated with his or her behavior or simply not interested in doing anything about it. The reasons for this indifference are many and varied but could include denial, ignorance, or demoralization. Of course, acknowledging

**principles**   general guidelines for action

**concepts**   major components of a theory

**constructs**   concepts developed or adopted for use in a particular theory

**variables**   operational definitions of concepts that specify how the concept is to be measured

**model**   a subclass of theory used to represent processes and relationships among variables

significant problems can be a threat to self-esteem. Examples include the obese individual who enjoys consuming large amounts of high-calorie foods and disdains exercise or the young excessive drinker who might consume five or six beers every day. Neither of these individuals believes there is a problem, or both actually may resist being informed of a problem. It is not surprising that the risk of failure, loss of self-esteem, loss of control, and possible loss of values that have maintained the previous pattern often result in defending against admitting there is a problem. Behaviors that have serious but delayed negative consequences, such as smoking cigarettes, physical inactivity, and poor diets, are frequently and easily defended in the precontemplation stage. Precontemplators who enter programs or therapy are at high risk for dropping out (Prochaska & DiClemente, 1984).

2.  During the **contemplation** stage, the individual becomes aware that a personal problem exists and considers behavior change. In this stage, the client recognizes that change often means having to give up something of value that was maintaining the problem behavior. The client struggles to understand the problem, its causes, and its remedies, and to find ways to regain control over his or her life. Clients seek accurate information and often are eager to talk about their problems. They also have a fear of failure. In this stage, the individual thinks about changing his or her health behavior at some point in the future. The first example above may perceive a link between his hypertension and his weight. The excessive drinker may perceive a connection between her marital problems and her overconsumption of alcohol. When a person perceives the costs and benefits of behavior change, he or she may become more ready for change. The obese person might seek dietary and exercise information; the heavy drinker might take steps to learn more about alcohol consumption and inquire about support groups. The contemplation stage could take months or years.

3.  The **preparation** stage merges with the contemplation stage so that the individual gets ready to experiment with the behavior change. The client undergoes psychological preparation in which he or she imagines behaving in a new way, shares the idea with others to see how they react, and tries on the behavior. This stage is often characterized by a lack of confidence and by perceived barriers that may thwart the attempt. On the other hand, the individual may gain skills that help achieve success.

4.  After a period of preparation, individuals may enter the **action** stage, changing their overt behavior and the environmental conditions that affect their behavior. For example, the obese person might try a healthier diet and begin some moderate regular exercise, and the heavy drinker might take steps to limit alcohol consumption and possibly join a support group. Although this stage may be somewhat experimental, self-esteem tends to rise because people are demonstrating their own **self-efficacy** through action. Individuals often let others know what they are doing, or other people may recognize it. This provides opportunities for others to reinforce the client's changes. More preparation and skill acquisition increases the likelihood of success.

5.  After a period of successful action, usually a few months, the individual turns to **maintenance**, a period of effort to prevent relapse to the troublesome behavior. Prochaska and DiClemente (1984) described maintenance as a continuance of change rather than an absence of change. Maintenance usually is a rather lengthy stage, often lasting years or months. Sustaining change and resisting temptation is neither immediate nor easy. In fact, relapse is not extraordinary, but rather a natural part of the change cycle (Prochaska et al., 1994). For example, smokers often have to work for the rest of their lives to avoid the temptation to relapse into the habit. When maintenance efforts fail, relapse occurs. **Termination** marks a point of total confidence that relapse will not occur and there is no temptation to return to unhealthy behaviors.

The transtheoretical model is not a straight line through the stages—it is a cyclical process (see Figure 10.1). Clients often drop out of the intervention at any one of the stages only to eventually re-enter.

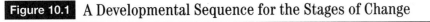

**Figure 10.1**  A Developmental Sequence for the Stages of Change

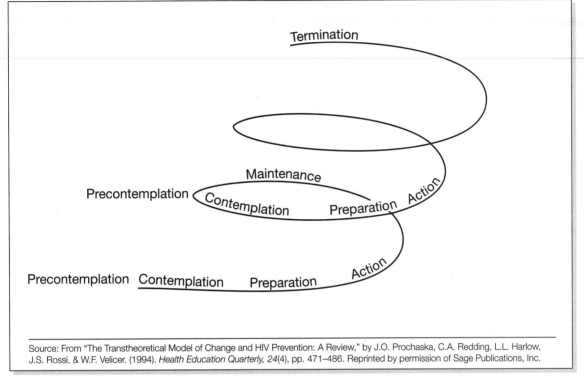

Source: From "The Transtheoretical Model of Change and HIV Prevention: A Review," by J.O. Prochaska, C.A. Redding, L.L. Harlow, J.S. Rossi, & W.F. Velicer. (1994). *Health Education Quarterly, 24*(4), pp. 471–486. Reprinted by permission of Sage Publications, Inc.

Others progress through the first four stages and relapse, requiring them to begin the cycle again. In our examples, the obese individual misses several exercise sessions, and the excessive drinker gets drunk at a party. From the action stage, both people may find themselves back at the precontemplation stage. In many cases, they may make many attempts to change before they achieve maintenance. The problem terminates only when the individual is not tempted to return to the negative behaviors and no longer has to make efforts to keep from relapsing. The duration of each stage varies with the behavior and the individual.

Although not in the business of psychotherapy, health educators/promoters can apply many of the processes identified in the stages of change model in their work with clients (Prochaska & DiClemente, 1982). Only the processes that are most open to use by health educators are included in this discussion. First, however, we will review four guiding principles

for applying this theory as a basis for health promotion design (Cowdery et al., 1995):

- The program must take a long-range view of health promotion and disease prevention.

- The program must respect individual rights and needs of employees (and other clients) and should respond to these needs.

- The program must be diverse in order to meet the varying needs of employees (and clients) and should be able to provide a variety of programs on demand, because this model requires programs to be offered upon request.

- The program must emphasize follow-up and relapse prevention.

**self-efficacy** the internal condition of experiencing competence to perform desired tasks that will influence the eventual outcome

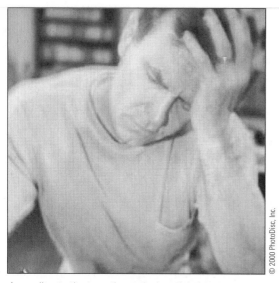

© 2000 PhotoDisc, Inc.

According to the transtheoretical model, the contemplation state is characterized by awareness of a problem and consideration of behavior change. This stage leads to preparation for change.

The theory offers a simple and effective way of categorizing a target population for programmatic attention and intervention components. Each stage presents distinct problems for health educators/promoters. The professional should recognize the importance of motivation, skills, successful experiences, and social and environmental supports in the various stages.

Research (Prochaska & DiClemente, 1983) has indicated that people in the precontemplation stage use the processes of change the least, suggesting that precontemplators have less information about their behavior, spend less time re-evaluating themselves, have fewer emotional reactions to the negative aspects of their choices, and do little to shift their attention or their environments away from the behavior. At this stage, health educators may initiate the consciousness-raising process by using attention getters, persuasive communication, broad-based community campaigns (e.g., bulletin boards, billboards, and messages on buses), and feedback. They also can help individuals become more aware of what they are feeling and thinking. Consciousness raising continues into the contemplation stage. Health educators and health promoters can provide

cues for action such as rewards, opportunities for nutritious snacks, easy access to exercise, and alternative activities to consuming alcohol. They can also use modeling and persuasive communication to alter beliefs, attitudes, and perceptions of social norms. However, professionals must be wary of using scare tactics and undue coercion. Decisions about health-related change must be made by the individual without force, intimidation, or pressure. Progress from precontemplation to contemplation can be attributable to developmental or environmental changes. Many people contemplate change because developmental processes or age milestones ("Oh my, I'm facing 40!") move them to new stages of life. Others encounter environmental changes, such as their children insisting that they stop smoking. During contemplation, family intervention may fortify awakening emotions about the need for change.

As the person moves to preparation and action, he or she may need assistance with how-to information and skill development as well as attitude change. There is usually a period of self–re-evaluation. This is both an affective and a cognitive appraisal of the problem and the kind of person the individual is able to be, given the problem. One's values and, therefore, one's sense of self may be in conflict with behaviors labeled problems. Health educators can help the client clarify his or her values and assist in accurate re-evaluation. The more accurately and openly people re-evaluate themselves prior to action, the less they may need to continue to re-evaluate themselves after taking action. In fact, continued self–re-evaluation may contribute to relapse.

The action stage is the busiest stage in the model. It involves choosing to liberate by applying counter-conditioning, stimulus control, and contingency control to the problem behavior. Individuals need to believe that they have autonomy to change their lives; thus, self-liberation is based partly on a sense of self-efficacy, the belief that one's actions have a significant role in achieving successful outcome. It involves becoming aware of new alternatives, some of which the health educator may offer; being committed to an alternative; and being willing to accept the consequences of that choice. Clients also must be effective with counter-conditioning—changing their experiences or responses to stimuli so they learn positive responses, such as relaxation. They also must be effective with stimulus control—restructuring their environments and thereby reducing the probability that a given stimulus will occur. For instance, if a person is more likely to smoke while drinking outside the home, this should be identified and eliminated.

Because action is a stressful stage of change, clients are particularly in need of helping relationships and reinforcement. This stage is ripe for opportunities for negative experiences—such as failure, guilt, coercion, and limits to personal freedom—to make it likely that relapse will occur. The individual may be more likely to continue if he or she attributes occasional backsliding to the natural process of change rather than weakness or failure (Hosper, Kok, & Strecher, 1990; DiClemente et al., 1991). This is one reason that sharing the behavior change through self-help groups, family exercise commitments, and worksite health promotion is often effective. Friends, classmates, and family members can provide excellent helping relationships, though they may require some education relating to their roles in the maintenance stage.

Preparation for maintenance is crucial. Successful maintenance builds on the processes that have gone before. Preparation for any individual's maintenance involves openly assessing the conditions under which that person is likely to be coerced into relapsing. Here, health educators can help by reviewing previous processes and examining with the client situations and conditions that present risks. Self–re-evaluation should continue, hopefully with the client discovering the kind of person he or she desires to be. As the person maintains, counter-conditioning and stimulus control continue to be effective. Controlling situations that trigger negative behavior is important. For instance, if gorging on snack food is related to gathering to watch sports on television, this stimulus should be recognized to prevent relapse.

Finally, health promoters should remember that relapse is more the rule than the exception. Neither the professional nor the client should despair over a relapse. The important thing is to return to the cycle at a point that is comfortable for the client.

The transtheoretical model can be applied to community change. Community coalitions are frequently used to create changes in community structures, policies, and programs (Brownson, Baker, & Novick, 1999). The ability of coalitions to create healthful changes depends on the coalition's ability to develop itself in a planned and organized manner. This would include developing a common vision of what they wish to accomplish and a common set of skills to engage in the change process together. It is also important that individuals within the coalition build relationships as individuals and as representatives of their respective community organizations. Building trust and long-term reciprocity builds **social capital**.

# THEORY OF REASONED ACTION AND THEORY OF PLANNED BEHAVIOR

Both the theory of reasoned action and the theory of planned behavior provide frameworks to study attitudes towards behaviors rather than behaviors themselves. Intent seems to be a splendid predictor of behavior, a measure of motivation to act. Beliefs are seen as basic components of attitudes.

## Theory of Reasoned Action

Two variables are prominent (see Figure 10.2) in the theory of reasoned action. First, the attitudes toward the behavior express the attitudes toward the expected net outcome or result of the behavior. They are important determinants of behavior. Marketers spend enormous sums of money to develop positive attitudes about their products through advertising. The theory isolates internal motivation from external influences. It also emphasizes the role of beliefs in building attitudes. Motivation is greatly influenced by the person's attitudes. If a person perceives, rightly or wrongly, that the outcome of the behavior will be favorable, he or she is more likely to pursue the action. This is highly motivating.

Second, subjective norms are the influences that others have on the individual's attitudes and

**social capital**   a sense of trust and long-term reciprocity among individuals and community organizations

**Figure 10.2** Diagram of the Theory of Reasoned Action

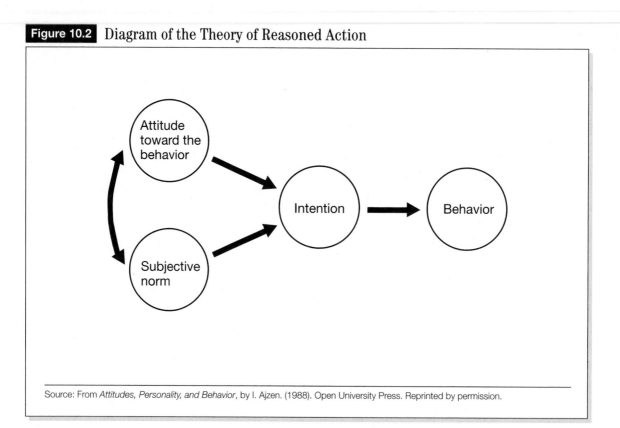

Source: From *Attitudes, Personality, and Behavior*, by I. Ajzen. (1988). Open University Press. Reprinted by permission.

behavior. What others—including parents, friends, teachers, star athletes, and musical performers—think, say, or do can greatly influence the individual's attitudes and behavior. This is important because people often have flawed perceptions of how others view the behavior. Adolescents typically overestimate their peers' acceptance of and use of drugs. Social norms tend to be more conservative than they are perceived to be (Hanson & Graham, 1991).

According to the theory of reasoned action (Ajzen & Fishbein, 1980), the person's intention to engage in a particular behavior is formed by three elements: (1) the person's own attitude toward the behavior, (2) the person's beliefs about what significant others think the individual should do, and (3) how important their opinions are to him or her. The intention includes the person's statement of intent as well as the probability that he or she will perform the behavior. Whether the person will actually perform the behavior is determined by the strength of the intention. For example, an adolescent

may be surrounded by peers who choose to predominately eat tasty, yet high-fat, foods. He may be interested in consuming a nutritious diet. If the peers taunt and tease him, the subjective norm toward the healthy diet may be a negative perception, and the intention to eat healthy may be weakened. If, however, friends and family support his intention, it may be strengthened. The theory of reasoned action states that, ultimately, behavior change is the result of changes in what people believe (Ajzen, 1988). Believing that eating cheeseburgers every day for lunch is normal for one's age group, the individual is unlikely to see the need to choose more healthy foods.

## Theory of Planned Behavior

The theory of planned behavior evolved from the theory of reasoned action. The theory acknowledges situations that are not totally under voluntary control, e.g., those involving addiction. This is the construct of perceived behavioral control, or one's attitudes about the ease or difficulty of performing the behavior. Some behaviors are more difficult than others, and the perceived difficulty of controlling the action is a crucial variable. This element is considered a result of past experience and anticipated problems that determine the person's perceived ease or difficulty in performing the behavior. Behaviors that are more difficult to execute are less likely to be attempted. Motivation is enhanced by personal confidence and restricted by lack of confidence.

As shown in Figure 10.3, the attitude toward the behavior, subjective norm, and perceived behavioral control govern the intention to behave in a certain way. The relative weights of the three variables may vary from person to person. Thus, one person may attach more weight to attitude, another to normative influences, still another to perceived control. Whatever the weights attached to the variables, the individual still controls the relationship between intention to act and the behavior.

## Applications to Health Promotion

Health promoters can utilize the theories in a number of ways. They should plan activities that produce the perception that favorable outcomes will accompany health-enhancing behaviors. Activities that refute some advertising claims could be effective strategies. They should also promote attitudes about positive social norms. For instance, through normative education they can demonstrate that most teens do not use drugs and find their use dangerous and unacceptable. Activities that cultivate skills and perceived confidence increase perceived control and, therefore, motivation. Perceived behavioral control can be affected by programming that allows for cognitive and behavioral changes to occur in small steps so that confidence about success is developed. If a health promotion program can change people's perceptions so that the population (1) has a positive attitude about changing behavior, (2) thinks important others believe it would

**Figure 10.3** Diagram of Theory of Planned Behavior

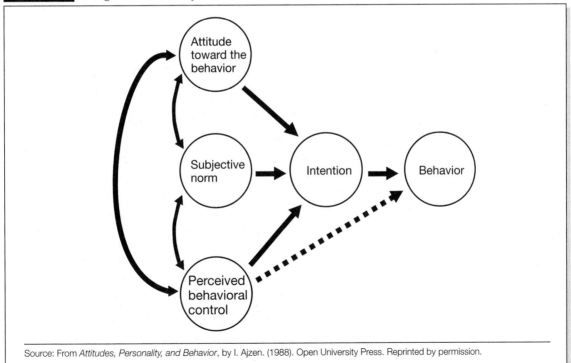

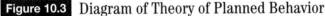

Source: From *Attitudes, Personality, and Behavior*, by I. Ajzen. (1988). Open University Press. Reprinted by permission.

be good for them to adapt their behaviors, and (3) feels like they have some control over making changes, individuals are more likely to change (Anspaugh, Dignan, & Anspaugh, 2000).

# HEALTH BELIEF MODEL

For over three decades, the Health Belief Model (HBM) has been one of the most influential and widely used psychosocial approaches to explaining health-related behavior (Rosenstock, 1991). The HBM explains and predicts preventive health behavior, concentrating on the relation of health behavior to the health and medical services available (Rosenstock, 1974). According to Creswell and Newman (1993), HBM is "the most extensive work done thus far in an effort to develop a theory and science of health behavior change." Originally developed to explain widespread failure to participate in programs to prevent or detect disease, it has been revised to include general health motivation, people's responses to illness, and behavior in response to diagnosed illness, particularly compliance with medical regimens. The HBM now provides an excellent means to analyze forces that influence health behavior. It also has applications in program planning and implementation.

Although the model deals with illness behavior and sick-role behavior, the discussion here will deal with health behavior only. Health behavior, as defined by Becker (1974), is any activity undertaken by individuals who believe themselves to be healthy, for the purpose of detecting and preventing disease in any asymptomatic stage. From the health educator's standpoint, we can emphasize the portion of behavior that has as its aim the prevention of disease and disability. The model postulates that health behavior of all kinds is related to general health beliefs that

- One is susceptible to health problems.
- Health problems have undesirable consequences.
- Health problems and their consequences usually are preventable.
- If health problems are to be overcome, barriers or costs have to be overcome.

The HBM consists of three distinct phases (see Figure 10.4) that lead to an action related to health: individual perception, modifying factors, and likelihood of action.

## Individual Perceptions

Individual perceptions are of two basic types: the individual's subjective perception of risk of contracting the health condition, called perceived susceptibility, and the perceived severity of the condition, such as disability or injury, dying, or other negative consequence. A good example is teenage sexual intercourse and the consequences of contracting a sexually transmissible disease (STD), such as AIDS, or producing a pregnancy. According to the model, the teen will be less likely to engage in sexual activity, especially unprotected sexual activity, if he or she perceives the effects of sexual activity as a threat to himself or herself and perceives that STDs and pregnancy are serious conditions. Further, the sexual activity must be perceived as causing or at least greatly increasing the likelihood of these outcomes. Both perceptions of personal susceptibility and severity of the condition are necessary to modify behavior or maintain (in this example) abstinence behavior. Many investigators label the combination of susceptibility and severity "perceived threat."

## Modifying Factors

If the individual perceptions of conditions are present, modifying factors now come into play. The ultimate decision to engage in the behavior is influenced quite heavily by modifying factors, which may include demographic variables, such as age, gender, and educational level; sociopsychologic variables, such as personality and peer pressure; and structural variables, such as knowledge about the condition or disease.

In the example of the teenager trying to make a conscious decision about sexual intercourse, the religious and moral values of the home may play a major role in the decision. Peers' actions and attitudes and the individual's perceptions of those actions and attitudes also may affect the decision. Individuals who perceive wrongly that all of their

**Figure 10.4**  The Health Belief Model

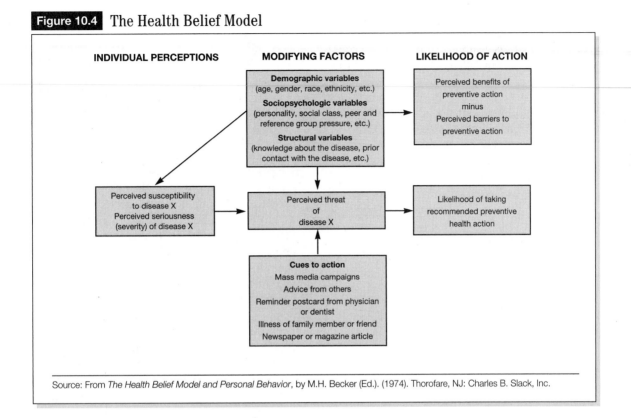

Source: From *The Health Belief Model and Personal Behavior*, by M.H. Becker (Ed.). (1974). Thorofare, NJ: Charles B. Slack, Inc.

friends are sexually active may be encouraged to be sexually active. Another modifying factor is the knowledge gained in health education class about the risk of contracting an STD or the fact that no part of the menstrual cycle is totally "safe" as far as pregnancy is concerned. Perhaps a greater modifying factor is the student's self-esteem, which allows him or her to have the confidence and independence to make important decisions without fear of being ridiculed. All of these factors and more can combine to influence the behavior.

Other modifying factors include the mass media and other sources that may act as calls to action (or inaction) based on how individuals interpret their messages in the context of perceptions. Media messages discouraging adolescent sexual activity may be consistent with messages from home, school, and church supporting the abstinence position. Many advertisements, music videos, and television programs may be seen as encouraging sexual activity but may be rejected because of their inconsistency with established perceptions related to the situation. Frequently, however, the media messages can be consistent with teens' attitudes of invincibility and exaggerated notions of prevalence of sexual activity and can therefore be a key factor in the decision to engage in sexual intercourse. Modifying factors can and often do provide both positive and negative values for the decision maker.

## Likelihood of Action

Individual action is determined by the balance or imbalance between the individual's perceived positive and negative forces affecting his or her health behavior (Creswell & Newman, 1993). In the example, the action of abstinence or at least the use of condoms gains positive feedback from family and friends. It also is consistent with the knowledge that the individual has acquired in the health education class.

Action is related to the appraisal of susceptibility. The individual acts only when he or she acknowledges personal susceptibility to undesirable consequences of the act or failure to act. The person also must desire to lower susceptibility or possess motives to reduce the threat. Action also depends upon the perceived severity of the health problem. Finally, the action is related to the individual's estimation of benefits of the action minus barriers to the action. This estimate can be a daunting task for young people to make without the help and guidance of concerned adults. The individual must estimate the effectiveness of the action and the potential negative aspect of the action. A nonconscious, cost-benefit analysis is thought to occur wherein the individual weighs an action's effectiveness against perceptions that it may be expensive, dangerous, unpleasant, inconvenient, time-consuming, and so forth (Rosenstock, 1991).

In 1977, Bandura introduced the concept of self-efficacy, or efficacy expectation as distinct from outcome expectation (Bandura 1977a, 1977b, 1986). This concept has been added to the HBM. Possessing self-efficacy, the person has "the conviction that one can successfully execute the behavior required to produce the outcomes" (Bandura, 1977a). For example, for an obese person to lose weight, he or she must believe not only that losing weight will benefit his or her health, but also that he or she is capable of losing weight.

An individual's perceptions are crucial to beliefs and actions. Beliefs are predicated on the perceived seriousness of the health problem or situation, the perceived susceptibility of the individual, the perceived benefits of taking the action, and the perceived barriers to taking action. Actions are predicated on all of these perceptions plus modifying factors such as demographic, sociopsychologic, and structural variables, as well as confidence that one can implement the action.

The effectiveness of the HBM is based upon three essential factors (Dignan & Carr, 1992):

(1) the readiness of the individual to consider behavioral changes to avoid disease or to minimize health risks; (2) the existence and power of forces in the individual's environment that urge change and make it possible, and (3) the behaviors themselves. Each of these factors is influenced by a complex set of forces that relate to the personality and environment of the individual, as well as past experiences with health services and providers.

One of the environmental forces that can influence change is the health educator.

Regardless of the abundant respect accorded to and massive research applications of the HBM, it has its critics. Some of these criticisms have merit and, in light of the frequency of the model's application, health educators should be aware of them. Janz and Becker (1984) asserted that the HBM is "limited to accounting for [only] as much of the variance in an individual's health related behaviors as can be explained by his attitudes and beliefs." Haefner and Kirscht (1970) said that altering beliefs about health may be sufficient to change actions that are motivated largely by health matters, but these alterations will be insufficient to change behaviors that satisfy a variety of motives simultaneously. Other efforts are required to influence personal practices that are habitual or that are determined by multiple motivational forces.

Perhaps the assumption most likely to be questioned is the one presuming that individuals will be receptive to messages aimed at changing their beliefs. Some research (Sorrentino, Short, & Raynor, 1984; Pezza, 1990) indicates that people are not uniformly receptive to new information about themselves. Most of us do some things we know might be harmful, risky, or dangerous. We do them for an assortment of reasons, including going along with the crowd for the fun and pleasure of the act. Nevertheless, the HBM has been a theoretical mainstay of health education and its application of structural models to explain the decision making that underlies health behavior.

## Health Belief Model and Health Education

The Health Belief Model has broad implications for health educators/promoters. Virtually every statement made thus far about the model provides opportunity for health educators to influence the behavior of young people. Programs should be based at least in part on how many and which members of the target population feel susceptible and believe the threat could be reduced by some action on their part at an acceptable cost. Programs also should be based upon the extent to which students, patients, or clients feel competent to carry out the prescribed actions over long periods (Rosenstock, 1991).

Perhaps the most obvious role of health educators lies in influencing the learners' perceptions. According to Bedworth and Bedworth (1992), before perception can take place, the individual must be exposed to an educational experience that deals with perceptions as its outcome. Susceptibility and seriousness have strong cognitive components that are partially dependent upon knowledge. Even though youngsters frequently understand the seriousness of health situations, they may not perceive themselves as susceptible. Teenagers are notorious for their feelings of invulnerability. This is a difficult perception to overcome, but overcoming it is a prerequisite to healthy lifestyles. This perception is related to attitudes, knowledge, and beliefs. Educators should address this point in curriculum development and in everyday instruction—not to impose scare tactics on students, but to help them face reality. A positive way of attaining this goal is to emphasize the benefits of the behavior. When a young person internalizes the benefits of action, logic leads to the perception of personal susceptibility.

We must recognize, however, that experiences and messages that reinforce negative perceptions also are a form of education. The plethora of advertising and media that seem to invite indiscriminate sexual behavior is an example of a message that says, "Do what you want; there is no risk!" One lucky, intoxicated trip home behind the wheel of a car provides an experience that may encourage repetitions of that behavior. Experiences such as this further strengthen the sense of invulnerability.

The health educator is a modifying force in the learner's environment. By providing knowledge, the educator is affecting a structural variable. By providing advice and support for the decision, the professional is acting as a cue to action. The health educator can organize peer support for the action. Research indicates that peer-led school-based substance-use prevention (Black, Tobler, & Sciacca; 1998, Bosworth & Sailes, 1993) and sexuality education (Milburn, 1996) curricula are superior to lecture programs led by teachers. The proliferation

of Students Against Driving Drunk and similar organizations show the popularity of peer modeling. The quality of the interaction with models and the group support are the critical elements.

Self-efficacy may be increased in a number of ways. One well-documented method is to set short-term rather than long-term goals (Bandura & Schunk, 1981). The teacher or provider should give reinforcement as the client or student moves toward the goals.

# HEALTH PROMOTION MODEL

Pender (1982, 1987) described two complementary aspects of healthy lifestyles that may have different underlying motivation: health protection or prevention, with avoidance of illness or injury as the incentive for action; and health promotion, with the desire for exuberant well-being as the primary stimulus for behavior. Pender and associates (1990) described the Health Belief Model as an example applied to the protection aspect and proposed the Health Promotion Model (HPM) (Pender, 1982, 1987) as a wellness-oriented framework for explaining and predicting the health-promoting component of life. Although many similarities exist between the HBM and the HPM, the latter is based on social cognitive theory, in which cognition, affect, actions, and environmental events operate interactively to determine behavior (Bandura, 1986). Figure 10.5 depicts the HPM.

The HPM contains the following seven cognitive/perceptual factors, which collectively influence the likelihood of engaging in health-promoting behaviors. These factors are considered amenable to change—an important and rather remarkable consideration for variables of any model proposed as a basis for structuring interventions to promote healthy lifestyles.

1. Importance of health reflects the value placed on health in relation to other personal life values (Wallston, Maides, & Wallston, 1976). Health educators and promoters can be heartened by the noted changeability of this factor. It suggests that attitudes and possibly values can be altered.

2. Perceived control of health is the belief that health is self-determined, is influenced by powerful

**Figure 10.5** The Health Promotion Model

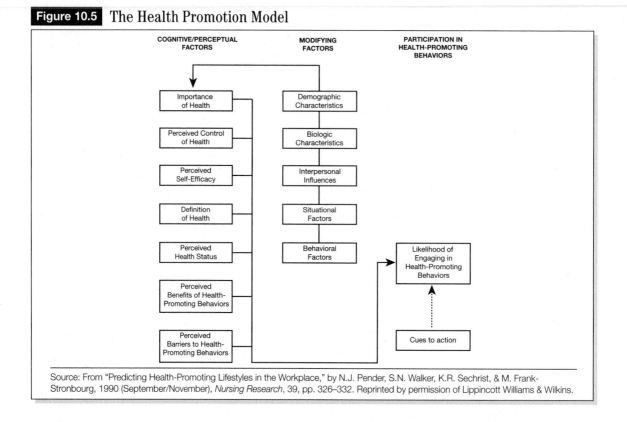

Source: From "Predicting Health-Promoting Lifestyles in the Workplace," by N.J. Pender, S.N. Walker, K.R. Sechrist, & M. Frank-Stronbourg, 1990 (September/November), *Nursing Research*, 39, pp. 326–332. Reprinted by permission of Lippincott Williams & Wilkins.

others, and is the result of chance and/or fate in some combination (Wallston, Wallston, et al., 1976). It is fair to assume that, to the extent the individual perceives that his or her health is controlled by chance or fate, interest in engaging in health-promoting behaviors will diminish. A health educator should try to assist the client/student to recognize that, at least to some extent, control of health resides with the individual. Patient educators should be attuned particularly to the person's need to understand that, by complying with treatment regimens and lifestyle changes, he or she may exercise some control over personal health.

3. Closely related to perceived control of health is perceived self-efficacy, the belief that one has the skill and competence to carry out specific actions. The specific actions the person may need to carry out may indeed affect his or her level of well-being. Confidence in one's skills in

carrying out these actions can enhance the likelihood of attempting them. In addition, self-efficacy is an important component of hardiness, the ability to withstand stress and change.

4. Definition of health reflects the personal meaning of health to an individual (Smith, 1983). For instance, does the person view health as the absence of physical illness, or does he or she see it as a vibrant condition, involving the spiritual, social, emotional, mental, and physical dimensions? No doubt, well-planned and -implemented health education can instill a holistic and positive meaning to health.

5. Perceived health status is the self-evaluation of current health as a subjective state. Various methods—such as health risk appraisals, counseling, and medical examinations—can be used to objectify health status. This, however, will not necessarily replace subjective perceptions of health status totally.

6. Perceived benefits of health-promoting behaviors reflect the perceived desirability of behavioral outcomes (Pender et al., 1990). Benefits may come in many forms—feeling better, social acceptance, more complete and open expression of love and affection, fewer days off from work, longer life expectancy—and effective health promotion can alter the perception of benefits. They also can be reinforced by gradual improvement in health status, such as through measurement of health-related components of fitness brought about by exercise.

7. Perceived barriers to health-promoting behaviors are perceived blocks to action. Examples are peer pressure—which may be lessened through refusal skills and self-concept development—or a lack of resources, which may be reduced by acquainting the individual with agencies in the community or by developing resources as part of a community health promotion program.

The HPM identified the following five modifying factors as affecting the cognitive/perceptual process and, therefore, indirectly determining health-related behaviors (Pender et al., 1990):

— **demographic characteristics**—age, ethnicity, education, and gender

— **biologic characteristics**—inherited predisposition to certain conditions, body composition, body type, and body weight

— **interpersonal influences**—things such as expectation of peers and family and social norms

— **situational factors**—health-promoting options available within one's environment

— **behavioral factors**—prior experiences with health actions, such as results of previous attempts to stop smoking

**Cues to action** are stimuli that provoke a health-related event. They may be internal or external. Internal cues include changes in attitudes or clarification of values. They may also be manifestations of illness. External cues can come from others such as family, friends, or health educators. According to the HPM, when a compelling group of modifying factors affects the cognitive/perceptual factors and cues to action are present at opportune times,

the likelihood of an individual engaging in health-related behaviors increases. Health educators can help to change or reinforce some precepts and cognitions while influencing some modifying factors. Perhaps the most significant single action the health educator/promoter can take is to provide an effective cue to action at the most propitious moment.

# SOCIAL COGNITIVE THEORY

Social learning theory was first introduced by Miller and Dollard (1941) and later refined by Bandura (1965), who more recently (1986) relabeled it social cognitive theory (SCT). SCT is especially attractive to health educators because it approaches the explanation and prediction of human behavior in terms of a continuous interaction among personal, behavioral, and environmental determinants. In determining behavior, SCT goes beyond knowledge and attitudes to include environmental reinforcement, the individual's expectations of the consequences of behavior, and social skills. Further, it addresses the behavior of the social groups and interaction of the individual within a larger social context (Resnicow, 1997).

An underlying assumption of SCT is that behavior is dynamic and depends on the environment and personal constructs that influence each other simultaneously. A continuing interaction, called **reciprocal determinism,** occurs among (1) a person, especially his or her cognitive processes, (2) the behavior of that person, and (3) the environment within which the behavior is performed. This interaction is depicted in Figure 10.6. Because the three components are interacting constantly, a change in one may result in a change in the others (Bandura, 1978, 1986, 1995). For example, personal conditions such as outcome expectations and self-efficacy may influence the likelihood that an individual may

> **cues to action**   stimuli that provoke a health-related event
>
> **reciprocal determinism**   a foundation of social learning theory; the interaction occurring among a person, the person's behavior, and the environment within which the behavior is performed

enact a behavior; the behavior may alter the social norms of his or her group; the change in norms may alter outcome expectations, thereby influencing personal motivation and subsequent behavior.

In SCT, personal factors include prior history, knowledge, attitudes, self-efficacy, expectations, and expectancies. Behavioral factors are a learned set of processes based on self-observation, self-judgment, and self-reaction as well as those related to the individual's ability to exert self-control. Behavior has a reciprocal impact on the environment and may exert effects on subsequent actions. Environmental factors center on feedback, including reinforcement, from outside the individual.

Reinforcement can be used to change behavior directly, vicariously by observing others and copying their rewarded behavior, or by self-management. Direct reinforcement can take the form of a facilitator providing positive feedback for a job done well. Bandura and Walters (1963) concluded that children also learn vicariously by watching other children and, to learn a new type of behavior, they do not have to be rewarded directly. Individuals change their behaviors because they desire to emulate role models who are being rewarded for their behaviors. The individual also can monitor and provide self-rewards, thus applying SCT through self-management. Important variables in SCT are self-efficacy, expectancies, expectations, and self-control.

Self-efficacy refers to the internal condition that the person experiences as feeling "competent" to perform desired tasks (Parcel & Baranowski, 1981) or to execute a specific behavior—"I can do this!" Obtaining a new set of skills and implementing them in real-life situations is highly dependent upon self-efficacy (Bandura, 1977b). Self-efficacy is the most important prerequisite for behavior change (Bandura 1977b, 1978) and a good predictor of behavior (Kok et al., 1991). It means the individual knows what the behavior is and how to do it and depends on cognitive processes. It influences how much effort an individual applies to a task and what levels of performance he or she attains (Ewart

**Figure 10.6** Reciprocal Determinism: The Underlying Assumption of Social Cognitive Theory

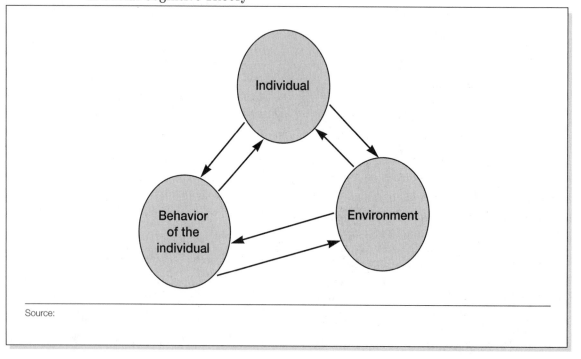

Source:

et al., 1983). Successful behavior change requires that individuals have a strong belief in their ability to exercise personal control over behavior (Stevens-Smith & Remley, 1994). Self-efficacy is task-specific, tied to specific behaviors. For example, an adolescent may be self-efficacious in sports but not in interactions with the other gender. In addition, self-efficacy generally declines with increasing complexity or difficulty of the task.

Self-efficacy information derives from four sources: (1) enactive or performance attainments, (2) vicarious experience, (3) verbal persuasion, and (4) physiological or emotional states. Performance attainments are the most influential sources of efficacy information, because they are based on the individual's own personal mastery experience. Moreover, one's perception of performance success is more predictive of future behavior than the performance itself.

The environment is considered critical in SCT because the environment provides models for behavior. According to SCT, expectations may be learned by observing others in similar situations. This is called "observational learning" or "vicarious experience." It takes place without any real reward for the learner, although he or she observes outcomes of others' behaviors. Observational learning sometimes can be a shortcut to learning, because the learner uncovers rules for behavior without the trial-and-error of personal experience. It is the basis for modeling. By purposefully observing others, we may determine whether a certain behavior or response is socially acceptable or reinforcing and base our decision to adopt that behavior on that information. In this way, behavior may be established rather than changed.

Observational learning and modeling have been used to explain why some children become involved in illegal activities and become less interested in school. They see neighborhood toughs gaining respect and the trappings of wealth by engaging in behaviors such as selling drugs, promoting prostitution, joining gangs, and gambling. Positive role models, such as those provided by mentors, are needed to depict positive social behaviors and illustrate the rewards gained from these behaviors.

Verbal persuasion, encouraging the individual to attempt a behavior or providing assurance that he or she has the skills necessary to do so, is frequently used in health education. When used alone, it is less powerful than performance attainment or vicarious experience. Nevertheless, it can be a powerful adjunct to those two sources.

Emotions and physiologic states play a role in behavior change. Bandura (1977a) noted that emotional arousal for learning can have both positive and negative effects. Stimulation and physical enjoyment may encourage future endeavor; however, excessive emotional arousal, depression, anger, or anxiety can inhibit performance. Certain stimuli can cause fearful responses that lead to emotional arousal that, in turn, can lead to defensive behavior. In this way, performance is affected by a stimulus-aversion outcome relationship. Although it is not recommended that fear techniques be utilized by health educators, learners often develop their own fears.

**Expectancies** denote value placed on an anticipated outcome, positive or negative. People will choose to perform the activity they perceive to be capable of maximizing positive outcome and minimizing negative outcome.

Expectancies differ from expectations. As a thinking organism, the human expects or anticipates certain events to occur in a particular situation. These are his or her **expectations**. For example, a teen may have the expectation that she will be offered a drink of alcohol at a party. However, recall that expectancies are values placed by the individual on what is expected to occur. The same teen may value sobriety and the avoidance of arrest—an expectancy. According to SCT, reinforcement works because the person performs the behavior consciously to obtain the desired outcome (expectancy). The individual may perform the action because of anticipated physical effects, such as pleasure or health benefits, or choose not to engage in the behavior because of anticipated pain or health risk. Social effects may include approval from family, recognition, tokens, and improved

**expectancies**    values placed by the individual on what is expected to occur

**expectations**    certain events that the individual expects to occur in a particular situation

status or such discouraging elements as disapproval, rejection, or financial loss. The social effects are particularly important with adolescents, because their identity is linked largely to peer behavior and group norms. Perceptions regarding peer behaviors and group norms are strong predictors of teen substance use, diet, and sexual habits (Botvin et al., 1993; Wulfert & Wan, 1993).

The construct of **self-control** holds that individuals may gain control of their own behavior through monitoring and adjusting the behavior (Clark et al., 1992). It also indicates that the person can gain some command of controlling reinforcers. The person's skills and choice of actions, not chance, are the critical determinants. The perception of this control is linked to self-efficacy. Developing assertiveness skills is integral to self-control. The concept of resilience, the ability to overcome negative experiences, is a part of self-control.

## SCT and Health Education

A number of techniques based on SCT have been shown to be effective in inducing behavior change. Depending on the characteristics of the individual or the population and the behavior sought, techniques may be combined. The trio of factors that interface with each other in reciprocal determinism—the individual, his or her behavior, and the environment—have implications for health educators. Professionals should recognize that any action that addresses any of the factors singly is likely to affect the others. They should also appreciate that learning usually occurs in a social context where interpersonal relationships play a role.

As an example, think about a young man who considers reducing his heavy alcohol consumption. Drinking has become an integral part of his life. He drinks heavily with many meals, drinks heavily during recreational outings, drinks when he enjoys a televised sports event with friends and at most other social occasions. A dramatic event, such as the death of a friend in an alcohol-related accident, may occur suddenly in the man's life, forcing him to consider his own drinking. Having decided to reduce his consumption of alcohol, the man is still faced with all his old drinking buddies in his old

locations. These environmental settings exert negative pressure on his decision, forcing him to seek out new friends, places, and activities. His attitude and actions may influence some of his old chums to make a similar decision.

**Revising Expectations**    Revising outcome expectations is an important fundamental of health education/promotion. Including information about the positive and negative outcomes of substance abuse, food selection, and sexual activity are examples of this process. Health educators should recognize, however, that adolescents may not be developmentally capable of seeing long-range health problems in their future. Focusing on immediate rather than delayed consequences seems to be more effective with youth (Glynn et al., 1990). Altering perceived social effects may have an even greater impact on health behavior than does improving knowledge of physical consequences (Resnicow, 1997). Social effects include perceptions of how engaging in a behavior will alter social status. The "normative education" approach, which combats adolescents' overestimations of prevalence and acceptability of drug use and sexual intercourse, is an attempt to apply this notion.

**Modeling**    Observing others executing a particular behavior is an effective way for the learner to begin the process of behavior change. This process of modeling successfully provides knowledge of what to do and a concrete example of how to do it. It can be done through demonstrations, role playing, videotapes, and films. A number of curricula on the market offer these opportunities. A key to application of modeling and vicarious reinforcement in health education is to identify the persons to emulate and discuss the parts of the behavior. These examples can be a well known person or an anonymous person in a videotape. Young people can be influenced greatly by a healthy successful senior citizen or middle-aged person. Elementary and middle school children are influenced by slightly older peers. Adults in treatment can be swayed by former patients who live vigorous lives. Behavioral capability can be developed and strengthened through modeling. Blomquist (1986), with some adaptation by Simons-Morton, Greene, and

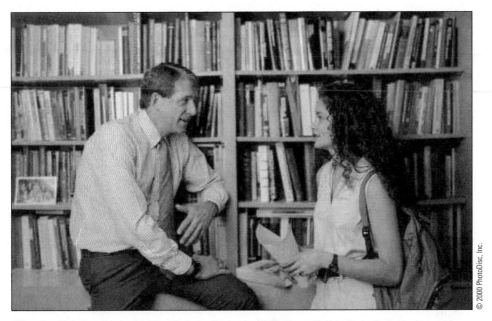

When health educators model health behavior and satisfaction with it to their students, it provides an effective way for students to learn how to begin the process of change.

Gottlieb (1995), provided useful points regarding modeling:

- The attention that the learner gives both to the model and the target behavior is crucial. It is best to select models who are similar to the learners in age, gender, race, and competence. Such qualities as likability, prestige, and status also enhance appeal as do models who already occupy the learners' aspired station in life. The use of multiple models helps increase the odds of including qualities that will impress individual learners. Also, the behavior modeled should not seriously conflict with the values of the learners. Modeling has been shown to be effective when presented with live models as in dramatizations, role playing, or, when practical, in real-life situations; film and videotape presentations are also effective as are puppets and clearly illustrated stories for children.

- Once learners have taken a positive view of the target behavior, the next step is to encourage its acquisition and retention. It is often helpful if the model describes the target behavior as it is demonstrated. Also, discussions following the modeling event that can clarify and put the behavior into words are helpful. When it is not feasible to practice the desired behavior in the learning situation it may be useful to provide for its mental rehearsal.

- The direct practice of the behavior following the modeling event can be very important even for simple actions that require no appreciable skill development. The motor reproductive process provides an additional way of remembering the behavior. When some degree of skill is required, e.g., as in breast self-examination, then instruction and practice will increase both the odds that the practice will be used and the effectiveness with which it is applied.

- The consequences of behavior learned through modeling provide the same reinforcing or inhibiting effect as behavior resulting from other sources; thus both artificial incentives and efforts to provide positive interpretations to natural consequences are recommended. Also, according to SCT, vicarious rewards or negative outcomes produce potent effects; thus, observations of models experiencing positive results can encourage the learner to make the initial effort. However, there is considerable evidence that overly dramatic scenes of models experiencing unhappy or tragic consequences for unfavorable behavior, as with drugs or unprotected sex, tend to be blocked out and ignored.

Health educators have a remarkable opportunity to present themselves as role models for children.

**self-control**    the condition in which the individual can gain control of his or her own behavior and controlling reinforcers

By exhibiting the kind of lifestyles we encourage in our pupils, we provide the model for their behavior. Educators who exhibit negative behavior such as drinking too much, smoking, using tobacco, and driving without buckling safety belts cannot realistically expect their pupils to behave any differently. On the other hand, teachers who maintain a trim, strong body through regular exercise and proper diet present the kind of image young people can emulate. Expressing satisfaction with healthy lifestyles is important to the potential of the motivational processes.

**Building Self-Efficacy**   Utilizing self-efficacy requires understanding people's perceptions about their ability to succeed. Building self-efficacy is often done best by setting very short-term achievable goals and providing practice in reaching them. Practice is usually necessary to learn skills and behaviors, particularly complex behaviors. Greater complexity requires more skills to attain efficiency in performance. Setting unattainable goals may produce feelings of failure and decrease efficacy. Taking small steps in successive increments may produce performance indicators that can enhance the learner's self-efficacy as well as acquisition of the skill. For example, setting modest but measurable goals in reducing body fat and increasing vital capacity through exercise can be useful in heightening self-efficacy. Self-efficacy is related closely to behavioral capacity. As health educators, we must strive to enhance individuals' capacity to behave in healthy ways. To know the most healthy behavior is not enough: A person also must know *how* to perform that behavior. Part of the responsibility of health education is to help the learner develop the coping skills and decision-making skills, comprehend the physical action required for the behavior, and generate the belief that he or she has the capacity to perform the action that will allow him or her to attain the goals.

Within a classroom setting, developing skills and self-efficacy associated with their use is a pressing concern. One method of accomplishing this is to incorporate simulated situations or role plays that address different risk behaviors in combination with interaction among classmates that enhances learners' ability to handle a given situation in reality

(Bandura, 1989). Skills training generally follows the pattern of describe-demonstrate-practice-feedback-practice.

**Contracting**   Contracting is a useful technique for acquiring behavioral capacity and self-efficacy. In this methodology, two or more people agree in writing to some combination of points. The contract should specify which two or more parties are involved in the agreement; what specific behaviors each will perform to, for, or with the other; some measure and criterion (goal) for success; some self-identified contingency, or reward, for successful performance; signatures of the participant or some combination of those elements (Parcel & Baranowski, 1981). The individual must feel personally capable of achieving the criterion. Contracts can be between the health educator and the client, patient and provider, family members, or any two or more people where change is dependent on the behaviors of more than just the client. Contracting is a valuable method because

— a written record is maintained of what behaviors each party expects to perform (thereby avoiding memory problems in the behavioral capability to perform)

— the person is committed publicly to performing a behavior, making other people expect those behaviors of the person

— the expectancies of the participant are taken into account by providing appropriate contingencies

— the environment is involved to the extent that these two people will do something to and for one another (thereby promoting social support)

Contracting requires some means of keeping track of whether or how frequently the desired behaviors are performed.

**Self-Monitoring**   One useful form of monitoring behavior is self-monitoring. Change processes require thinking through the intended change, setting specific goals, and providing feedback; self-monitoring is one method. In effect, it is a contract with self where the client/student keeps track of the significant action, such as food selection and exercise. Combined with contracting, self-monitoring can produce self-control.

As an example of the combination of contracting and self-monitoring, consider the sedentary individual who, with the support of her husband, wishes to begin exercising regularly. The contract is to begin at a certain level, say 15 minutes of walking three times a week for one month. After one month, the length of time is to increase, followed by the frequency until an agreed-upon target is achieved and maintained. According to the contract, the woman is to record her activity with each session. Her husband is to encourage her and provide services to make her tasks easier, such as making sure that her exercise clothes are clean and laid out in a convenient place. Rewards could be written into the contract, too, such as dinner at a favorite restaurant after one successful month and a new exercise suit after two months. This example also demonstrates the construct of reciprocal determinism. The individual's behavior can affect her by improving the way she feels and looks. For a brief period, this regimen may cause soreness and stiffness. As part of the environment, her husband can affect the woman and her behavior with positive reinforcement. Her activity also may affect the husband, possibly causing him to consider an exercise program himself.

SCT lends itself to inappropriate applications if the planner of interventions is careless. To be effective, planners should first identify the behavioral outcome and the SCT variables most likely to influence change in the behavior. At that point, the intervention methods can be matched to SCT variables to influence the behavioral outcome. The last step is to translate the theory into practical and effective strategies that help change people's lives.

## KEY POINTS

1. No single theory or model dominates research or practice in health education/promotion. The professional is best advised to apply the most relevant theory to the situation and setting.

2. The three domains of learning are the cognitive, referring to acquisition of knowledge and information; the affective, consisting of emotions, personal interests, values, and attitudes; and the psychomotor, which is concerned with human movement and acquisition of skills.

3. Change can occur in three ways: maturation, learning, or a combination of maturation and learning.

4. Theory can be applied to explain relationships; serve as a basis for research, needs assessment, and interventions; predict outcomes; and aid in measuring the impact of interventions.

5. The transtheoretical model provides a description of a logical series of decision stages of change.

6. In the theory of reasoned action, attitudes toward a particular behavior and subjective norms form the person's intention to engage in the behavior. The strength of the intention determines if he or she will actually perform the behavior. The theory of planned behavior adds the construct of perceived behavioral control as a variable determining behavior.

7. The Health Belief Model (HBM), one of the most widely used approaches to explaining health-related behavior, postulates that health behavior is related to beliefs that one is susceptible to health problems, health problems have undesirable consequences, health problems and their consequences are usually preventable, and barriers and costs must be overcome if health problems are to be overcome.

8. The Health Promotion Model contains seven cognitive/perceptual factors that collectively influence the likelihood of engaging in health-promoting behavior.

9. Social cognitive theory goes beyond knowledge and attitudes in determining behavior to include environmental reinforcement, the individual's expectations of the consequences of behavior, and social skills. An underlying assumption is that behavior is dynamic and depends on the environment and personal constructs. The concepts of modeling, self-efficacy, and reciprocal determinism are the foundations of SCT.

# REFERENCES

Ajzen, I. (1988). *Attitudes, personality, and behavior*. Chicago: Dorsey.

Ajzen, I., & Fishbein, M. (1980). *Understanding attitudes and predicting social behavior*. Englewood Cliffs, NJ: Prentice-Hall.

Anspaugh, D.J., Dignan, M.B., & Anspaugh, S.L. (2000). *Developing health promotion programs*. Boston: McGraw Hill.

Bandura, A. (1965). Influence of models' reinforcement contingencies on the acquisition of initiative responses. *Journal of Personality and Social Psychology, 1*(6), 589–595.

Bandura, A. (1977a). *Social learning theory*. Englewood Cliffs, NJ: Prentice Hall.

Bandura, A. (1977b). Self-efficacy: Toward a unifying theory of behavioral change. *Psychological Review, 84*(2), 191–215.

Bandura, A. (1978). The self system in reciprocal determinism. *American Psychologist, 33*(4), 344–358.

Bandura, A. (1986). *Social foundations of thought and action: A social cognitive theory*. Englewood Cliffs, NJ: Prentice-Hall.

Bandura, A. (1989). Self efficacy mechanism in physiological activation and health-promoting behavior. In J. Madden, IV, S. Matthysee, & J. Barchas. (Eds.), *Adaptation, learning and affect*. New York: Raven.

Bandura, A. (1995). *Self-efficacy: The exercise of control*. New York: Freeman.

Bandura, A., & and Schunk, D.H. (1981). Cultivating competence, self-efficacy, and intrinsic interest through proximal self-motivations. *Journal of Personality and Social Psychology, 41*(3), 586–598.

Bandura, A., & Walters, R.H. (1963). *Social learning and personality development*. New York: Holt, Rinehart & Winston.

Becker, M.H. (Ed.). (1974). The health belief model and personal health behavior. *Health Education Monographs 2*(4), 404–419.

Bedworth, A.E., & Bedworth, D.A. (1992). *The profession and practice of health education*. Dubuque, IA: Wm. C. Brown.

Black, D.R., Tobler, N.S., & Sciacca, J.P. (1998). Peer helping/involvement: An efficacious way to meet the challenge of reducing alcohol, tobacco, and other drug use among youth? *Journal of School Health, 68*(3), 87–93.

Blomquist, K.B. (1986). Modeling and health behavior: Strategies for prevention in the schools. *Health Education, 17*(3), 8–11.

Bloom, B.S. (Ed.). (1956). *Taxonomy of education objectives, handbook I: Cognitive domain*. New York: David McKay.

Bosworth, K., & Sailes, J. (1993). Content and teaching strategies in 10 selected drug abuse prevention curricula. *Journal of School Health, 63*(6), 87–93.

Botvin, G.J., Baker, E., Botvin, E.M., Dusenbury, L., Cardwell, J., & Diaz, T. (1993). Factors promoting cigarette smoking among black youth: A causal modeling approach. *Addiction and Behavior, 18*(4), 397–405.

Brownson, R.C., Baker, E.A., & Novick, L.F. (1999). *Community-based prevention: Programs that work*. Gaithersburg, MD: Aspen.

Clark, N.M, Janz, N.K., Dodge, J.A., & Sharp, P.A. (1992). Self-regulation of health behavior: The "take PRIDE" program. *Health Education Quarterly, 19*(3), 341–354.

Coleman, J.C. (1969). *Psychology and effective behavior*. Palo Alto, CA: Scott, Foresman and Company.

Cottrell, R.R., Girvan, J.T., & McKenzie, J.F. (1999). *Principles of health promotion and education*. Boston: Allyn & Bacon.

Cowdery, J.E., Wang, M.Q., Eddy, J.M, &. Trucks, J.K. (1995). A theory driven health promotion program in a university setting. *Journal of Health Education, 26*(4), 248–250.

Creswell, Jr., W.H., & Newman, I.M. (1993). *School health practice* (10th ed.). St. Louis: Times Mirror/Mosby College Publishing.

DiClemente, C.D., Prochaska, J.O., Fairhurst, S., Velicer, W.F., Velasquez, M.M., & Rossi, J.S. (1991). The process of smoking cessation: An analysis of precontemplation, contemplation, and preparation stages of change. *Journal of Consulting and Clinical Psychology, 59*(2), 295–304.

Dignan, M. & Carr, P.A. (1992). *Program planning for health education and health promotion* (2nd ed.). Philadelphia: Lea and Febiger.

Ewart, C.K., Taylor, C.B., Reese, L.B., & Debusk, R.F. (1983). Effects of early post-myocardial infarction exercise testing on self-perception and subsequent physical activity. *American Journal of Cardiology, 51*, 1076–1080.

Glanz, K., Lewis, F.M., & Rimer, B.K. (Eds.). (1997). *Health behavior and health education: Theory, research, and practice* (2nd ed.). San Francisco: Jossey-Bass.

Glynn, T.J., Boyd, G.M., & Gruman, J.C. (1990). Essential elements of self-help/minimal intervention strategies for smoking cessation. *Health Education Quarterly, 17*(3), 329–345.

Green, L.W., & Lewis, F.M. (1986). *Evaluation and measurement in health education and health promotion*. Mountain View, CA: Mayfield.

Haefner, D., & Kirscht, J. (1970). Motivational and behavioral effects of modifying health beliefs. *Public Health Reports, 85*(6), 478–484.

Hanson, W.B. & Graham, J.W. (1991). Preventing alcohol, marijuana, and cigarette use among adolescents: Peer pressure resistance training versus establishing conservative norms. *Preventive Medicine, 20*(3), 414–430.

Hochbaum, G.M., Sorenson, J.R., & Lorig, K. (1992). Theory in health education practice. *Health Education Quarterly, 19*(3), 295–313.

Hosper, H.J., Kok, G, & Strecher, V.J. (1990). Attributions for previous failures and subsequent outcome in a weight reduction program. *Health Education Quarterly, 17*(4), 409–415.

Janz, N., & Becker, M. (1984). The health belief model: A decade later. *Health Education Quarterly, 11*(1), 1–47.

Kerlinger, F.N. (1986). *Foundations of behavioral research* (3d ed.). New York: Holt, Rinehart & Winston.

Knutson, A.L. (1965). *The individual, society, and health behavior*. New York: Russell Sage Foundation.

Kok, G., deVries, H., Mudde, A.N., & Strecher, V.J. (1991). Personal health education and the role of self-efficacy; Dutch research. *Health Education Research, 6*(2), 231–238.

Krathwohl, D.R., Bloom, B., & Masia, B. (1964). *Taxonomy of educational goals, handbook II: Affective domain*. New York: David McKay Co.

McKenzie, J.F., & Smeltzer, J.L. (1997). *Planning, implementing, and evaluating health promotion programs: A primer* (2nd ed.). Boston: Allyn & Bacon.

Milburn, K. (1996). A critical review of peer education with young people with special preference to sexual health. *Peer Facilitation Quarterly, 14*(1), 6–17.

Miller, N.E., & Dollard, J. (1941). *Social learning and imitation*. New Haven, CT: Yale University Press.

Parcel, G.S., & Baranowski, T. (1981). Social learning theory and health education. *Health Education, 12*(3), 14–18.

Pender, N.J.(1982). *Health promotion in nursing practice.* New York: Appleton-Century-Crofts.

Pender, N.J. (1987). *Health promotion in nursing practice* (2d ed.). Norwalk, CT: Appleton & Lange.

Pender, N.J., Walker, S.N., Sechrist, K.R., & Frank-Stromborg, M. (1990). Predicting health-promoting lifestyles in the workplace. *Nursing Research, 39*(6), 326–332.

Pezza, P. (1990). Orientation to uncertainty and information seeking about personal health. *Health Education, 21*(2), 34–36.

Prochaska, J.O., & DiClemente, C.C. (1982). Transtheoretical therapy: Toward a more integrative model of change. *Psychotherapy: Theory, Research and Practice, 19*(3), 276–288.

Prochaska, J.O., & DiClemente, C.C. (1983). Stages and processes of self-change of smoking: Toward an integrative model of change. *Journal of Consulting and Clinical Psychology, 51*(3), 390–395.

Prochaska, J.O., & DiClemente, C.C. (1984). *The transtheoretical approach: Crossing traditional foundations of change.* Homewood, IL: Dorsey.

Prochaska, J.O., Reading, C.A., Harlow, L.L., Rossi, J.S., & Velicer, W.F. (1994). The transtheoretical model of change and HIV prevention: A review. *Health Education Quarterly, 24*(4), 471–486.

Prochaska, J.O., & Velicer, W.F. (1997). Introduction: The transtheoretical model. *American Journal of Health Promotion, 12*(1), 6–7.

Resnicow, K. (1997). Models of health behavior change used in health education programs. In D. Allensworth, E. Lawson, L. Nicholson, & J. Wyche (Eds), *Schools & health: Our nation's investment.* Washington, DC: National Academy Press.

Rogers, C. R. (1967). The interpersonal relationship in the facilitation of learning. In Association for Supervision and Curriculum Development, *Humanizing education: The person in the process.* Washington, DC: National Education Association.

Rosenstock, I.M. (1974). Historical origins of the health belief model. *Health Education Monographs, 2*(4), 328–335.

Rosenstock, I.M. (1991). The health belief model: Explaining health behavior through expectancies. In K. Glanz, F.M. Lewis, & B.K. Rimer (Eds.), *Health behavior and health education: Theory, research, and practice.* San Francisco: Jossey-Bass.

Rudd, J., & Glanz, K. (1991). How individuals use information for health action: Consumer information processing. In K. Glanz, F.M. Lewis, & B.K. Rimer (Eds.), *Health behavior and health education: Theory, research, and practice.* San Francisco: Jossey-Bass.

Shirreffs, J.A. (1984). The nature and meaning of health education. In L. Rubinson & W.F. Alles (Eds.), *Health education: Foundations for the future.* St. Louis: Times Mirror/Mosby.

Simons-Morton, B.G., Greene, W.H., & Gottlieb, N.H. (1995). *Introduction to health education and health promotion* (2nd ed.). Prospect Heights, IL: Waveland.

Smith, J.A. (1983). *The idea of health: Implications for the nursing professional.* New York: Teachers College Press.

Sorrentino, R., Short, J., & Raynor, J. (1984). Uncertainty orientation: Implications for affective and cognitive views of achievement behavior. *Journal of Personality and Social Psychology, 46*(1), 189–206.

Stevens-Smith, P., & Remley, Jr., T.P. (1994). Drugs, AIDS, and teens: Intervention and the school counselor. *The School Counselor, 41*(3), 180–183.

van Ryn, M., & Heaney, C.A. (1992). What's the use of theory? *Health Education Quarterly, 19*(3), 315–330.

Velicer, W.F., & Prochaska, J.O. (1997). The transtheoretical model of health behavior change. *American Journal of Health Promotion, 12*(1), 38–48.

Wallston, K.A., Maides, S., & Wallston, B.S. (1976). Health-related information seeking as a function of health-related locus of control and health value. *Journal of Research in Personality, 10*(2), 215–222.

Wallston, K.A., Wallston, B.S., Kaplan, G.D., & Maides, S.A. (1976). Development and validation of the health locus of control (HLC) scale. *Journal of Consulting Clinical Psychology, 44*(4), 580–585.

Wulfert, E., & Wan, C.K. (1993). Condom use: A self-efficacy model. *Health Psychology, 12*(5), 346–353.

# Needs Assessment, Planning, and Program Implementation

D
eveloping a program of health education or health promotion is not a simple endeavor. Done properly, it requires considerable expertise and effort. Figure 11.1 presents a useful way to visualize the process of program development. The key elements in achieving the final desired product are needs assessment, development of the program plan, implementation of the plan, and evaluation of the program and its outcomes.

As discussed in Chapter 5, (page 109) the Role Delineation Project identified seven responsibilities defined by competencies and subcompetencies that entry-level health educators should have (these are

**Figure 11.1**  Planning Paradigm

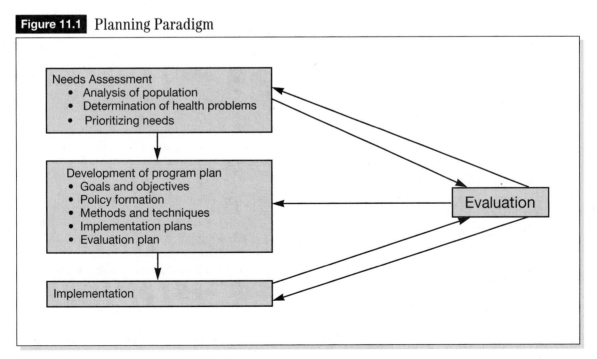

listed in Appendix B). Among them are needs assessment, planning, implementation, and evaluation. Recall, however, that the separate identification of these responsibilities does not mean they are independent of one another in this process. It is both logical and useful to consider needs assessment, particularly the determination of health problems, to be part of the planning process. To envision implementation and evaluation as part of the planning process is equally logical. This text takes the approach that the lines separating the four competencies are not concrete and that the overall planning process consists of needs assessment, program planning, planning for implementation, and planning for evaluation. It also takes the position that, as long as a program is active, these four responsibilities—needs assessment, planning, implementation, and evaluation—never end.

A detailed description of the four responsibilities can be so demanding that entire texts and courses are needed to cover them comprehensively. Nevertheless, needs assessment, program planning, and implementation are introduced in this chapter and the responsibility of evaluation in Chapter 12.

Simons-Morton and associates (1995) defined planning as "the process of making decisions as to what topic to address or what problems to attack, and where to direct time and resources." Reeves, Bergwall, and Woodside (1984) defined planning as "making current decisions in the light of their future effects." Given that health educators/promoters see their work as an effort to improve the future, such important tasks should not be undertaken without a well–thought out plan of action. Planning, however, is an endless process. The organizational environment can be turbulent, and an effective planning process can help cope with the confusion. Therefore, the successful planner must continually seek information about new developments and incorporate these data into the plan. Flexibility is a major asset in planning.

Just as separating needs assessment and planning is difficult, so is finding the point at which planning ends and implementation commences. Many experts see implementation as a continuation of the needs assessment/planning process. Certainly, selecting appropriate methods, media, and materials for carrying out a program is an important part of

the process of planning and implementation. Applying what is selected to the learner/client in meaningful ways is just as critical. Description of these competencies is more suitable to the many "methods" textbooks and, therefore, will not be addressed thoroughly here.

**Planning** for health education is contingent upon a number of factors, including size of the population, results of the needs assessment process, and resources available. A number of paradigms help clarify the planning process. Some of them will be discussed in the latter half of this chapter under "Planning Models."

Breckon, Harvey, and Lancaster (1998) set forth seven general principles of planning that serve as a useful way to introduce the topic:

1. **Plan the process.** Plan for planning, complete with timetable for planning and for the plan. Determine who is to be involved in planning, the best time to plan the program, what data are needed, where the planning should occur, what resistance is expected, and what will enhance the project's success.

2. **Plan with people.** Involve clients and consumers of the project to give them ownership in the activity and to avail the planning group of clients' knowledge of subtleties of the problem. Involve administrators, health educators, and others who will be providing the services to generate more ideas.

3. **Plan with data.** Seek out the necessary information on relevant diseases, disorders, and behaviors and analyze those data by age, gender, and other applicable variables. Knowledge of the community's problems, people, and programs is necessary to determine the context at the beginning of the process.

4. **Plan for permanence.** Plan for an ongoing, long-term program. Most health problems do not go away and require education for generations. Include planning for long-term staffing.

5. **Plan for priorities.** Spend your time developing programs of highest need and greatest opportunity for success. Prioritize your list of needs and revise them periodically. This implies

an overall assessment of community needs and agency opportunities.

6. **Plan for measurable outcomes in acceptable formats.** Commit your energy to planning programs that will change undesirable behaviors to desirable actions. Plan to measure and evaluate behavior change and to measure and evaluate reduction of the major problem the behavior caused. Think in terms of both immediate and long-term results. It is important to report measures of change in terms that are acceptable to the health education/promotion community. A useful approach would be to use the health indicators of *Healthy People 2010* (U.S. DHHS, 2000).

7. **Plan for evaluation.** Build evaluation into the program design. Develop a plan for evaluating the short- and long-term results. In planning the evaluation process, it is important to emphasize internal validity—assurance that the program, not something else, caused the change that was measured. Another important consideration is external validity—the assurance that the results of the evaluation can be generalized to other people and settings. Plan to evaluate the planning process.

The critical practice of including community members and recipients of the program in planning and implementing that program (indicated in the second principle above) is often lost on professionals. Stewart (1993) wrote

> The tendency of the professional health worker to feel his mandate has been given, and that his expertness entitles and indeed obligates him to make all the expert decisions for his own expert reasons, is not unnatural. . . . But it is a serious handicap particularly when those he serves are of a different social class from himself (which they almost always are) and sometimes reach almost crippling extremes when they belong to a markedly different culture as we frequently [find] in our communities.

People are naturally resistant to change. Nix (1978) defined five kinds of changes people frequently resist:

— changes they do not understand clearly

— changes they or their representatives had no part in bringing about

— changes that threaten their vested interest and security

— changes advocated by those they do not like or trust

— changes that do not fit into the cultural values of the community

This underscores the necessity of establishing relationships in the community—getting to know the people and allowing them to get to know you—and of involving clients and constituencies in the process. Skills-oriented training of community members can achieve these ends by breaking down resistance to change and giving participants confidence in their ability to contribute to the team.

## NEEDS ASSESSMENT

**Needs assessment** is a planned process that identifies the reported needs of an individual or group (Gilmore & Campbell, 1996). It is an attempt to understand a setting and its people in relation to each other and to the external environment. Needs assessment requires the abilities to analyze the population and to determine the health problems of that population. This analysis of the community allows for both a general overview and a collection of detailed information. Information gathered during needs assessment may be either quantitative or qualitative. This is a vital responsibility for planners of health promotion programs, especially community or worksite health promotion. Just as good physicians get to know their patients and make diagnoses before undertaking treatment, good planners must get to know the population under study and define its problems before recommending actions.

Health professionals have various reasons for conducting needs assessment. The one most

**planning**    the process of making decisions as to what topic to address, what problems to attack, and/or where to direct time and resources

**needs assessment**    a planned process that identifies the reported needs of an individual or a group

frequently cited—to use the results of the assessment as a logical starting point for program planning—is the orientation of this chapter. Assessments also can be used with the same target population on a continuing basis to detect changing needs over time. In this case, services and programs can be adjusted to fit the changing needs. Individualized assessment, which has recently emerged and proven valuable in health maintenance and health promotional efforts (Gilmore & Campbell, 1996), can help the individual detect risk factors that may threaten his or her health. Finally, there is a growing emphasis on capacity analysis or asset analysis, which addresses the capacities, skills, and assets of a community (Kretzmann & McKnight, 1993). The latter's focus on positive attributes makes it a useful complement to the needs assessment process.

Health education/promotion planners must be skilled at obtaining demographic information about people, such as education level, income level, ethnic background, average household size, and occupation. Planners also must be adept at obtaining health-related information about a group of people, such as live birth rate, infant mortality rate, death rate, causes of death, incidence of infectious diseases, hospital admissions, and access to health care. Sources of health-related data include the Centers for Disease Control and Prevention, the National Institutes of Health, Bureau of the Census, local health department, and other governmental offices. Each school district keeps records of immunization, chronic diseases and conditions, absenteeism, and ethnic makeup of the population. Other public records contain information about social issues, such as housing and average family income. Local community health organizations and hospitals constitute excellent sources of information about specific health issues and problems. Researching other sources, such as medical records, health department records, school nurse reports, and news articles, do not require direct contact with individuals within the population.

Professionals also must be skilled in gathering information about individuals' behaviors, identifying those that foster well-being and those that hinder it, and inferring needs for health promotion from the data. Finally, the health education/promotion planner must be proficient in determining the resources within a community. The major criterion in choosing data to collect and analyze is the extent to which the data will help guide decisions about planning, implementation, and evaluation. Collection and analysis of data are not the ends in themselves; they are means to the ends.

The methods and technology of needs assessment can be simple and inexpensive or highly complex and costly, depending on the purpose of the data collection. Perhaps the best starting place in assessing needs is to determine how the trait or problem has been measured in the past. Some characteristics associated with health may be difficult to measure in a functional way. Once the means to express the existence of a problem have been established, standards or other criteria can be determined to indicate the extent of the problem. The next step is to determine what information is desired, including where those data can be found and how they can best be collected. Actual data collection and analysis make up the next step.

Frequently, articles from local newspapers can help identify health problems and reach conclusions about their occurrence. This technique is relatively inexpensive and may yield qualitative information. Use of news articles, however, is a crude method and probably is useful only in obtaining general information. It is inferior to the other methods because its validity is questionable. Newspapers tend to print sensational stories and frequently omit "mundane" information important to health.

Information may be collected from individuals, groups, or from existing data sources. If from individuals or groups, data should be collected from at least a representative sample of the population under study, preferably a group chosen at random. Depending on the type of data collected, the intended use of this data, and the standard of accuracy desired, statisticians may be required to determine statistical significance. After analysis, the assessor should be able to describe the nature and extent of the health problem. The various methods of collecting information from individuals include surveys (mail, face-to-face, telephone), medical examinations, and interviews. Each has its own advantages and disadvantages, as shown in Table 11.1.

**Table 11.1**  Advantages & Disadvantages of Individual Data Collection Techniques

|  | Advantages | Disadvantages |
| --- | --- | --- |
| **Mail survey** | Low cost in money and personnel | Low rate of return (response) |
|  | Easy to reach diverse groups and wide geographic area | Some persons will respond if only to express complaints |
|  | Privacy, leading to honest answers, even to threatening or embarrassing questions | Delay in receiving responses |
|  | Encourage completion by respondents | Usually requires simple questions |
|  | Convenience to respondent, leading to more thoughtful responses | Cannot clarify questions to respondent |
|  | Eliminates interviewer-induced bias | No control over who answers survey; risk of collaboration |
|  | Validity | No interaction |
|  |  | Requires accurate mailing list |
| **Face-to-face survey** | Can easily use open-ended or complex questions | Costly |
|  | Control of time expended | Requires training of interviewer |
|  | Can encourage answering all questions | Difficult to ask and answer threatening or embarrassing questions |
|  | Assurance of identity of respondent | May get only socially desirable answers |
|  | High response rate; very representative results | Loss of privacy/anonymity |
|  | Can be a morale builder in the community |  |
| **Telephone survey** | Quick data collection | Time limitations |
|  | High response rate | Invades respondents' home privacy |
|  | Can use complex, open-ended questions | May not get accurate answers to threatening or embarrassing questions |
|  | Better able to identify respondent than mail | May be contaminated by interviewer bias |
|  | Sample may not be representative |  |
| **Medical examination** | Highly accurate results | Costly |
|  | Able to identify respondent | Requires much time |
|  | Yields quantitative information about groups that, when taken as a whole, can yield qualitative information | Some tests require interpretation |
| **Interview** | Uniqueness of experience encourages participation | May not get accurate answers to threatening or embarrassing questions |
|  | More flexible than face-to-face survey | Scheduling may be difficult |
|  | Allows for building trust between interviewer and interviewee | Requires skilled interviewer who can make split-second judgments |
|  | Allows for getting more complete information | Requires thorough training of interviewer |
|  | May record for more thorough analysis | Difficult to analyze data |

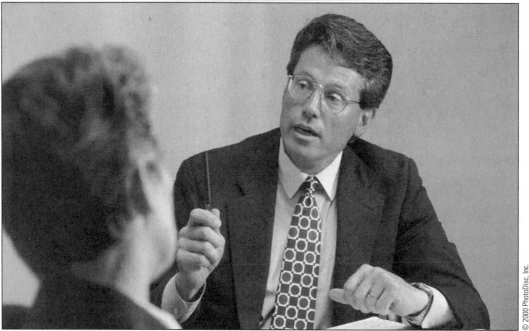

Interviews and face-to-face surveys are useful methods of collecting data from individuals.

## Research Techniques

**The Delphi Process**   The Delphi technique is a special multistep survey method that uses a series of questionnaires to generate a consensus on an issue. It can be used to identify goals and objectives, examine possible alternatives, establish priorities, reveal group values, gather information, and educate a respondent group (Moore, 1987). The questionnaire, consisting of a few broad questions, usually is sent by mail to a small (10–15) group of participants. After the responses are analyzed, a second questionnaire is developed, this time with more specific questions. The same respondents' feedback is analyzed again, and a third questionnaire is developed and sent out. Usually, three to five questionnaires are necessary to arrive at consensus.

The Delphi process uses subjective responses and is appropriate in situations where objective information is not available from other sources (Gilmore & Campbell, 1996). Because it requires a substantial commitment on the part of participants, this method usually produces ample information of high quality. The technique also has the advantage of being useful in obtaining opinions from specific groups, such as experts or victims of a health problem, when assembling people in one location is difficult.

The process has its drawbacks. For instance, a large amount of administrative time and cost are necessary. The participants also must commit a considerable amount of time. Results can be vague because there is no face-to-face discussion to allow for clarification of comments.

Health promoters may occasionally be required to assess needs in ways that involve several people at a time. There are several exceptional methods of accomplishing this task, including nominal group process and focus groups.

**Nominal Group Process**   The highly structured nominal group process allows researchers to qualify and quantify specific needs of a target group. Since its development by Delbecq and Van de Ven (Delbecq, Van de Ven, & Gustafson, 1986), it has been used by a variety of professionals, including those in health care, human service agencies, voluntary organizations, university extension services, and educational settings (Baily, 1973; Gilmore, 1979; Delbecq, Van de Ven, & Gustafson, 1986; Sarvela et al., 1991; Queeney, 1995). It utilizes small (5–7) groups of individuals who have some involvement with and understanding of the issues in question. Group members are asked to write their answers to a question without discussing it. Each participant then shares one of his or her responses in round-robin fashion until each response from every person has been recorded. Responses then are discussed so they are all clear to the group. Participants then vote to select and rank a prescribed number of items they think are most important.

The process may stop at this point, or this vote may be treated as preliminary, with ensuing discussion followed by a final vote. The nominal group process provides both quantitative data, in the sense of voted-upon priorities, and qualitative data, in terms of descriptive discussion of the problem (Delbecq, Van de Ven & Gustafson, 1986).

The nominal group process has a number of advantages. People who are most affected by a health or social problem can participate in its identification. All participants have equal opportunity to share their ideas. Because ideas are not evaluated until the end and the process is highly structured, diverse and minority opinions are tolerated. This can lead to discovery of "common ground" among those present.

The process also has its disadvantages. Because it requires a commitment of at least an hour, finding enough willing participants often is difficult. Biases may enter into the process because it encourages expression of personal opinions, beliefs, and experiences. The responses actually may differ from the intended direction of the questions, causing the participants to focus on issues different from those originally presented.

## Focus Groups

The focus group originated in the group depth interview that was developed as a form of group therapy (Boyd, Westfall, & Starch, 1981). It evolved into a marketing technique that attempts to understand consumer behavior (Folch-Lyon & Trost, 1981). Focus groups have also been used successfully in education, government, social change, and diversity arenas to identify attitudes related to the item being studied. Frequently, the technique is applied to gain introductory information to direct the design of more powerful research.

Focus groups typically are used in an exploratory manner to generate hypotheses, uncover attitudes and opinions, and test new ideas. The group usually consists of 6 to 12 people who are homogeneous on relevant characteristics and selected because they are representative of a larger group. The group gathers in an unstructured interview designed to allow participants to discuss the topic and share their feelings, attitudes, and ideas in a relaxed, informal setting. The moderator must guide the discussion skillfully so interaction occurs and participants feel free to share their opinions and attitudes while focusing attention on a single area or issue. Often, focus groups are videotaped or viewed by administrative staff through a one-way mirror. After the session is finished, the opinions, behaviors, and reactions of the group members are analyzed to draw conclusions about the attitudes and practices of the larger group the focus group represents.

Advantages of focus groups are many. First, the process is relatively low-cost. A group is easy to arrange and usually requires no more than two hours of the participants' time. Because the atmosphere of the process is not rigid, groups usually display a great deal of spontaneity and a wide range of ideas, emotions, perceptions, thoughts, and attitudes. Often, the group deviates from the direction originally intended. Rather than being viewed as a negative, these deviations may lead to insights that are relevant to the issues and should be analyzed as carefully as the other responses. The moderator, however, must be sensitive to the range of the deviation and direct the group back to the topic if necessary.

Focus groups are quite small and, for that reason, generalizing from their interactions to larger groups is not easy (Schechter, Vanchieri, & Crofton, 1990). Focus groups yield data that are exclusively qualitative, making decoding, tabulating, and analyzing difficult (Gilmore & Campbell, 1996). They also are dependent on the moderator's skill, experience, and objectivity.

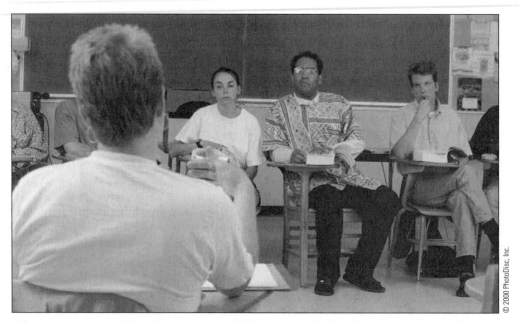

© 2000 PhotoDisc, Inc.

A focus group is conducted with students to obtain their input on the health needs in their school district.

Regardless of the methodology chosen for data collection, four essential characteristics of the process are

- **Validity**. The instrument used to gather information reveals the information for which it is used or measures what it purports to measure.

- **Reliability**. The instrument yields the same or similar results if it is administered to the same people again.

- **Representativeness of the sample.** The properties measured are characteristic of the population at large. The sample of respondents typifies the entire population regarding the issues being studied.

- **Generalizability**. The conclusions drawn from the sample can be applied to the population at large.

These methods of gathering information produce data that can be analyzed to determine the needs that health education/promotion will strive to meet. The actual process of analyzing data and exposing specific needs depends upon many factors, including the nature of the information-gathering techniques and level of the data.

Regardless of the needs-assessment methodology, once the specific needs have been reported, results of the assessment should be reported to the target group. This gives the target group the opportunity to clarify and acknowledge the extent to which the identified needs reflect the needs of the group accurately. Then the health professional and the target group can reach a joint resolution regarding needs to address and how best to address them (Gilmore & Campbell, 1996).

## DEVELOPMENT OF A PROGRAM PLAN

The individuals who will be involved in the program also must be involved in planning the program. This necessitates the formation of a committee or planning team. Members of the committee should be people who represent all facets of the population to be served as well as health professionals. It is a principle of education programming that individuals are more likely to act when their needs are being met and when they are involved in making decisions. A committee to develop a school health education program (usually referred to as "curriculum development") should include health educators, administrators, nurses, physicians, parents, community members (including representatives of community organizations), and possibly students. A committee to develop a community health education program should include citizens in the target population, health educators, physicians, members of community health organizations, and others interested in the targeted problem. Roles of the various members of the group should be discussed and agreed upon.

The successful planner understands the parts of programs and how they are expected to interact to produce an outcome. Successful planning also requires understanding how behavior is formed and changed. The framework for both kinds of knowledge is theory. Theory is the unifying thread that not only explains the condition that exists but also the action that can change that condition. Several theories of behavior change and learning that are useful in development of a program plan are discussed in Chapter 10.

## Prioritizing Needs

After analysis of the data collected, needs must be identified and prioritized. A single program or curriculum usually cannot attack all of the problems of its constituents. Therefore, setting priorities is necessary. This can be done in a number of ways, including the techniques already discussed.

If the collection techniques are planned appropriately, the data they generate also can indicate the relative importance of the needs of the target group. For instance, a survey question might ask, "In order, what are the three most important barriers to successful childrearing in your community?"

Another method is to have the identified needs ranked by a sample of the target group, not necessarily the individuals who provided the data. The group first is asked to select the five most important needs. Second, the group is asked to rank the five needs listed most often in the first step on a 1–5 scale with a rank of 1 having a weight of 5, a rank of 2 having a weight of 4, and so on. The weights then are added together for each need, and the totals present the highest priorities in order.

Another method developed by Sork (1982) and summarized by Gilmore and Campbell (1996) includes the following basic steps:

1. Select appropriate criteria. The two general categories of importance and feasibility are suggested. Examples of the former are number of people affected, magnitude of the difference between present and future status, and alignment with organizational goals. Examples of the latter are efficacy level of health education and promotion intervention, resource availability, and perceived ability to change.

2. Assign relative importance to each criterion. Criteria are weighted equally or by degree on a scale of 1 to 10, with criterion of least weight (i.e., 1) identified first, and then each subsequent criterion compared against it so the criterion weighted 10 is 10 times the weight of 1.

3. Apply each criterion to each need. A separate list of priorities is established for each criterion used, with priority values expressed numerically or through descriptors such as high, medium, and low.

4. Combine individual values to yield a total priority value for each need. One approach here is to add weighted ranks and establish mean ranks for each identified need.

5. Arrange needs for highest to lowest total priority value and indicate how priorities will be used. Resource alignment with the identified needs can be established in this step.

Green and Kreuter (1999) used another prioritization approach. Their technique is based upon a series of questions during their phase of epidemiological assessment:

1. Which problem has the greatest impact (e.g., death, disease, lost work days, and the like)?

2. Are certain subpopulations at special risk (e.g., related to age, race, ethnicity, and the like)?

3. Which problems are most susceptible to intervention?

4. Which problem is not being addressed by other agencies?

5. Which problem, when addressed appropriately, has the greatest potential for an attractive yield in benefits?

6. Are any of the health problems ranked highly as a regional or national priority?

This approach is helpful in allowing the planner to see the big picture of external forces and resources when more delimited issues for a given area are being assessed and reviewed for resolution.

## Goals and Objectives

Formulating goals and objectives is a major step in any planning process. The direction, day-to-day activities, and evaluation of a program are established by its goals and objectives. Designing goals and objectives is a major skill required of health educators.

Goals are broad statements of what is to be accomplished. They form the foundation of the remainder of the planning process. Therefore, they must be written in language that is so clear and so precise that all members of the planning committee, as well as other observers, understand the exact intention and direction of the project. Goals must deal in real terms with the problems of the target population and realistic solutions to those problems.

Goal statements should have unanimous agreement. In the absence of consensus, the nature of the planning task should be re-examined, the composition of the planning group should be questioned, and a solution for the dilemma should be decided before any further activities take place (Dignan & Carr, 1992).

Some situations may be aided by developing **program goals**, proclaiming the program's intended achievements. Usually the program goals do not describe the various program services.

The goals that are most critical to health education are **educational goals.** According to Dignan and Carr (1992), educational goals may reflect the program's effect on the agency or on the learner/client. We are most concerned with goals relating to effects on the learner/client, which may consist of anticipated changes in health status of the target population or changes in behavior of the target population. Goals may be long-term or short-term; in some instances, identifying both long- and short-term goals is useful.

**Objectives** are precise statements that map out the tasks necessary to reach a goal. Objectives are composed of two parts: content and behavior. They should be fashioned so as to make clear the content of the intervention, the type and direction of behavior change facilitated in the target population, the magnitude or degree of change, and a precise explanation of the way the change will be measured. Including the time frame within which the change will take place is useful in most situations. The reader of an objective should have a clear understanding of the requirements for its successful completion. This type of objective is a **behavioral objective.**

Each objective should be written in a complete sentence with a precise verb. Examples of precise verbs are list, discuss, define, diagram, and apply. When objectives use verbs such as these, the planner, implementer, and learner/client gain a clear understanding of what will constitute achievement of the objective.

Objectives should also indicate the methods with which attainment will be measured. Knowledge can be measured with tests, programmed texts, structured interviews, and self-reporting. Changes in attitudes, feelings, and emotions can be measured in similar ways, although these affective objectives are more difficult to state precisely and are harder to measure specifically. Behavioral changes can be measured by direct observation, portfolios, self-reporting, and reports from others. Nonetheless, objectives for all of these three domains—cognitive, affective, and behavioral—should be developed.

Sometimes, constructing **educator objectives** is helpful. This type of objective can guide the teacher by describing what he or she hopes to achieve in the area of health being examined. Educator objectives should be written only after learner behavioral objectives have been developed. Examples of educator objectives are

— to show a video on exercise
— to assign students to list the major points of the video
— to discuss the major points listed
— to demonstrate proper methods of stretching and warm-up

Educator objectives must reflect methodology within the educator's competency.

## Policy Formation

Once a clear statement of intent and direction has been established, the existing policies in the institutions and agencies that will be responsible for effecting change must be analyzed. Policies are governing principles, usually accompanied by written limitations on employee behavior and organizational action. At this point, administrators may be added temporarily to the planning committee, or at least consulted. Policies should be examined so program plans can work within the existing policies when possible.

Establishing new policies or altering existing policies may become necessary. The planner should not assume that a policy is cast in stone and cannot be changed. The process may require educating administrators, but if the program is justifiable in terms of learner/client needs, change is usually possible.

Policies should have substantial support of the planning committee and the target population, should be fair and nondiscriminatory, and should be developed to allow flexibility and creativity on the practitioner's part. Flexibility will allow for dealing with unforeseen occurrences. Policies should include a mechanism for altering the policies themselves if they are later found to be detrimental to the program.

## Methods and Techniques

The planning committee must determine how the objectives will be obtained. Once again the committee may be expanded temporarily to include consultants with special expertise in teaching methods or community organization. Methods are general descriptions of how change within the target population is to be accomplished. Examples of methods are classroom instruction, mass media, writing legislation, coalition building, and community development. Techniques or activities, in contrast, are specific strategies, such as field trips, lectures, pamphlets, public service announcements, small-group discussions, debates, and simulations.

Deciding which methods and techniques will be most effective in reaching the program goals and objectives is the key element of the process. A good deal of information already exists regarding the advantages and disadvantages of several methods and activities. Members of the target population should be consulted in selecting the methods, when feasible. The success of the method depends in large part on its acceptance by the target population.

## Implementation Plan

The logistics for implementing the program vary according to the scope of the program, characteristics of the target population, number of institutions or organizations involved, resource requirements, and a number of other factors. Implementation of a new program or service should be well planned, and the roles of the various organizations and individuals delineated carefully.

Frequently a pilot project, in which the program is implemented on a small scale, is helpful as part of the implementation plan. A small-scale beginning can reveal gaps in service and other deficiencies that can be corrected before the entire project is put in place. For instance, school health education instructional programs can be tried in one or two grades or in a single school before implementing them in the entire school district. Community or worksite health education/promotion programs might be tried out in a single site or department before being implemented throughout an area.

**program goals**   broad statements of the program's intended achievements

**educational goals**   broad statements of the program's effect on the agency or on the learner/client

**objectives**   precise statements that map out the tasks necessary to reach a goal

**behavioral objective**   a statement of desired outcome that indicates who is to demonstrate how much of what action by when

**educator objectives**   objectives that address the methodology, techniques, informational content, and other aspects the instructor determines to be necessary to achieve the behavioral objectives

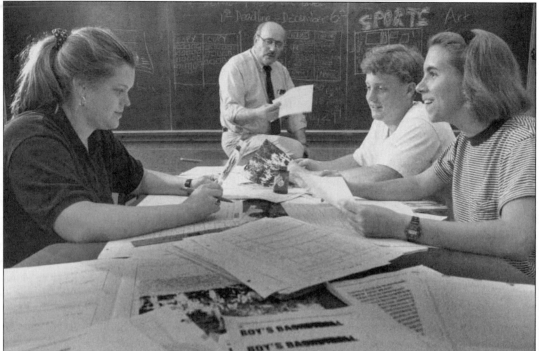

Planning for implementation and evaluation is critical for successful health promotion programming.

Developing the strategies for implementing the program can be as critical as the program itself. Care should be taken to develop a thorough plan.

At some point, it must be determined if the program actually is plausible. According to Smith (1989), a program is plausible if

— it intends to bring about some change

— its intentions are clear

— its planned activities are reasonable, i.e., they are of the right nature to influence the expected outcomes

— its activities are sufficient in quantity and quality to exert that influence

— its resources are present in sufficient amount and type for the activities to be implemented as planned

These items may be addressed at various points during the planning process, and they require some rudimentary evaluation. To commit resources, any program requires some appraisal of the plan, in terms of these requirements, for plausibility.

## Evaluation Plan

Evaluation means comparing something with a preset standard. For instance, suppose you were to measure the height of every person in your class. How would you determine which individuals are "tall," "short," or "medium?" To make this determination, you must have a preset standard defining the three classifications. For instance, you might say that a male whose height is more than 6 feet is "tall," and a male whose height is less than 5½ feet is "short." Anyone between these two points is considered to be "medium" height for males, and you would develop a separate standard for females.

Have you ever regarded one person as tall and another person as medium height only to observe them to be the same height when they are standing together? Maybe you have seen a basketball player on television and evaluated his height as "short" only to learn that he is 6½ feet tall. Certain extraneous variables—such as body type, shoe sole or heels, or (as in the basketball example) context—can lead to mistaken evaluations of height. Similarly, evaluation of the effect of programs and curricula can be contaminated by variables we do not wish to be a part of our evaluation. This is why a well-conceived plan of evaluation is so important.

Development of the evaluation plan should include those who will be conducting the evaluation and those whose work will be evaluated. Employing consultants with specific expertise in evaluation to assist in formation of the plan is certainly acceptable.

The actual processes that take place in the program should be evaluated. Likewise, the short- and long-term outcomes of the program should be evaluated. The ultimate standards by which performance of the program is evaluated are its goals and objectives. Program evaluation will be discussed in more detail in Chapter 12.

# IMPLEMENTATION

Putting a program or curriculum into action takes a good deal of preparation. Needs have been identified, goals and objectives finalized, and requirements of the program delineated. At this point, the people involved in the program must employ and train staff as well as obtain facilities, equipment, materials, and other resources. This involves contract negotiations, purchasing decisions, budgeting, and a multitude of other preliminary actions.

Green and Kreuter (1999) offered some interesting food for thought with the statement:

> In the final analysis, textbooks can offer little on implementation that will improve upon a well-thought-out plan, an adequate budget, solid organizational and policy support, constructive training and supervision of staff, and careful monitoring in the process evaluation stage. The keys to success in implementation beyond these five ingredients are experience, sensitivity to people's needs, flexibility in the face of changing circumstances, keeping an eye on long-term goals, and a sense of humor.

The essence of "quality staff" is embodied in this statement.

Workshops or training sessions often are conducted to acquaint staff with the project's plan and methods. This is especially useful when new school curricula are implemented. If teachers participate in the design and are kept abreast of developments as they occur, training is much easier. Nonetheless, workshops usually are a fruitful part of the implementation process.

At the implementation stage of the process and throughout the program's operation, individuals from the target population should be included. People are more likely to act when they can relate the educational situation to their own lives, and they should be involved in carrying out programs designed to address their needs.

However, no matter how carefully the plan is developed, the program or curriculum likely will have to be changed as it is implemented. This should be expected.

# PLANNING MODELS

Following are brief explanations of several models that are used in planning health promotion/education programs. The elements of the process of instituting a program that is depicted in Figure 11.1 (page 257) and described in the previous sections of this chapter—needs assessment, development of plan, implementation, and evaluation—can be seen in these models.

These models should not be confused with theories/models of learning and change presented in Chapter 10, which help explain how change takes place. The models presented in this chapter are used to offer structure to the processes of planning, implementing, and evaluating health education/promotion programs.

## The PRECEDE-PROCEED Model

The PRECEDE-PROCEED model, a planning model for health promotion, is an outgrowth of the professional disciplines of epidemiology, health education, and health administration (Green & Kreuter, 1999). These disciplines are dependent on the sciences of statistics, social and behavioral sciences, biomedical sciences, economics, and management sciences. It was designed to be acceptable to health promoters/educators having various philosophical and theoretical orientations and to be applicable to a variety of settings. This model is unique in that it begins with active engagement of the target population in defining the desired final outcome and works backward, asking what factors must precede that result (Gilbert & Sawyer, 1995).

PRECEDE is an acronym for **p**redisposing, **re**inforcing, and **e**nabling **c**auses in **e**ducational **d**iagnosis and **e**valuation. The PRECEDE framework, developed by Green et al. (1980), provides a highly focused target of intervention and renders insights concerning evaluation. PRECEDE was enriched and expanded in PROCEED, an acronym for **p**olicy, **r**egulatory, and **o**rganizational **c**onstructs in **e**ducational and **e**nvironmental **d**evelopment. PRECEDE and PROCEED (used in this order) provide a continuous series of steps or phases of planning, implementation, and evaluation. Identifying priorities and setting objectives in the PRECEDE phases

provide the objects and criteria for policy, implementation, and evaluation in the PROCEED phases (Green & Kreuter, 1999). The framework starts with the final consequences of behavior and conditions and works backward to the original causes. This forces the planner to begin the planning process from the outcome end, asking the *why* before the *how*. Figure 11.2 presents the PRECEDE-PROCEED framework. Phases occur in numerical order.

In *Phase 1*, the **social assessment**, the quality of life of the population is assessed, producing a picture of some of the general hopes or problems of concern to people. Social assessment is best accomplished by involving community members in a self-study. The subjective assessment of quality of life

---

**Figure 11.2**   PRECEDE-PROCEED Model for Health Promotion Planning

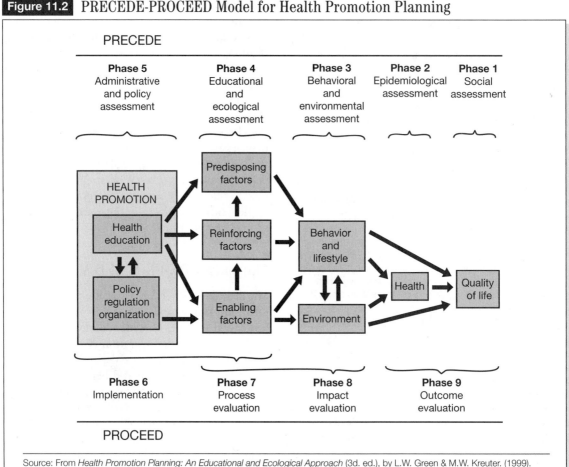

Source: From *Health Promotion Planning: An Educational and Ecological Approach* (3d. ed.), by L.W. Green & M.W. Kreuter. (1999). Mountain View, CA: Mayfield. Reprinted with permission of the publisher.

offers a view of a particular situation through the eyes of the community residents themselves, showing where health lies in the context of their lives. Among the means to accomplish this task are the Delphi technique, nominal group process, and focus groups. General social problems—for instance, unemployment, hostility, and crime—are strong indicators of the quality of life. Many quality-of-life indicators and factors associated with them can be expressed numerically as population density, crime rates, and dropout rates. These are obtainable readily from government offices, behavioral sciences literature, and similar sources. Quality-of-life concerns must be considered before assigning priority to problems because planning is enhanced if goals are known. This practice conserves resources, informs the client (learner) of expected outcomes in advance, and strengthens evaluations. Phase 1 relies on epidemiological and social sciences methods and information.

Three steps are foundations of the first four phases of PRECEDE. These steps are

- Self-study by the community (with or without technical assistance) of its needs, aspirations, and resources or assets

- Documentation of the presumed causes of the needs or determinants of the desired goals

- Decision on the priorities to be assigned among the problems, needs, or goals based on perceived importance and presumed changeability, and formulation of quantified goals and objectives

*Phase 2*, the **epidemiological assessment**, involves identifying health goals or problems associated with the quality of life. It is also dependent upon epidemiology and social sciences. In this phase, the planner must (1) identify the specific goals or situations contributing to the social problems, and (2) select the specific health problems most deserving of attention. In order to accomplish these tasks, the planner must gain access to epidemiological data, combine those data with information documenting the social concerns and needs of the population, and use both as the basis for discussion and negotiation to establish program priorities and strategies. The epidemiological data can show, for instance, the total number of active or existing cases of a disease (its **prevalence**), the number of new cases of a disease in a certain period of time (its **incidence**), and how health problems are distributed in a population. These types of information can suggest the importance of the health problems in relation to quality of life. This is essentially needs assessment.

Setting priorities for health promotion is often a challenging exercise. Among several issues to include in the decision are the degree of impact the health problem causes, its susceptibility to intervention, and the presence of existing interventions by other agencies. **Program objectives** should now be developed, based upon the risk factors of the specifically defined health problem. Objectives should specify who (target population) will receive the program, what health benefit they will receive, how much of that benefit should be received, and by when it should be received.

*Phase 3*, the **behavioral** and **environmental assessment**, identifies specific health-related behaviors

**social assessment**   the application, through broad participation, of multiple sources of information designed to expand people's understanding of their own quality of life and aspirations for the common good

**epidemiological assessment**   the delineation of the extent, distribution, and causes of a health problem in a defined population

**prevalence**   total number of active or existing cases of a disease

**incidence**   number of new cases of a disease in a certain period of time

**program objectives**   precise statements that address who will receive the program, what health benefit they will receive, how much of that benefit should be received, and when that benefit should be achieved

**behavioral assessment**   a systematic analysis of the behavioral links to the goals or problems identified in the epidemiological and social assessments

**environmental assessment**   (also called ecological assessment) a systematic analysis of factors in the social and physical environment that interact with behavior to produce health effects or quality-of-life outcomes (adapted from Green & Kreuter, 1999)

and environmental factors linked to the health problem selected. The Phase 3 planner should be familiar with social and behavioral theory and concepts. This phase calls for an analysis of the personal and collective actions most pertinent to controlling the determinants of health or quality-of-life issues selected in Phases 1 and 2. In addition, it calls for analysis of the immediate environmental circumstances that may be constraining or conditioning behavior or that may be directly influencing health or quality-of-life issues. Nonbehavioral factors such as age, genetics, climate, residence, mental impairment, and gender were identified in Phase 1 as possible contributors to health problems. Being aware of environmental factors and nonbehavioral factors helps reinforce the limitations of programs that consist only of health education directed at changing personal behavior. It helps keep perspective on the multiple determinants of the health problem, helps identify high-risk population groups, allows for recognition of the powerful social forces that can be influenced by organizational strategies, and identifies factors for which strategies other than health education (perhaps political, social, or economic) may be developed.

Failure to identify and rank the lifestyle and **environmental factors** influencing the desired outcomes will result in disintegration of the planning process. The planner establishes cause-and-effect relationships between health of the population and behavioral and environmental factors. Target behaviors are selected, and an approach to changing them is stated in the form of behavioral objectives.

Behavioral assessment is a five-step process:

1. Delineating the behavioral and nonbehavioral causes of the health problem

2. Developing a classification of behaviors, i.e., dividing the list of behavioral factors into preventive factors and treatment procedures, so that highly specific actions can be used as a basis for specifying the behavioral objectives of the program

3. Rating behaviors in terms of importance (based upon demonstrating a clear link between the behavior and the health problem) and frequency of occurrence

4. Rating behaviors in terms of changeability

5. Choosing behavioral targets based upon importance and changeability

After completing the five-step process, the final procedure for the health education planner in the behavioral assessment step is to prepare precise behavioral objectives.

Environmental assessment is also a five-step process:

1. Identifying which environmental causes of the health problem are changeable

2. Rating environmental factors' relative importance based on strength of the relationship of the factor to the health or quality-of-life goal or problem and on the incidence, prevalence, or number of people affected by the environmental factor

3. Rating environmental factors' changeability; narrowing down the list based on relative changeability

4. Choosing environmental targets

5. Stating objectives for environmental change in quantitative terms

In *Phase 4,* **educational and ecological assessment,** factors that have the potential to effect behavioral and environmental change are identified and sorted. The three kinds of factors most responsive to health promotion are

1. Antecedents to behavior that provide the rationale or motivation for the behavior, called predisposing factors, including knowledge, beliefs, attitudes, values, genetic predispositions, and early childhood experiences

2. Antecedents to behavior that allow a motivation to be realized, called enabling factors, such as presence of and accessibility to community resources, transportation, skills, laws and statutes, or barriers

3. Factors following a behavior that provide the continuing reward or incentive for the persistence or repetition of the behavior, called reinforcing factors, which may be tangible or imagined; may be delivered by self, family, peers, teachers, or others; and may include praise from others, the pleasure of an action, or demeaning attitudes of peers

At the center of educational assessment is selecting the factors—from among the predisposing, enabling, and reinforcing factors above—that, if modified, will help to bring about the desired changes. After identifying and sorting factors into the above three categories, the planning team sets priorities among the categories and establishes priorities within the categories.

Criteria for setting priorities are importance and changeability. Importance is estimated by judging prevalence, immediacy (how urgent or compelling the factor is), and necessity (whether the factor must be present for change to occur). Changeability is often estimated based on the results of previous programs or predictions made from examining relevant theories.

Finally, learning and resource objectives are formulated. Learning objectives define the targeted predisposing factors and skills to be developed in the targets of intervention at the end of the program. Resource objectives define the environmental enabling factors that should be present at the end of the program.

*Phase 5*, the **administrative** and **policy assessment**, involves assessing organizational and administrative capabilities and résources for developing and implementing a program. Limitations of resources, policies, abilities, and time are assessed (as discussed in "Policy Formation" above). These limitations can be defeated by collaboration with other agencies or development of coalitions and political alliances. The policies you can use to support your program or that need to be changed should also be identified. Administrative assessment is a three-step process:

1. Assessment of resources needed, including time, personnel, and money

2. Assessment of available resources

3. Assessment of factors influencing implementation, including staff commitment and attitudes, previously accepted goals and objectives, community circumstances, training, supervision, and political issues

Policy assessment is the appraisal of conditions that are "locked in" by existing policies and regulations because of legal, political, or environmental conditions. It includes (1) assessment of the organizational mission, policies, and regulations; and (2) assessment of political forces. Policies and regulations can be used to implement programs or obstruct them. Utilizing political forces and understanding the system can greatly enhance the chances of implementing a program successfully.

At some point in the process, educational strategies must be selected to affect the predisposing, reinforcing, and enabling factors. In the PRECEDE-PROCEED framework, it is mentioned after Phase 5. Obviously, a wide selection of methodologies is available. Some examples of educational strategies are simulations and games, programmed learning, educational television, audiovisual aids, and mass media. A variety of educational strategies is preferable to a single method. All three categories of factors should receive attention. Other health promotion tactics include community organization, political action, and coalition building. The more complex the cause of the behavioral problem, the greater is the range of strategies required.

Implementation, *Phase 6*, and planning are functionally merged. This is the point at which PRECEDE and PROCEED meet. Knowledge of political, education, and administrative theory are requisite to success.

Three types or "levels" of evaluation make up Phases 7, 8, and 9. Evaluation may be viewed as the comparison of an object of interest against a standard

---

**environmental factors**   determinants outside the person that can be modified to support behavior, health, or quality of life

**educational and ecological assessment**   the delineation of factors that predispose, enable, and reinforce a specific behavior or that, through behavior, affect environmental changes

**administrative assessment**   an analysis of the policies, resources, and circumstances prevailing in an organization that facilitate or hinder the development of the health promotion program

**policy assessment**   appraisal of conditions that are presumed unchangeable in existing policies and regulations

of acceptability. Process evaluation is that of professional practices. Impact evaluation assesses the immediate result of the program on knowledge, attitudes, and behavior. Outcome evaluation (which may not be completed for years) is the evaluation of long-term effects of the program—the outcome as measured by the change in quality of life. Although evaluation appears near the end of the PROCEED framework, it should be continuous, an integral part of the model from the outset. Making it so requires skills in political and administrative sciences and in community organization.

The PRECEDE-PROCEED framework is founded upon two fundamental propositions (Green & Kreuter, 1999):

- Health and health risks have multiple determinants.
- Because health and health risks are determined by multiple causes, attempts to effect behavioral, environmental, and social change must be multidimensional or multisectoral.

All health educators would be wise to hold these two propositions in the forefront of their planning and execution of their art.

## Planned Approach to Community Health (PATCH)

PATCH is a process designed to help communities achieve their own objectives. The PATCH approach is an adaptation of the PRECEDE model. PATCH was developed by the Centers for Disease Control and Prevention staff as a way of reconciling the federal funding requirements (that were locked into specific disease categories) with the community development principles of local planning for the needs that communities identify themselves. PATCH helps communities establish a health promotion team, collect and use local data, set health priorities, and design and evaluate interventions. Figure 11.3 illustrates the circular philosophy of PATCH, starting with mobilizing the community. The community is

**Figure 11.3**   The Five Phases of PATCH

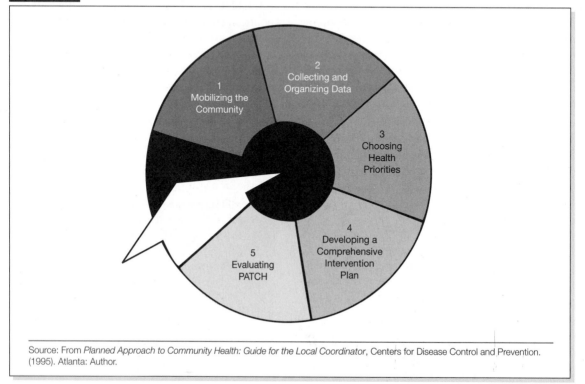

Source: From *Planned Approach to Community Health: Guide for the Local Coordinator*, Centers for Disease Control and Prevention. (1995). Atlanta: Author.

involved in data collection, which leads to choosing health priorities for action and developing intervention plans. Finally, evaluation is used to continue community involvement. The evaluation provides information about continuing problems and encourages a search for alternative interventions, thus refreshing the process.

PATCH is based on the postulate that the most effective center for health promotion is the community and that decisions for social change affecting the more complicated lifestyle issues can be made best collectively and in close proximity to those affected. It is a networking model of planning. Vertical networks include local, state, and national levels of government and nongovernmental agencies. Horizontal networks function at local, state, and national levels and form connections among the broad range of agencies that serve the target population. This often leads to creation of coalitions of local organizations. Figure 11.4 illustrates this networking approach.

Multisectoral collaboration is a key to PATCH. Support is modeled to emanate from central levels, including federal offices and national organizations, to local levels, linking local, state, and federal public health agencies in efforts applied at the local level. This support often comes in the form of limited start-up funding, information, technical assistance, and direct leadership. Often, local planners are brought into contact with state and federal agencies stationed to provide support to health promotion endeavors. Horizontal communication is encouraged among central-level organizations that have local counterparts who need support to collaborate. This improves communication among several agencies at the federal level, among statewide public and private organizations, and among local groups and individuals.

The guiding principles behind PATCH are (CDC,1995)

- *Community members participate in the process.* Fundamental to PATCH is active participation

**Figure 11.4** Mobilizing Vertical and Horizontal Communications and Support Among the National, Regional, and Community Levels

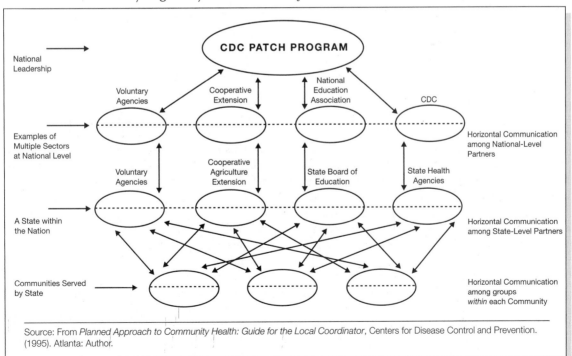

Source: From *Planned Approach to Community Health: Guide for the Local Coordinator*, Centers for Disease Control and Prevention. (1995). Atlanta: Author.

by a wide range of community members. These people analyze community data, set priorities, plan intervention activities, and make decisions on health priorities in their communities.

- *Data guide the development of programs.* Many types of data can describe a community's health status and needs. These data can also help community members design appropriate interventions.

- *Participants develop a comprehensive health promotion strategy.* Community members analyze the factors that contribute to an identified health problem. They review community policies, services, and resources and design an overall community health promotion strategy. Interventions —which may include educational programs, mass media campaigns, policy advocacy, and environmental measures—are conducted in various settings, such as schools, health care facilities, community sites, and worksites. Participants are encouraged to relate intervention goals to the appropriate national health objectives.

- *Evaluation emphasizes feedback and program improvement.* Timely feedback is essential to the people involved in the program. Evaluation can also lead to improvements in the program.

- *The community capacity for health promotion is increased.* The PATCH process can be repeated to address various health priorities. PATCH aims to increase the capacity of community members to address health issues by strengthening their community health planning and health promotion skills.

The PATCH goals are (1) creating a practical mechanism through which effective community health education action could be targeted to address local level health priorities and (2) providing a means wherein state health education agencies would work with local leaders to establish community health education programs through a skills-based program of technical assistance (Nelson et al., 1989). Using the guiding principles above, these goals are achievable. Community intervention—including elements such as a strong core of local support and participation in the process; collection of local data and analysis of health issues; multiple intervention strategies designed to meet objectives developed from community analysis; continuous monitoring of problems and evaluation of strategies; and acquisition of public health system support—was organized within the PRECEDE framework (Green et al., 1980; Green & Kreuter, 1999).

## Mico's Model for Health Education Planning

Mico's (Ross & Mico, 1980) model for health education planning (also applicable to health promotion) is designed in two dimensions, as shown in Table 11.2. The model is divided into six phases, from bottom to top:

1. Initiation of the planning activity
2. Needs assessment
3. Goal setting
4. Planning or programming the activity
5. Implementing the activity
6. Evaluating the activity's effectiveness

The three columns identify the

— activity's content or subject matter
— steps and techniques (methods) associated with each horizontal phase
— process or interactions involved in each phase

Success or failure of the activity often depends upon what happens in Phase 1 (Initiate). The key elements are understanding the clients' problems and the clients' system, devising an entry strategy, making an initial contract, and making the clients aware that a problem exists so they are ready to change. Obviously, the health educator's credibility is pivotal to initial success of the project.

The contract (item 2 in the method dimension) is an initial commitment from the client and does not necessarily have to be in writing. It is used to build trust and to develop readiness in the client. It also clarifies what is expected of each party, describes the scope and conditions of the activity, identifies the resources needed, and carries provisions for change if conditions warrant.

**Table 11.2** Mico's Model for Health Education Planning

| | Content Dimension | Method Dimension | Process Dimension |
|---|---|---|---|
| **Phase 6: Evaluation** | 4. Knowledge of problem and client systems | 4. Redefine problem and standards | 4. Consensus of new definitions |
| | 3. Technology of feedback systems | 3. Feedback to activity, accountability | 3. Communication, threat reduction |
| | 2. Language and systems | 2. Data collection and analysis | 2. Learning assimilation |
| | 1. Nature of evaluation | 1. Clarify evaluation measures | 1. Agreement |
| **Phase 5: Implementation** | 4. Writing skills | 4. Reporting | 4. Communications |
| | 3. Dynamics of problem solving | 3. Problem solving | 3. Creative conflict resolution, win-win |
| | 2. Knowledge of subject and content T & TA[3] being provided for | 2. Training and technical assistance | 2. Skill development, helping |
| | 1. Knowledge of plan, how it is to work | 1. Initiate activity | 1. Communications, orientations |
| **Phase 4: Planning/ Programming** | 3. Nature of political process | 3. Negotiate commitments, MOAs[2] | 3. Negotiation |
| | 2. Systems analysis and management science | 2. Design management systems and tools | 2. Role clarification, communications |
| | 1. Techniques of planning | 1. Develop implementation plan | 1. Understanding and commitment |
| **Phase 3: Goal Setting** | 5. Theory of change | 5. Determine strategies for implementation | 5. Consensus |
| | 4. MBO[1] technology | 4. Select goals and objectives | 4. Decision making, consensus |
| | 3. Forecasting | 3. Alternative goals statement, force-field analysis | 3. Reality testing, creative problem solving |
| | 2. Nature of policy | 2. Link to policy development | 2. Understanding of process and rules |
| | 1. Role of goals, how to set them, measure | 1. Establish criteria for goals | 1. Agreement |
| **Phase 2: Needs Assessment** | 4. Relevance of data | 4. Describe nature and extent of problem | 4. Reduce fantasy by fact |
| | 3. Language of systems | 3. Data collection and analysis | 3. Open communications, sensitivity to data sources |
| | 2. Data sources | 2. Determine data to be collected | 2. Agreement |
| | 1. Standards and criteria | 1. Identify and review present criteria | 1. Agreement on starting point |
| **Phase 1: Initiate** | 3. Power and influence structures community organization, culture | 3. Organize concerned | 3. Involvement, leadership, values clarification |
| | 2. Contract terminology and resources | 2. Develop initial contract | 2. Legitimacy, commitment, trust, readiness |
| | 1. Knowledge of problem and client system | 1. Entry or intervention strategy, force-field analysis, interviewing | 1. Unfreezing, threat reduction, credibility, awareness of need |

[1] MBO: Management by objective     [2] MOA: Memoranda of agreement     [3] T & TA: Training and technical assistance

Source: H.S. Ross, and P.R. Mico, *Theory and Practice in Health Education* (Mountain View, CA: Mayfield Publishing, 1980). Reprinted by permission.

Leaders in the community or organization must be identified in Phase 1. The leadership's knowledge of health education must be adequate to ensure success. Values of those involved—leaders, consumers, and providers—must be clarified to lessen the possibility of later conflict.

Phase 2 of the model is Needs Assessment. Mico pointed out that the technology for needs assessment can be simple and inexpensive or highly refined and costly, depending on the purpose. This phase has four steps:

1. Identify how the problem has been measured in the past. This can help bring the problem into focus. All the major performers should agree on the starting point of the assessment, the standards and criteria, and the nature and extent of the problem. A good starting point is the methods used to measure the problem in the past.

2. Determine what data to collect and how to collect them. The planning committee must agree on approaches and on why each is important.

3. Collect and analyze the data. Planning for this step requires becoming familiar with the technical approaches and methods, costs, practicality, and effectiveness of various data collection and analysis methods so sensible decisions can be made. The approach taken by the committee must be agreed upon. Therefore, open communication among the committee, the health educator, and the client (learner) is essential.

4. Describe the nature and extent of the problem, based upon accurate data and expert analysis of those data.

Phase 3 is Goal Setting. Mico defined "goal" as a future event toward which a committed endeavor is directed. He defined objectives as steps to be taken in pursuit of a goal. Objectives often carry built-in indicators of success. Phase 3 entails a five-step operation:

1. Establish criteria for goals. As an example of criteria, goals must be measurable events and they must be framed in a reasonable time.

2. Ensure that goal setting is linked to the organizational or community policy development. This is important because policy is the driving force behind the organization of systems necessary to carry out the plan.

3. Make a comprehensive statement of alternative goals and the effects or consequences of each. This requires the ability to project into the future to anticipate changes that are likely to occur.

4. Select goals to pursue from the list of alternatives. Several models of decision making can be applied to this step. Mico strongly recommended total group support in decision making.

5. Develop strategies for implementing goals.

In Phase 4 of the Mico model, Planning/Programming, an implementation plan is established, systems and tools for managing the activity are designed, and commitment from those involved is negotiated. This is a three-step phase:

1. Develop written plans. This may take concentrated study of planning methods and requires understanding and commitment.

2. Design management systems and tools. The design must: (a) ensure continuity of effort as an activity proceeds toward its goal, (b) monitor the activity's implementation, (c) keep communication open among the plan's elements and people, and (d) institute a prevention/intervention system to determine if a problem is developing. If a problem is apparent, the problem can be overcome by dealing with its indicators. Mico endorses management by objectives (MBO), a system of management based on establishing specific actions to be carried out or end results to be attained. MBO includes information regarding the resources and time frames necessary to carry out the tasks, as well as the identity of those responsible for implementation.

3. Negotiate commitments. This can be done through written documents called memoranda of agreement or through the contract mentioned in Phase 1. Sometimes this requires considerable political and negotiating skills.

Phase 5, Implementation, has four steps:

1. Initiate the activity. This involves providing assistance to participants, problem solving, and reporting progress. (One could argue that the

actual initiation began with the first entry or intervention by a health educator or the planning committee.)

2. Provide ongoing training, technical assistance, and consultation. Helping people to do a better job enhances the learning value of the activity. Frequently, training courses and technical manuals must be developed.

3. Deal constructively with problems as they arise.

4. Report or document the activity's ongoing progress so everyone is informed.

Phase 6, Evaluation, is a four-step procedure that is crucial to success of the new program.

1. Clarify the evaluation measures. If the objectives initially had built-in measurement indicators, evaluation can begin by identifying and reviewing those measures. This step includes accountability for funds and other resources. Some members of the team may have expertise in interpreting measurement indicators and results; others may not. Everyone must understand the measures.

2. Collect and analyze data. This will reveal the results of the activity and the reasons for them.

3. Report the evaluation so participants will have feedback on the extent of success of the activity.

4. Use what was learned in evaluation to redefine the problem, and refine measures and standards to determine its nature and extent. Well planned and well executed evaluation can contribute to the self-renewal of a program and give it continual energy.

## Multilevel Approach To Community Health (MATCH)

MATCH (Simons-Morton et al., 1988) is a socioecological health promotion framework. As a conceptual model, it can be useful in situations where extensive local needs assessments are not possible due to the rapid pace of contemporary health education and health promotion practice (Simons-Morton, et al., 1995). Figure 11.5 depicts the levels of MATCH as well as the five phases that assist planners in developing programs and establishing

links among health outcomes, intervention objectives, and intervention approaches.

MATCH is ecological because it is an integrated whole, recognizing that the factors that influence health and health behavior are interrelated and occur at multiple societal levels. The MATCH planner takes into account the many determinants of health and focuses on specific local actions to address them. The approach is designed to be applied when behavioral and environmental risk and protective factors for disease and injury are generally known and when general priorities for action have been determined. Thus, much of the needs assessment function has already been completed before MATCH is implemented.

Interventions can be directed at five societal levels—individual, interpersonal, organizational, societal, and governmental—and at different practice settings, including schools, worksite, health care, and community.

1. Individual-level behaviors, while substantially controlled by the individual, are also influenced by environmental factors.

2. The interpersonal level includes friends, family, and health care providers.

3. Organizational factors include policies, resources, and programs to affect health and behavior; churches, schools, and businesses are influential organizations.

4. Societal perspectives, trends, and support for programs, practices, and policies can be serious influences on health. The societal level includes any group of people, often unknown to the target population, with whom that population interacts.

5. Government factors include resources, programs, policies, legislation, and environmental controls.

Many factors within the five societal levels are possible targets for health promotion programming within many different practice settings.

MATCH consists of five phases: goals selection, intervention planning, program development, implementation preparations, and evaluation. Each phase consists of several steps.

## Figure 11.5   MATCH: Multilevel Approach to Community Health

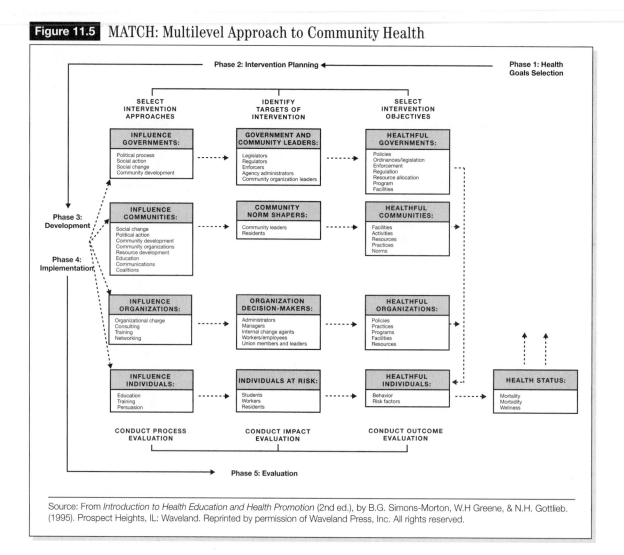

Source: From *Introduction to Health Education and Health Promotion* (2nd ed.), by B.G. Simons-Morton, W.H Greene, & N.H. Gottlieb. (1995). Prospect Heights, IL: Waveland. Reprinted by permission of Waveland Press, Inc. All rights reserved.

*Phase I* is Goals Selection, whose four steps are (1) select health status goals, (2) select high-priority target population(s), (3) identify health behavior goals, and (4) identify environmental factor goals. Each step in Phase I includes several considerations.

Selection of health status goals are normally based on the prevalence of the health problem and risk, status of the target population, the perceived and actual importance of the health problem in relation to other problems facing the target population, the health problem's potential for change, and other considerations unique to the mission and priorities of the program (Simons-Morton et al., 1995).

What amounts to the needs assessment at this step is identifying the most prevalent and important health needs as demonstrated by local health data or deriving conclusions from national published data. The importance of the problem and its potential for change should be central considerations.

Selecting high-priority population(s) identifies the group of people who will be addressed by the intervention. The target population is likely to be one at high risk for the health problem. It may be people for whom the planner is normally responsible, such as nursing home residents or teenagers, making accessibility an important variable. Given that programs reflect the mission and goals of the funding organizations, programmatic considerations are important in the identification of the target population.

Identifying health behavior goals means pinpointing those health behaviors that are most closely associated with the health goals of the population, most prevalent, and changeable.

Selecting environmental goals is the listing of environmental factors that are targeted for attention —factors that place the target population at risk, protect them from the health problem or from damaging behaviors, or promote healthful behaviors.

*Phase II* of MATCH, Intervention Planning, involves matching intervention objectives with intervention targets and actions. The four steps are (1) identify the targets of the intervention actions, (2) select intervention objectives, (3) identify the mediators of the intervention objectives, and (4) select the intervention approach.

The targets of the intervention actions (TIAs) are those who control or have influence over the intervention objective with which they are matched. The TIAs may be people close to the target population such as friends, family, or teachers; they may be organizational leaders such as administrator or nurses; they may be community leaders or government officials. The objectives of the intervention also affect the selection of the TIAs. It is important to identify those who can influence the intervention objective and target each for the intervention objectives over which they exercise control.

Intervention objectives are directed toward changing the target health behavior and environmental factors, so their selection is crucial. Great attention should be given to their selection. Programs that target multiple objectives at one or more societal levels are more likely to be successful and to be funded. The prevalence of the environmental or behavioral risk or protective factor, the societal level (individual, interpersonal, societal, organizational, or governmental) and TIA, the practice setting, and programming considerations are all criteria for selection.

Mediators (such as knowledge, perceptions, attitudes, values, skills, experiences, and reinforcement) are factors that are causally associated with the target behavior. Therefore, altering them appropriately,

usually through education, is likely to lead to desired behavior change. Identifying the mediator related to the intervention objective is, therefore, necessary to success.

Selecting an intervention approach depends on the specific intervention objective. If the approach is proper and effective, the TIAs respond to or act upon the intervention objective by learning, deciding, or behaving. Thus, the intervening is the most important health education/promotion activity. Approaches include teaching, consulting, training, organizing the community, **social marketing,** and advocating for a particular cause.

*Phase III*, Program Development, consists of four steps: (1) create program units or components, (2) select or develop curricula and create intervention guides, (3) develop session plans, and (4) create or acquire instructional materials. It is the link between planning and action.

Health promotion/education programs usually have several components. They may focus on different behaviors or environmental goals, intervention targets, settings, approaches, or even target populations, but they all are fixed on the same health status goals. In some cases, each component of a program may focus on a special part of the problem.

The blueprint for each program component is a curriculum or intervention guide describing how the component is meant to work. A great deal of effort and expertise is required to complete this step.

Each session of the curriculum or intervention guide has educational objectives, learning activities, and learning materials. All must be directly related and clearly described.

In some cases, health educators/promoters create their own instructional materials, products, and resources. In others, they acquire materials already developed and evaluated. Several effective programs and program components are available for purchase and/or adoption. (Chapter 9 describes some examples and numerous sources of products, and program components are available from resources cited in Appendix E.)

---

**social marketing**  the planning and implementation of programs to bring about social change using concepts from commercial marketing

*Phase IV* is Implementation Preparation. The health educator/promoter is now ready to plan implementation and conduct the interventions. The steps in this phase are (1) facilitate adoption, implementation, and maintenance; and (2) select and train implementers.

Implementation planners know that implementing a program requires cooperation from others. Planners must develop a specific proposal to document the need for change, describe the intervention, obtain input and approval from decision makers, resolve conflicts, and obtain authorization for resources. They must also develop the need, readiness, and environmental supports for change by building enthusiasm about the new program. To overcome TIAs' doubts, planners should demonstrate the efficacy of the intervention either by providing a relevant model of the use of program components or documenting the success of similar programs in other areas. Often a pilot study of the program is effective. To ensure success, planners might select change agents and opinion leaders and convince them of the need for change. Their support can mean the difference between success and failure. Establishing constructive working relationships with decision makers, participants, other professionals, and the target population is necessary for successful implementation.

Using experienced health educators/promoters is one way of enhancing chances for success. Another option is to train less-qualified individuals so that they can promote the mastery of relevant skills by the participants.

*Phase V*, Evaluation, consists of process evaluation, impact evaluation, and outcome evaluation. These will be discussed in detail in Chapter 12.

Process evaluation is concerned with utility of the implementation plan and procedures, the extent and quality of implementation, and the effects of implementation on immediate learning outcomes. It includes evaluation of the recruitment, session and program implementation, quality of the learning activities, and immediate learning outcomes that were the objectives of the sessions.

Impact evaluation is concerned with changes in the targeted mediators, health behaviors, and environmental factors. Generally, impact evaluation is short-term examination of changes in knowledge, attitudes, and practices.

Outcome evaluation is focused on long-term maintenance of changes in behavior or environmental factors and on health outcomes, such as reduced incidence of disease, decreased death rates, or lowered rates of teen pregnancy.

The MATCH process allows health educators/promoters to utilize a logical, systematic approach to program planning. It is most useful when the bulk of the needs assessment has been completed.

## KEY POINTS

1. The overall planning process includes needs assessment, program planning, planning for implementation, and planning for evaluation. It is important to include community members and program recipients in planning and implementing a program.

2. Needs assessment identifies the reported needs of an individual or group. Survey, medical examinations, interviews, reviews of news articles, the Delphi technique, nominal group process, and focus groups are examples of needs assessment techniques.

3. Steps in planning include prioritizing needs, developing goals and objectives, forming appropriate policies, designing methods and techniques to effect change, developing a plan for implementing the program, and planning for evaluation.

4. PRECEDE-PROCEED is a nine-phase model that provides a framework for planning from the outcome and through three levels of evaluation.

5. PATCH is a networking model based on the postulate that the most effective center for health promotion is the community.

6. The Mico model for health education planning is two-dimensional. A fundamental component of the model is a contract between the client and the planner.

7.  MATCH is an ecological approach to health education planning that recognizes that factors influencing health and health behavior are interrelated and occur at multiple societal levels. It is more useful when most of needs assessment has been completed.

## REFERENCES

Baily, A.R. (1973). Who should set health priorities? *Journal of Extension, 11*(1), 20–27.

Boyd, H.W., Westfall, R., & Starch, S.T. (1981). *Marketing research text and case.* Homewood, IL: Richard D. Irwin.

Breckon, D.J., Harvey, J.R., & Lancaster, R.B. (1998). *Community health education: Settings, roles, and skills for the 21st century.* Gaitherburg, MD: Aspen.

Centers for Disease Control and Prevention. (1995). *Planned approach to community health: A guide for local coordinators.* Atlanta, GA.

Delbecq, A.L., Van de Ven, A.H., & Gustafson, D.H. (1986). *Group techniques for program planning: A guide to nominal group and Delphi processes.* Middleton, WI: Green Briar Press.

Dignan, M.B., & Carr, P.A. (1992). *Program planning for health education and promotion* (2nd ed.). Baltimore: Williams & Wilkins.

Folch-Lyon, E., & Trost, F. (1981). Conducting focus group sessions, Part I. *Studies in Family Planning, 12*(12), 443–449.

Gilbert, G.G., &. Sawyer, R.G. (1995). *Health education: Creating strategies for school and community health.* Boston: Jones and Bartlett.

Gilmore, G.D. (1979). Planning for family wellness. *Health Education, 10*(5), 12–16.

Gilmore, G. D. & Campbell, M.D. (1996). *Needs assessment strategies for health education and health promotion* (2nd ed.). Madison, WI: Brown & Benchmark.

Green, L.W., & Kreuter, M.W. (1999). *Health promotion planning: An educational and ecological approach.* Mountain View, CA: Mayfield.

Green, L.W., Kreuter, M.W., Deeds, S.G., & Partridge, K.B. (1980). *Health education planning: A diagnostic approach.* Palo Alto, CA: Mayfield.

Kretzmann, J., & McKnight, J. (1993). *Building communities from the inside out.* Chicago: ACTA Publications.

Moore, C.M. (1987). *Group techniques for idea building.* Newbury Park, CA: Sage.

Nelson, D.J., Sennet, L., Lefebvre, R.C., Loisell, L, McClements, L., & Carleton, R.A. (1989). A campaign strategy for weight loss at worksites. *Health Education Research, 4*(1), 79–85.

Nix, H.L. (1978). *The community and its involvement in the study planning action process.* (HEW Publication Number CEC 78-78355). Washington, DC: Government Printing Office.

Queeney, D.S. (1995). *Assessing needs in continuing education: An essential tool for quality improvement.* San Francisco: Jossey-Bass.

Reeves, P.N., Bergwall, D.F., & Woodside, N.B. (1984). *Introduction to health planning* (3rd ed.). Arlington, VA: Information Resources Press.

Ross, H.S., & Mico, P.R. (1980). *Theory and practice in health education.* Palo Alto, CA: Mayfield.

Sarvela, P. D., Holcomb, D.R., Huetteman, J.K., Bajracharya, S.M., & Odulana, J.A. (1991). A university employee health promotion program needs assessment. *Journal of Health Education, 22*(2), 116–120.

Schechter, C., Vanchieri, C., & Crofton, C. (1990). Evaluating women's attitudes and perceptions in developing mammography promotion messages. *Public Health Reports, 105*(3), 253–257.

Simons-Morton, B.G., Greene, W.H., & Gottlieb, N.H. (1995). *Introduction to health education and health promotion.* Prospect Heights, IL: Waveland.

Simons-Morton, D.G., Simons-Morton, B.G., Parcel, G.S., & Bunker, J.F. (1988). Influencing personal and environmental conditions for community health: A multilevel intervention model. *Family and Community Health, 11*(2), 25–35.

Smith, M.F. (1989). *Evaluability assessment: A practical approach.* Boston: Kluwer Academic Publishers.

Sork, T.J. (1982). *Determining priorities.* Vancouver: University of British Columbia.

Stewart, G.W. (1993). Community health education: Principles and problems. *Health Education Quarterly* (Supplement 1), S29–S47.

U.S. Department of Health and Human Services. (2000). *Healthy people 2010* (Conference edition). Washington, DC: U.S. Government Printing Office.

# Evaluation

E valuation is an often-misunderstood part of the planning and implementation of health education/promotion. Students often view evaluation as a test for which they must cram to get a good grade. Educators sometimes see evaluation as the laborious task of filling out forms that only result in meetings with a supervisor to discuss their deficiencies. Supervisors, planners, and teachers may see evaluation as a way of enforcing discipline on employees and students. Evaluation is none of these.

When done properly, evaluation is a form of inquiry and self-analysis. Rather than being ruled by edict, it should be flexible. Only when evaluation is viewed as a positive force, set on improvement rather than on blame, is it welcomed by all those involved.

When acknowledged to be part of the planning process, evaluation can be a method of determining whether objectives are being met and can provide feedback that may ease or improve the attainment of objectives. Hindsight, after all, is usually more accurate than foresight. Although evaluation does not appear until the end of the health education process in many schematic depictions, it should encourage revisions throughout the implementation phase and inspire professionals to consider new beginnings. In short, evaluation should be a nonthreatening, positive force in health education, regardless of setting.

## THE PURPOSES OF EVALUATION

There are many perspectives on the purposes of evaluation in educational settings. Creswell and Newman (1993) placed evaluation in a positive light by stating that its purpose is not to prove or disprove, but to *improve*. Certainly, the quality of programs and individual performance should ultimately be improved by effective evaluation.

Some of the most important purposes of evaluation are the diagnosis and/or classification of schoolchildren who need special assistance and the determination of the specific kind of help they need. This helps ensure that school health services will be used in appropriate ways for all children.

Practiced appropriately, evaluation can provide feedback to professionals about the strengths and limitations of their programs. It can be a means of making informed decisions about performance, persons, activities, or programs and a means of improving service and instructional delivery. By indicating the quality of their performance against certain criteria, evaluation can be a source of motivation to clients and students. It also can alert parents and students to problems before those problems become impossible to avert or difficult to correct.

When health educators/promoters demonstrate the effectiveness of their programs through evaluation, it improves the credibility of the program and of health education/promotion in general—important considerations in the modern age of educational accountability. Educators and their programs must demonstrate their excellence on a regular basis.

A distinction should be drawn between evaluation of programs and evaluation of individuals. Many health educators, particularly those who practice in school settings, are required to determine the progress of individual learners against preset standards. Health educators and health promoters also frequently must evaluate a program against the goals and objectives of that program. The purposes of evaluating individuals and programs may differ, as seen in Box 12.1. Although a great deal of overlap exists between the two—and sometimes the results of individual evaluations can be applied to program evaluation—at other times the competencies involved are quite different, even though the principles are the same.

An important aspect of program evaluation is its ability to judge a program's merit against the values of stakeholders (Stake, 1975). Understanding how different people perceive the program is more than just a fascinating exercise: Community leaders, target population, government officials, program administrator, the public, the program evaluator, and funding agencies may all see the program in very different ways.

Evaluation can be made clear and precise by careful planning of the evaluation itself. Instruments for measuring various characteristics must be designed or selected so they yield complete and accurate information. To be useful, the data obtained from those measurements should be organized in the clearest and most helpful way possible.

---

**Box 12.1**    The Purposes of Evaluation

**We evaluate individuals to**

determine present knowledge, attitudes, and practices related to health, thereby to obtain a foundation for constructing objectives for instruction

find out if learning difficulties are present

ascertain the rate at which learning is taking place

ascertain the degree to which learning is taking place

determine the level of achievement for each individual student/client (as well as for the group)

assess the differences between actual performance and commonly accepted standards

determine what progress can be reported to students and families

**We evaluate programs to**

determine if a prospective program is plausible

assess the rate and level of attainment of desired outcomes, goals, and objectives

assess accomplishments of the program, i.e., compare the actual effects of a program with demonstrated population needs

identify limitations or weaknesses of the program

identify strengths of the program

identify areas to emphasize in staff development

identify unintended effects of the program

determine the value of learning experiences, teaching strategies, and individual program components

assess the value of learning aids and materials and of the ways in which they have been used or are being used

determine the quality of the total health education curriculum

determine if a program has been implemented as planned

identify modifications that must be made in any element of the program (e.g., goals, objectives, processes)

determine the generalizability of a program or program elements to other populations

promote positive public relations and community awareness

justify the program and its expenditure of resources and garner favorable attention

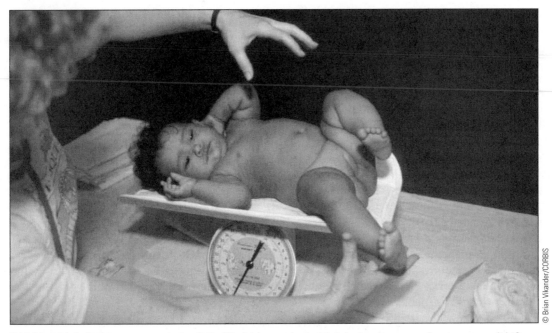

Weighing this baby is a measurement activity. Would you evaluate this infant as heavy, medium, or overweight? Criteria other than the number on the scale—including age, length, and physical appearance—may influence your evaluation.

## MEASUREMENT VERSUS EVALUATION

Dignan and Carr (1992) wrote, "We cannot evaluate if we do not have the ability to measure." Evaluation is done to arrive at a judgment of value, worth, merit, or effectiveness (Payne, 1992). Green and Kreuter (1999) defined **evaluation** as the comparison of an object of interest with a standard of acceptability. The standard of acceptability is expressed in well-written objectives; the comparison must be based upon data. These data are collected by the process of **measurement,** which is the determination of quantity or quality of an object of interest—or, in the words of McDermott and Sarvela (1999), "the set of rules used to assign numbers to different objects, events, issues, or people." Measurement provides a means for learning something about a program that can be used for evaluation (Veney & Kaluzny, 1991). It also can be used to learn something about an individual student, client, or professional. Therefore, measurement is the basic tool of evaluation.

Recall the example given in Chapter 11 (see page 268). The task was to classify the heights of a group of people as tall, medium, or short. The standards of acceptability for males were 6 feet tall or taller is "tall"; 5½ feet tall and shorter is "short"; and between 5½ feet and 6 feet is "medium." To apply these standards of acceptability, one must measure—that is, determine the height, in feet and inches, of each individual being evaluated.

Similarly, we may need to measure the percentage of teens who engage in a certain risk behavior. This can be done in a number of ways. One possibility is a self-report questionnaire of a random sample of teens in the population. If we find an unacceptably high percentage of the behavior, we may implement a health promotion program with the objective of reducing to 5 percent the number of

**evaluation** comparison of an object of interest against a standard of acceptability

**measurement** determination of quantity or quality of an object of interest

teens who engage in this behavior. By administering another self-report questionnaire, we can obtain information to use to evaluate our program's effectiveness. We would rate it satisfactory if it met the standard of acceptability: 5 percent or less of teens in the sample engage in the risk behavior at the conclusion of the program. We could repeat the measurement at other intervals of time.

Many instruments are available for measuring an entity, and measuring may be of different types. For instance, a shopper may find Dungeness crabs priced by the dozen or by the pound. Because quantity and pounds are different units of measure, we may be frustrated and confused shoppers (evaluators). In a similar vein, we may choose to measure the success of a program by increased knowledge, number of observed behaviors, or many other ways. Dignan and Carr (1992) stated, "The type of measurement chosen depends on the criteria selected for evaluation, the need for precision, and the opportunity to collect information."

We cannot overemphasize the role of objectives in guiding evaluation. They establish the criteria upon which measurement and evaluation are based. Oberteuffer, Harrelson, and Pollock (1972) stated

> Specification of instructional objectives in behavioral terms not only facilitates but assumes the validity of related evaluation procedures. . . . Objectives provide a blueprint for what is to be evaluated and how it might be done.

Frequently, we measure and evaluate only the cognitive domain, because the cognitive domain is easier to measure than either the affective or the action domain. Just as objectives should emphasize all three domains, however, all three domains should be included in measurement and evaluation.

Program evaluation involves the collection and analysis of information to determine the relevance, progress, efficiency, and effectiveness of program activities (Veney & Kaluzny, 1991). "Relevance" is the degree to which the service is needed. "Progress" refers to tracking program activities and assessing whether program implementation complies with the plan developed to meet *the objectives.* The "efficiency" question asks whether the program results could be obtained less expensively. "Effectiveness" refers to meeting predetermined needs.

# MEASUREMENT INSTRUMENTS

Measurement instruments are the tools we use to collect data. Examples are achievement tests; attitudinal inventories; behavioral inventories, including self-report questionnaires and observation; biomedical instruments; and health risk appraisals.

## Tests, Inventories, and Questionnaires

Achievement tests are commonly used to measure the degree to which an individual has mastered a body of knowledge, including health-related knowledge. They are routinely used in classrooms. The two basic forms of achievement tests are **criterion-referenced** and **norm-referenced tests**. Criterion-referenced tests have an absolute pass or fail score, or criterion score. The exam for the Certified Health Education Specialist is a criterion-referenced test. A norm-referenced test is one in which an individual's score is compared to a group score. Examples include college entrance examinations and classroom tests where individual student scores are compared with the class mean.

Attitudinal inventories measure a person's attitudes, beliefs, values, or opinions about issues, objects, or events. Components of the inventories usually indicate if the individual feels positively or negatively, or agrees or disagrees, about the issue being studied.

Behavioral inventories measure the behavior of individuals. Self-report questionnaires are usually believed to provide useful information if they are confidential. Examples include surveys about eating habits or sexual behavior. Observations of the individual's behaviors are a second type of behavioral inventory.

Biomedical instruments are used to measure physiological functions or characteristics such as blood pressure, cholesterol level, weight, and blood sugar level.

In health risk appraisals, individuals provide information about their personal habits, physiological status, and medical history. These provide a measure of the person's health status at that time. They also provide a personalized risk estimate, usually with explanations, and frequently with estimates of "health age." They are very useful in developing individualized health improvement programs and in evaluating the effectiveness of health promotion programs.

## Kinds of Measurement

### Qualitative Versus Quantitative    **Qualitative measurement** attempts to provide statements that describe processes or experiences resulting from exposure to a program or an activity. Being descriptive, it may refer to how well something is done. Often, qualitative evaluation is based on the need to discover information about the acceptance of programs rather than to test the impact of programs. Qualitative information usually is grouped according to similar characteristics, such as drinkers/nondrinkers, male/female, or different age groups. Analyzing qualitative data such as that gained from interviews is a creative process; different people may approach it in different ways. It is based more on the examiner's experience and knowledge of a given subject than on tried-and-true analysis methods (Patton, 1980). It can produce results showing how much or, sometimes, how many. One of the goals of qualitative evaluation is to develop understanding of the processes by which programs reach intended audiences, the impact produced, and the changes that may take place thereafter (Patton, 1982).

**Quantitative measurement** yields numerical values such as how many questions were answered correctly, how often a person engaged in a specific behavior, how many pounds a person weighed, or how many people composed a household. It usually is easily explained and defensible.

Kreuter and Green (1978) recommend the simultaneous use of both quantitative and qualitative evaluation:

> Quantitative and qualitative methods can be used together in evaluation, permitting the collection of information that describes the program in greater depth than would be possible through use of either method alone.

Whereas quantitative evaluation is primarily useful to determine program efficacy, qualitative evaluation can be used to explain why the effects occurred.

### Objective Versus Subjective    Measurement instruments may be objective or subjective. Both can be of service to health promoters in evaluating

the fulfillment of specific objectives. Objective instruments provide consistent scoring, regardless of who is doing the measurement. The evaluator does not need to apply personal judgment to interpret responses procured with an objective instrument. These instruments are good at measuring recall or recognition of facts and at counting observations. Quantitative measures are more likely to be taken using objective instruments—which frequently fail to measure comprehension, application, or attitudes.

Subjective instruments, on the other hand, require that the evaluator have training and skill at interpreting the responses obtained with the instrument. Different people may arrive at different determinations or scores from the same subjective instrument. Therefore, establishing validity and reliability of subjective instruments is more difficult. Qualitative measures more frequently use subjective instruments.

For measurement instruments to be useful, they must have several important qualities: validity, reliability, sensitivity, objectivity, discrimination, and administrability.

## Validity

**Validity** is a test's tendency to measure what it's intended to measure. Following are different types of validity:

- **Content validity** indicates how well the instrument samples the unit being measured (Creswell

**criterion-referenced tests**    tests that have an absolute pass or fail score

**norm-referenced tests**    tests where an individual's score is compared to a group score

**qualitative measurement**    that which attempts to provide statements describing processes or experiences resulting from exposure to a program or an activity

**quantitative measurement**    that which yields numerical values such as how many, how much, or how often

**validity**    the tendency of a measurement instrument to measure what it is intended to measure

& Newman, 1993). It demonstrates the degree to which the sample of items, tasks, or questions are representative of the defined universe or domain of content (American Education Research Association et al., 1985).

- **Criterion-related validity** demonstrates that test scores are systematically related to one or more outcome criteria (McDermott & Sarvela, 1999). For example, a college entrance exam has criterion-related validity if it can predict, and is related to, college grade point average. The two forms of criterion-related validity are predictive and concurrent. Predictive validity is the degree to which a test can predict how well a student (or client) will do in a given situation (Anspaugh & Ezell, 1998). For example, if students who score well on a written test of skills to resist social and peer pressure to drink alcohol are actually less likely to drink, the test has good predictive validity for future drinking behavior. Concurrent validity is the degree to which the scores on the test in question relate to scores on another accepted performance criterion—perhaps an older, more established instrument. This is a central control issue in health education: how well a person's measures of knowledge, attitude, and practice obtained with a test actually compare to that person's behavior.

- **Construct validity** is the degree to which an instrument measures some hypothetical entity, such as intelligence, appreciation of health, or self-esteem. This kind of validity is based upon logical inferences as to whether the instrument actually measures what it is designed to measure.

- **Face validity** is the lowest level that an instrument can possess. An instrument is said to possess face validity if "on the face" of things, the instrument appears to measure the construct under consideration and appears to be appropriate for the audience for whom it is intended (McDermott & Sarvela, 1999). An instrument that can boast only of face validity is usually considered inadequate for wide distribution and its data inappropriate for inferring general conclusions.

Validity is the most important consideration in evaluation of measurement instruments. The appropriateness, meaningfulness, and usefulness of the instrument are all bound to its validity. The quality of the data it yields and the assertions made about the data are dependent on instrument validity. However, validity is dependent upon the context and purpose for which the instrument is being used (Smith & Glass, 1987). For example, instruments that measure attitudes about violence may of necessity be somewhat different in current times, when individuals committing violent acts in schools draw headlines, as opposed to times of war, or to situations wherein less attention is given to domestic youth violence.

## Reliability

**Reliability** is a test's ability to yield consistent results. A reliable instrument employs the same processes and generates the same types of information every time it is used. Carmine and Zeller (1979) described reliability as the degree to which repeated observations of the same characteristic (e.g., health knowledge) yield the same results. An instrument that is valid is always reliable, but a reliable instrument is not always valid. For example, a poorly calibrated scale may yield the same incorrect weight repeatedly. Similarly, a poorly worded self-report behavior questionnaire may also produce consistent, but incorrect, responses. If the scale is calibrated properly, and the questionnaire is worded properly, however, they will provide valid results repeatedly. Of course, total accuracy and total consistency do not exist in the real world.

Hopkins and Antes (1990) stated that generally reliability will be greater for

— a long test than for a short one

— a test over homogeneous content rather than heterogeneous content

— a set of scores from a group of examinees with a wide range of ability rather than from a group that has members much alike

— a test composed of well-written and appropriate items

— measures with few scoring errors than for measures that vary from test to test or paper to paper because of scoring procedures

— test scores obtained by proper conditions for testing students who have optimum motivation

## Sensitivity

**Sensitivity** is the ability to reflect changes in the state or amount of the phenomenon being measured. Can the test really measure changes in a person's attitudes or an increase in his or her knowledge? Can the self-report questionnaire accurately reflect, say, changes in use of snuff by the teenage males in a sample? Can the instrument correctly identify persons who have the trait being studied?

A corollary to sensitivity is **specificity,** or a test's ability to identify correctly those who do *not* have the disease or characteristic of interest (Lilienfeld & Stolley, 1994). An instrument that has high specificity reduces "false positives," or cases that appear to have the characteristics but do not.

## Objectivity

**Objectivity** is a test's ability not only to yield similar scores on successive occasions, but also to yield similar scores when administered by different people. This requires elimination of personal bias and self-interest. It also implies fairness in the way the test is constructed, such as its reading level, as well as the way in which it is scored. Instruments that yield qualitative information tend to be less objective, and analysis of their information by different people is less consistent than that of quantitative instruments.

## Discrimination

**Discrimination** is a test's ability to accurately provide different scores between the respondents who possess the quality being measured, such as knowledge, and those who do not. This is the foundation of the measurement/evaluation relationship.

## Administrability

**Administrability** is the ease with which the instrument can be utilized in appropriate ways. Does it meet time and resource requirements? How difficult is it to score? If a test requires a sophisticated scoring technology or several hours to administer, it may be impractical for a given situation. On the other hand, a test that is easy to administer and score may not be the best choice for assessing the content area.

# LEVELS OF PROGRAM EVALUATION

A comprehensive evaluation of programs consists of three levels of evaluation: diagnostic evaluation, formative evaluation, and summative evaluation of impact and outcome. Resources, time, complexity, and the program's dominant goal may make it difficult to evaluate well at all levels. (See Figure 12.1.)

## Diagnostic Evaluation

**Diagnostic evaluation** is a component of needs assessment. Its function is to analyze health problems and issues to determine which groups or individuals most need knowledge, attitude change, behavior change, or skill development. It provides specific knowledge of the health conditions that exist and

**reliability**   the ability of a measurement instrument to yield consistent results each time it is used

**sensitivity**   the ability of a measurement instrument to reflect changes in the state or amount of the phenomenon being measured

**specificity**   the ability of a test to correctly rule out those who do not have the characteristic of interest

**objectivity**   the ability of a measurement instrument to yield similar results on successive occasions and to yield similar results when administered by different people

**discrimination**   the ability of a measurement instrument to provide different scores between respondents who possess the quality being measured and those who do not

**administrability**   the ease with which a measurement instrument can be utilized in appropriate ways

**diagnostic evaluation**   evaluation to determine the needs of an individual or group prior to planning the program activities

## Figure 12.1   Levels of Evaluation

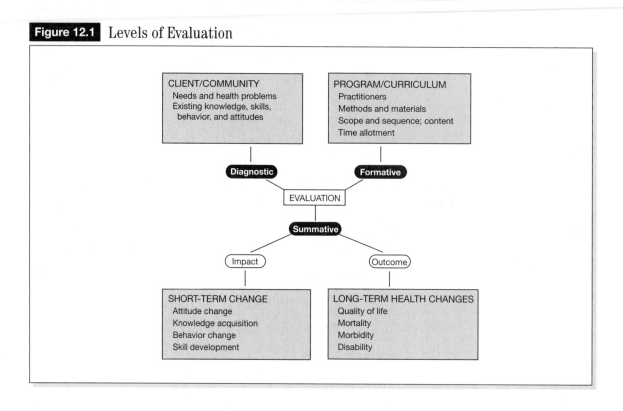

suggests actions to correct them. Later, when the effects of a program are being evaluated, the results of diagnostic evaluation provide a baseline for comparison.

## Formative Evaluation

**Formative evaluation** (often referred to as "process evaluation") is the ongoing evaluation while the program is being developed and implemented (McDermott & Sarvela, 1999). It focuses on the functioning elements of the program or curriculum, including educational methods, content, materials, time allotments, steps of implementation, achievement of the enabling objectives, and instructor performance. It is associated with ongoing operations of the program and helps to improve the program and its management. This ongoing type of program evaluation focuses on whether the program's content and materials match the program's objectives, what aspects of the program are working and what are not, and whether the program is being carried out as intended—all so that changes can be

made to increase its probability of success. Formative evaluation can also provide information on level of support from management, adequacy of resources, and whether the project is close to budget.

Process evaluation helps to explain the causes of a program's strengths or weaknesses and to indicate modifications needed to improve the program (National Task Force for the Preparation and Practice of Health Educators, 1985). Because this kind of information is often qualitative in nature, data collection may be done by observation, interviews, and open-ended survey questions. Client/student perceptions are an important indicator of process success. This level of evaluation frequently leads to change in methods, activities, techniques, and instructor performance. It should be continuous.

## Summative Evaluations of Impact and Outcome

In **summative evaluation**, we are interested in ascertaining the degree to which the program has met

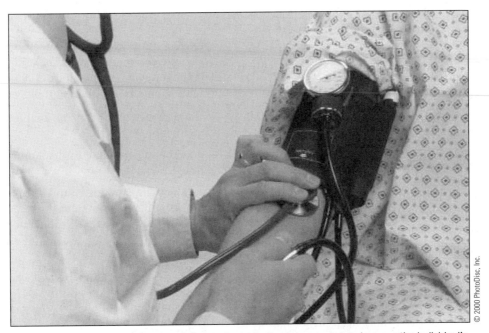

Measuring blood pressure is a part of diagnostic evaluation in a program to improve the individual's health status. Determining if students/clients can measure their own heart rate can be a diagnostic step in an education program.

some predetermined goals and objectives. This type of evaluation assesses the effect of the program on the target population. It is usually quantitative in nature, often obtaining data from a large sample of the population. Summative evaluation is carried out on two levels: impact and outcome.

**Impact evaluation** is based on measures of the immediate or short-term effects of the program or curriculum; it is used to determine if objectives are met. These effects usually are indicated by changes in knowledge, attitudes, beliefs, and skill development. Impact evaluation is highly dependent upon the quality of the measurement instrument and does not necessarily indicate that long-term goals have been attained. It is often used to evaluate the performance of educators.

**Outcome evaluation** is based on measures of the long-term or ultimate changes that come about as a result of the program or curriculum; it is used to determine if program goals have been achieved. These goals may include indications of behavioral change or changes in quality of life, health status, morbidity, or mortality. Outcome evaluation can be difficult and expensive because of the obstacles involved in following large groups of people for a long time. As Hochbaum (1982) observed:

> Such problems stem from 1) the usual inability to observe and measure behavioral outcomes when these do not manifest themselves until long after the program has ceased, for example in school health education, and, 2) the difficulty of identifying the role played by health education in producing behavioral outcomes when other

**formative evaluation**    the ongoing process of evaluation while the program is being developed and implemented; also called process evaluation

**summative evaluation**    evaluation done to ascertain if the program has met predetermined objectives

**impact evaluation**    evaluation of a program or curriculum in terms of its immediate, short-term effects

**outcome evaluation**    evaluation of a program or curriculum in terms of its long-term or ultimate effects

interventions, conditions, or events may have influenced such outcomes as much or more, either by adding to or by counteracting the educational efforts.

Tracking individuals to determine the permanence of behavior change is equally problematic. For these reasons, most evaluations conclude at the impact level. When done with population groups, outcome evaluation often focuses on changes in mortality, morbidity, or such group characteristics as teen pregnancy rate or self-reported drug use.

Under some circumstances, program evaluation should not be undertaken (McDermott & Sarvela, 1999). If there are no questions to be answered because the effect of the program is obvious, if the task of evaluation is merely an information-gathering exercise with no focus, or if evaluation is not likely to result in any change, evaluation serves no purpose. In many cases, such as a lack of will to change or unavailability of resources to implement changes, the evaluation may have little value. If there are no clear objectives, if they are ill-defined, or if the program boundaries are obscured, evaluation has little value. Of course, these situations indicate poor planning. If there are insufficient resources—human and monetary—to do the evaluation properly, it should not be undertaken. Therefore, it is important to assess the evaluability of a program before undertaking the actual evaluation.

# EVALUATION OF THE LEARNER/CLIENT

Most of the discussion of evaluation has centered thus far on program evaluation, mostly because of the emphasis the Role Delineation Project placed on program evaluation. Some health educators, particularly classroom teachers, evaluate individuals regularly, if not daily. Perhaps the outstanding omission of the Role Delineation Project is any specific emphasis on the competencies and skills necessary to evaluate students and clients. The various purposes of evaluating individuals and programs are contained in Box 12.1. However, in some cases, it is possible to use cumulative evaluations of individuals to evaluate the success of a program.

# Evaluation by Teachers

Competence in measurement and evaluation is essential for classroom teachers. The National Council on Measurement in Education (1990) stated that a teacher should be skilled in the following areas:

— choosing assessment methods appropriate for instructional objectives

— developing assessment methods appropriate for instructional decisions

— administering, scoring, and interpreting the results of both commercially produced and teacher-produced assessment methods

— using assessment results in making decisions about individual students, planning instruction, developing curriculum, and school improvement

— developing pupil grading procedures that use pupil assessment

— communicating assessment results to students, parents, other lay audiences, and educators

— recognizing and having knowledge about unethical, illogical, and inappropriate assessment

One of the most popular methods for teachers to evaluate student progress is through pretests and post-tests. By definition, pretests are given before instruction to determine the learner's specific knowledge, attitudes, behaviors, and skills. These tests are diagnostic in nature and can tell the teacher which learning activities are necessary and which can be omitted. They provide baseline information that is useful in evaluating the learner's progress and the effectiveness of the learning experience. Post-tests provide data relative to changes in the learner's knowledge, attitudes, behaviors, and skills. Post-test score minus pretest score on the same test may be an indication of change. Basically, pretest/post-test is diagnostic evaluation followed by impact evaluation. Cumulative results of pretests and post-tests can provide effective evaluation of program methodology as well as student performance. Outcome evaluation of individuals is difficult and expensive. It usually requires maintaining contact with a sample of participants for a long period of time, eliciting data from them occasionally. For this reason, most assessment of individuals is reported as impact evaluation.

### Tests and Test Items

Classroom measurement instruments may be standardized or teacher-made. *Standardized tests* are those that have been published after careful development and refinement. This careful development is designed to ensure that the tests consistently measure what they are supposed to measure (validity). Standardized tests, however, may not include the items necessary to evaluate a specific teacher's lessons. They also may have been normed with a target population somewhat different from the class being tested. If this is the case, comparisons of students' performance will be of poor quality, because they are not comparisons with the students' peers.

For these and other reasons, *teacher-made* tests are the most commonly used tests in classroom evaluation. Although they can be constructed to fit specific purposes and students, they may lack qualities such as validity and reliability. Teachers can improve their skills at generating tests by attending workshops and taking courses on test construction—both important ways to increase effectiveness. Although standardized tests have some attractive qualities, they probably will never replace teacher-made tests.

Regardless of the format of the test item, the following characteristics are universally acknowledged to be necessary:

- The item is worded clearly so the student understands the point of the item or the specific nature of the task.
- The item is stated as concisely as possible.
- The level of difficulty is appropriate to the educational and maturational levels of the pupils and the nature of the content being assessed.
- No irrelevant clues or other technical errors are included.
- The item is free of racial, ethnic, and sexual bias.
- The item does not trick the respondent into giving a wrong answer.
- The item is written in proper grammar without double negatives.

The following sections will present some basic concepts, guidelines, and examples of techniques of measuring knowledge, attitudes, and behaviors. However, measurement of these three entities should not be considered isolated from one another. According to Astin (1992), assessment is most effective when it reflects an understanding of learning as multidimensional, integrated, and revealed in performance over time.

## Measuring Knowledge

Several different forms of test items can be used to measure the knowledge possessed or gained by students/clients. They are typically employed in the type of summative evaluation of impact.

Knowledge levels are most frequently measured by *constructed-response* items, which require the respondents to develop their own answers, and *selected-response* items, which require respondents to choose from two or more possible answers. Examples of constructed-response items are the short-answer essay item, the extended-answer essay item, and the completion item. Selected-response items include multiple-choice and true-false items. Examinations take time to construct and time to grade. The general rule of thumb is that the easier the examination to construct, the more difficult it is to grade, and vice versa (Bender et al., 1997).

### Essay Items

Essay items can be used to measure skills and values as well as knowledge. Guidelines for using essay questions include

- Use essay questions to measure objectives, such as attainment of critical thinking skills, that cannot be measured well through other types of questions.
- Limit and define the scope of learner responses to essay questions by phrasing the questions specifically enough so students know the kind of response that is intended—that is, define the respondent's task as completely and specifically as possible.
- Elicit reactions to a situation, not a description of it.

- Instead of eliciting a restatement of facts, construct questions to elicit the how, why, or significance of a piece of information.
- Where possible, use several brief essays rather than one or two extended essays.
- Write model answers with specific points that should be included in learner's responses. Do not concentrate so narrowly that a listing of facts or items is required.
- Avoid giving a choice among optional questions unless special circumstances make such options necessary.
- When grading the papers, read the first question on all papers, then the second on all papers and so on, to increase uniformity and objectivity in grading.

Examples of essay items include

- Compare and contrast three studies on the effects of aerobic exercise versus anaerobic exercise in older citizens.
- Define the term "controlled substance" as described in the Controlled Substances Act and explain how it is applied under the law.

## Completion Items    Guidelines for writing completion items include

- Make the missing word or phrase a significant one that, if answered incorrectly, would invalidate the entire statement.
- Do not require the learner to make more than one or two completions in any one item.
- Write items in language and vocabulary appropriate to the respondents' reading level.
- Minimize reliance on rote memorization—do not simply lift items from the text with blanks inserted for key words.
- In general, place the blank near or at the end of the statement.
- Avoid using "a" or "an" before the blank, because this can tip off the correct answer. If this is unavoidable, insert "a/an."
- Try to provide blanks that represent only one correct answer by avoiding ambiguous or open-ended items.

- Avoid extraneous clues to the correct answers.
- Think of the answer first, then write a question wherein that answer is the only appropriate answer.

Examples of completion items are

1. According to the article in the *Journal of the American Medical Association,* the leading underlying cause of death in America is _____ _____.

2. The greatest risk factor in acquiring skin cancer is exposure to _____.

3. The blood alcohol concentration that constitutes legal drunkenness in this state is _____ _____.

## Short-Answer Items    The short-answer item has characteristics of both constructed-response essay items and completion items. This type of test item requires the respondent to provide an answer in only a few words. Examples include

1. What is the name of the type of exercise in which only a limited amount of oxygen is utilized?

2. Name three of the food groups in the Food Pyramid.

3. List the four chambers of the heart.

Many of the guidelines for writing completion items also apply to short-answer items.

## True/False Items    Guidelines for preparing true/false items include

- Avoid loosely worded and ambiguous statements—for example, those that use qualifiers such as "many" and "few."
- Use only items that test knowledge of important ideas.
- Use only a single idea in each item.
- Make the important element of the statement readily apparent to the student.
- Avoid using terms such as "usually," "always," "no," "never," and "all." These provide extraneous clues.

- Make approximately half of the items true and approximately half false.
- Base true/false items on statements that are absolutely true or false without qualification or exception.
- Do not take sentences directly from the textbook.
- Do not make true statements consistently longer than false statements and vice versa.
- Avoid statements that are partly true and partly false.
- Avoid long and involved statements with many qualifying clauses.
- Do not use trick questions; make items clear, simple, and concise.
- Avoid negative questions wherever possible, and double negatives in any case.

Examples of true/false items are

T    F    1. Lung cancer is most often caused by cigarette smoking.
T    F    2. The most powerful chamber in the heart is the left atrium.
T    F    3. Alcohol is a depressant drug.

## Multiple Choice Items

Multiple choice items contain the item stem, which asks the question or starts the statement, the correct answer, and the incorrect answers, or distractors. Multiple choice items can be used to measure knowledge, understanding, judgment, problem solving, methods of appropriate action, and ability to make predictions (Ebel & Frisbie, 1986). They generally have greater reliability than true/false items and do not need homogeneous material (as matching items do). In writing multiple choice items,

- Avoid exact textbook wording for items.
- Focus on a single important idea, concept, or problem, rather than multiple foci or trivia.
- Test higher levels of understanding, not just memorization.
- Use either a direct question or an incomplete statement, whichever seems more appropriate and effective. If using an incomplete statement, the responses should come at the end of the sentence.

- Make sure each item has one and only one correct or best answer.
- Base each item on a single central problem that is stated clearly and completely in the stem.
- Avoid negative statements whenever possible. If they must be included, underline or capitalize the negative word so the student will not overlook it.
- Whenever possible, make all choices approximately the same length. In no case should the correct answer become obvious by its length.
- Keep the choices short whenever possible.
- Make responses grammatically consistent with the stem and parallel to one another in form.
- Arrange the responses in logical order, if one exists.
- Whenever there is no reason for the answers to be arranged in order, position the correct answers randomly throughout the test.
- Make the responses independent and mutually exclusive.
- Make items independent of each other so that items do not contain clues to each other.
- Use the "none of the above" and "all of the above" with caution.
- Avoid using lists of options such as "A, B, and C, but not D" and "C and D only."
- Make all responses plausible and attractive to learners who lack the information or ability that the item tests.
- Group items by content area or sequence of instruction.
- For future tests, change incorrect responses that attract no or few answers.

Examples of multiple choice items are

1. The chamber of the heart that pumps blood to the lungs is the
   a. right atrium
   b. left atrium
   c. aorta
   d. right ventricle
   e. left ventricle

2. An example of a "gateway" drug for teens is

   a. heroin

   b. crack

   c. methamphetamine

   d. nicotine

   e. PCP

## Matching Items
Matching items are a special form of multiple-choice items. Some guidelines for using matching items are

- Explain clearly in the instructions the basis on which items are to be matched and the procedure to be followed.
- Limit the test to one subject area or topic.
- Word the items and responses clearly and precisely.
- Keep the lists of items to be matched relatively short, especially for young children.
- Arrange the list of items for maximum clarity and convenience to the learner.
- Place all items and responses on a single page.
- Avoid extraneous clues.
- Provide for extra responses to reduce guessing.
- Provide only one possible correct response for each item.

- If responses can be used more than once, make this clear to the student in the oral and written instructions.
- Arrange the responses in random order except for numerical responses, which should be arranged from low to high.
- Provide clear directions.

An example of matching items are

___ 1. The addictive          a. cocaine
       drug in tobacco        b. alcohol
       smoke                  c. nicotine

___ 2. The drug that is       d. methamphetamine
       used medically
       as an anesthetic

Regardless of whether the evaluation is objective or subjective, the measurement techniques should be designed or selected on the basis of their capacity to measure qualities or entities that are relevant to the objectives. Each type of test item has its strengths and weaknesses. Knowledgeable educators select the test item on the basis of its applicability to the learners, content, objectives, and setting. A few advantages and disadvantages of the various types of test items are provided in Box 12.2.

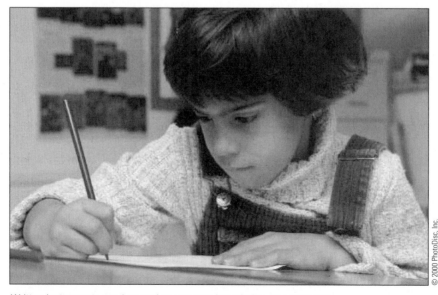

Written instruments can be used to measure knowledge and attitudes.

## Box 12.2   Advantages and Disadvantages of Types of Test Items

### ESSAY QUESTION TESTS

The essay question test requires the student to organize information in a systematic fashion. Use of the essay question allows the teacher to gain insight into the amount of understanding students have developed from instruction.

### Advantages

This type of test is relatively easy to prepare.

Essay questions can be written on the chalkboard or even dictated, thus eliminating the expense of duplicating materials.

Originality and creativity on the part of the student are encouraged.

Essay questions stimulate students to organize their thinking.

Chances of cheating are minimized because of the amount of writing involved.

Essay questions can be used to evaluate organizational ability and expression of ideas.

Answers to essay questions help reveal the individuality of students. Questions can invoke a variety of responses that reflect personal attitudes, values, habits, and differences.

Guessing at answers is reduced to a minimum.

Essay questions are the best-known way of evaluating an individual student's ability to express him- or herself.

### Disadvantages

Determining reliability is difficult because different teachers will score essay answers in different ways.

Scoring is rather subjective and is unconsciously influenced by such factors as legibility, neatness, grammar, spelling, word choice, and bluffing; grading is difficult.

Scoring is time-consuming.

Students with poor writing skills are at a disadvantage.

Writing essay answers is time-consuming, and students may feel pressured by this type of test. Slow writers are not necessarily slow thinkers, but this may be the impression given.

Younger children have particular difficulty in formulating and writing answers to essay questions.

An essay question test can sample only a limited amount of material covered.

### COMPLETION ITEMS AND SHORT ANSWER

Completion, or fill-in, tests consist of a number of statements that have certain key words or phrases omitted. This type of test measures the student's ability to select a word or phrase that is consistent in logic and style with the other elements in the statement. If students understand the implications of the sentence, they should be able to provide the answer that best fulfills the intent of the item.

Short answer items can be written as questions or statements. Respondents must provide the answers in only a few words. Many of the advantages and disadvantages of short answer items are the same as those for completion items.

### Advantages

It is easy to construct.

It has wide applications to testing situations presented in the form of charts or diagrams.

It minimizes guessing because the answer must come from the student.

It does not require student writing ability as a major factor.

It allows for objective scoring.

Students supply the answers, reducing guessing.

### Disadvantages

This type of test stresses factual information. The result may be a collection of items calling for unrelated facts or isolated bits of information.

It places a premium on rote memory rather than on real understanding.

It is unsuitable for complex learning tasks.

Phrasing an item so that only one correct response is elicited is often difficult. Alternative answers provided by students may be very close to correct, making scoring problematical.

In a poorly formatted completion test, answers may be scattered all over the page, as on a diagram, making scoring time-consuming.

Clues within an item can allow students to respond correctly without understanding the concept being assessed.

(continued)

**Box 12.2**    Advantages and Disadvantages of Types of Test Items (continued)

## TRUE/FALSE ITEMS

A true/false test consists of declaratory statements that are either true or false. Students must decide about each test item and answer accordingly.

### Advantages

It is familiar to students because it is so widely used.

It is easy to construct, which is one reason it is used extensively.

It can be used to sample a wide range of subject matter. Because the items can be answered in a short time, a large number can be included on a simple test.

The test is easy to score, and the score is quite objective.

It can be used as an instructional test to promote interest and introduce points for discussion.

The test is versatile and can be employed for short quizzes, lesson reviews, and end-of-chapter tests.

Items may be constructed either as factual statements or as questions that require reasoning.

It can have items that are especially useful when there are only two logical choices concerning an issue.

### Disadvantages

A simple true/false item is of doubtful value for measuring achievement.

It is mainly limited to cognitive knowledge areas.

The true/false test encourages guessing. Even without any knowledge of the subject matter, a student has a 50 percent chance of getting the item right, and if the item is poorly written, perhaps a higher chance.

Constructing items that are completely true or completely false without making the correct response obvious can be difficult.

Avoiding ambiguities, irrelevant details, and clues is difficult.

Unless the test consists of a large number of items, reliability is likely to be low.

Items that test for minor details receive as much credit as items that test for major points.

If the material is in any way controversial, true/false items are difficult to construct. For example, the following statement, although false, can give students a wrong perception: "Marijuana is not a harmful drug."

Sometimes the relative degree of truth in an item is debatable. Such items should be avoided, because students may try to guess what is in the teacher's mind instead of making their own decisions.

## MULTIPLE CHOICE ITEMS

Items on multiple choice tests require the student to recognize which of several suggested responses is the best answer. This kind of test provides an opportunity to develop thought-provoking questions and cover a great deal of material. It is considered the best short answer test format.

### Advantages

Items can measure simple to complex levels of knowledge.

Items can be written to measure inference, discrimination, and judgment.

Items can be constructed to measure recall as well as recognition.

They are very versatile.

Guessing is minimized when there are three or four alternate choices.

Sampling of material covered can be extensive. Many questions can be included on a test because a response can be made quickly.

Scoring is objective. In a properly constructed item, only one possible response is correct.

Scoring is rapid.

Students who choose certain distractors let teachers know where corrections are needed.

### Disadvantages

Developing a multiple choice test is time-consuming and difficult.

Items are too often factually based, unduly stressing memory.

More than one response may be correct or nearly correct.

It may be difficult to find adequate responses.

(continued)

## Box 12.2 Advantages and Disadvantages of Types of Test Items (continued)

It is difficult to exclude clues to the correct response.

Incorrect, but plausible, alternative answers are often difficult to develop.

Items can take up a considerable amount of space.

The student must do a lot of reading.

The format does not allow students to express their own thoughts.

The format may not be appropriate for very young students.

**MATCHING TESTS**

Matching tests call for answers in one column to be paired with the premise in another column. This kind of test is, in effect, a form of multiple choice test, except that the number of choices is compounded.

**Advantages**

It allows coverage of broad subject matter, enhancing content validity.

It is adaptable to many subject areas.

It is especially useful for maps, charts, or pictorial representations.

The test can be developed fairly quickly and easily.

Its format uses space economically.

It is easy to score.

**Disadvantages**

It does not assess the extent to which meaning has been grasped.

It increases in difficulty as the number of items to be matched increases.

The format tests only factual information.

It permits guessing.

It is likely to include clues to the correct answers.

Source: Adapted with permission from *Teaching Today's Health* (4th ed.), by D.J. Anspaugh & G. Ezell, 1995, Boston: Allyn & Bacon.

## Measuring Attitudes

Health education has the perplexing problem that measuring knowledge does not necessarily transfer to the attitudes and behaviors that are its primary goals. In addition, health promoters/educators are often required to justify program activities in terms of attitude change. Teacher-made tests usually lack the ability to assess attitudes or behavior. In addition, few standardized attitude tests appropriate for elementary school students are available (Pollock & Middleton, 1994). Essay exams provide better means for assessing attitudes than do the other items mentioned, but even essay questions can be contaminated if students give responses they think the teacher would favor rather than their true feelings. To remedy this situation, attitude scales have been developed that are quite effective. These frequently are based upon either the forced-choice format, the Likert scale, or the semantic differential format.

### Forced-Choice Format

This format, also called "paired comparisons," allows the respondent to select the more favorable of two choices. A score is derived, usually the median of the respondent's favorable choices. A disadvantage of the forced-choice instrument is its often-obvious presentation of the response the teacher prefers. Students who are interested in pleasing the teacher may make this choice rather than express their true feelings. Samples are shown in Box 12.3.

### Likert Scale

The Likert scale is probably the tool most commonly used by health educators to measure attitudes (McDermott & Sarvela, 1999). It provides a greater range of choices than does the typical forced-choice scale. When ranking people with regard to a particular attitude, the Likert scale is highly reliable (Miller, 1977). Likert scales for young children should provide only a few choices, such as those in Box 12.4.

For respondents who are more mature, several choices can be utilized, such as those in Box 12.5. The responses may be weighted: For instance, in items 1 and 2, "Strongly Agree" may be given a value of 5, "Agree" a 4, "Undecided" a 3, "Disagree" a 2, and "Strongly Disagree" a value of 1. Depending on the wording of the item, the values may be

**Box 12.3    Forced-Choice Attitude Items**

|  | AGREE | DISAGREE |
|---|---|---|
| 1. Regular exercise is important to health. | _____ | _____ |
| 2. Abortion is acceptable only if the mother was raped or her life is in danger. | _____ | _____ |
| 3. Drinking alcohol can result in problems with the law. | _____ | _____ |
| 4. I like to laugh at other people's mistakes. | _____ | _____ |

**Box 12.4    A Likert Scale with Three Choices**

|  | AGREE | NOT SURE | DISAGREE |
|---|---|---|---|
| 1. It helps to talk to someone about my problems. | ___ | ___ | ___ |
| 2. Smoking can lead to serious illness. | ___ | ___ | ___ |
| 3. I have no sympathy for drug users who get AIDS. | ___ | ___ | ___ |
| 4. A few minutes of quiet time to myself every day makes me feel good. | ___ | ___ | ___ |

**Box 12.5    A Likert Scale with Five Choices**

|  | STRONGLY AGREE | AGREE | UNDECIDED | DISAGREE | STRONGLY DISAGREE |
|---|---|---|---|---|---|
| 1. Regular exercise is good for the heart. | _____ | _____ | _____ | _____ | _____ |
| 2. Cigarettes contain an addictive drug. | _____ | _____ | _____ | _____ | _____ |
| 3. I would rather watch TV than play outside. | _____ | _____ | _____ | _____ | _____ |
| 4. People who get AIDS have only themselves to blame. | _____ | _____ | _____ | _____ | _____ |

reversed for some items, such as items 3 and 4. The total numerical score provides a rough measure of attitude. Just as with the forced-choice, the fact that students may respond in ways that reflect their perceptions of the teacher's wishes is a disadvantage.

**Semantic Differential Format**    The semantic differential is a means of measuring a respondent's feeling toward or value placed on a concept. It is useful for measuring changes in attitude after instruction. A set of bipolar adjectives is provided with spaces between them, as shown in Box 12.6.

The respondent is asked to rate the concept (in Box 12.6, the concept is "Health Education") by checking the space corresponding most closely to his or her feelings about the word or concept. Some word sets may appear irrelevant to the concept, but the respondent should provide a response based on a quick reaction to the words themselves. These seemingly irrelevant words make the responses less vulnerable to answering as the respondent thinks the administrator favors. A middle space allows for neutral responses, and other spaces reflect the degree of positive or negative feelings. Pairs of words

**Box 12.6**    A Semantic Differential Model

**Health Education**

| Good | ___ : | ___ : | ___ : | ___ : | ___ : | ___ : | ___ : | Bad |
|------|-------|-------|-------|-------|-------|-------|-------|-----|
| Caring | ___ : | ___ : | ___ : | ___ : | ___ : | ___ : | ___ : | Uncaring |
| Unfair | ___ : | ___ : | ___ : | ___ : | ___ : | ___ : | ___ : | Fair |
| Fast | ___ : | ___ : | ___ : | ___ : | ___ : | ___ : | ___ : | Slow |
| Smooth | ___ : | ___ : | ___ : | ___ : | ___ : | ___ : | ___ : | Rough |
| Awful | ___ : | ___ : | ___ : | ___ : | ___ : | ___ : | ___ : | Nice |
| Strong | ___ : | ___ : | ___ : | ___ : | ___ : | ___ : | ___ : | Weak |
| Sad | ___ : | ___ : | ___ : | ___ : | ___ : | ___ : | ___ : | Happy |
| Pretty | ___ : | ___ : | ___ : | ___ : | ___ : | ___ : | ___ : | Ugly |
| Clean | ___ : | ___ : | ___ : | ___ : | ___ : | ___ : | ___ : | Dirty |

should be mixed so the positive word is not always on the same side. Possible scoring could be 7 points for most positive, 4 points for neutral, and 1 point for most negative. The total score represents the respondent's feelings toward the concept.

## Guttman Scale

The Guttman scale, also called cumulative scale, is comprised of a set of items that are ordered based on difficulty or value-loading (Rubinson & Neutens, 1987). Although they can be used to measure knowledge, they are more frequently used to measure attitudes toward a single variable. Scales are designed by arranging a set of items by their degree of positiveness or favorableness towards the variable under study. A respondent whose score on a Guttman scale places him or her at a particular point on the attitude continuum must agree with all items below his own scale position and must disagree with all items above his scale position (Mueller, 1986). Box 12.7 contains a Guttman scale measuring attitudes about abortion. In this example, an individual who agrees with the first statement will also probably agree with all other statements, while a person who agrees with only statements 4 and 5 will probably not agree with statements 1, 2, or 3.

The Guttman scale allows for attitudes and psychological constructs to be narrowly defined. Therefore, scale scores have a very precise interpretation, allowing for comparison among individuals.

## Interviews

Interviews have been discussed as part of needs assessment (see Chapter 11). They are also very useful in determining individuals' attitudes about certain issues or groups of people. They have the advantages of being useful when the respondent cannot read or write or when the questions are long and complex. They are also expedient when the content of the study is not specified or well defined. However, they can allow bias to occur if the respondents feel that the interviewer has expectations of them. There is also the possibility that variation will be introduced by multiple interviewers or by one interviewer's differing reactions to multiple respondents.

The teacher-student conference is a special type of interview. By establishing a rapport with the

**Box 12.7**    The Guttman Scale

1. Abortion should be given on demand.
2. Abortion is OK for family planning.
3. Abortion is OK in cases of rape.
4. Abortion is acceptable if the fetus is malformed.
5. Abortion is acceptable when a mother's life is in danger.

Source: From *Measuring Social Attitudes*, by D.J. Mueller, 1986, New York: Teachers College Press. Reprinted by permission of the publisher.

individual student, the teacher can become a confidant. This is conducive to learning about both the student's health behavior and his or her attitudes. Students who are embarrassed to discuss feelings in class often find it easier to open up in individual conferences.

## Measuring Behavior

Determining health-related behavior is often difficult. Health instruction and health promotion programs usually have establishment of behavior or behavior change as central objectives. For example, a first aid class may require the proper performance of CPR. Other programs may be geared to increasing frequency of condom use or selection of healthier foods.

Observation   One way to measure behavior is through observation. By critically observing typical situations, teachers can determine if instruction has had significant impact on students' behavior. This is usually done by the instructor, although it could be done by some neutral party. For example, a teacher could observe and note the food choices made by children at the lunch counter. An evaluator could be employed to observe college students' drinking behaviors at bars or nightclubs. This type of evaluation requires a consistent number of observations during a consistent time period with detailed descriptions of behaviors observed and noted with a planned method of recording. Reliability among raters and among rating instances is dependent upon adequate training. Another problem, called "social desirability response bias," occurs when subjects know they are being observed and change their behavior to behave more socially desirably.

Methods of conducting and recording observations include checklists and records that count the number of times the behavior is observed. It is also possible for the evaluator to rate the quality of the behavior through numerical rating scales, graphic rating scales using lines or bars, or through forced-choice scales that allow the evaluator to rate the individual in terms of a set of alternatives.

Teacher observation sometimes can be an effective method of gauging behavior. However, this method is clouded because teachers can observe students only in the school environment, when children may be on their best behavior or may not have the freedom to engage in some behaviors, such as drinking and smoking. Discretion must be exercised so as not to violate student privacy.

Students can be trained to observe their peers. In order to be effective, students should work together to establish the criteria or standards for judging their peers' work and behavior. Instruments, such as checklists, can be developed to assist students to observe peers.

Similar to and supplemental to teacher observation is a technique called "anecdotal record keeping," which is usually performed by the teacher, but could also be done by parents. This technique should be a simple, objective report of a specific event and preferably be used only with behaviors that cannot be evaluated by other means. The reports should contain all relevant information (including time, date, setting) and the incident, along with the signature of the observer. All teachers should be encouraged to keep anecdotal records, because a collection of anecdotes from multiple sources and varying settings can indicate behavioral patterns. Including only relevant information and prompt recording encourages better understanding and accuracy. Positive as well as negative anecdotes should be reported. After all, no student exhibits only positive or negative behavior. Still, interpretation of observation depends a great deal on the eye of the beholder.

Self-Report Instruments   Behavior can also be measured by behavior inventories, diaries, or self-report questionnaires; all of these are forms of self-report instruments. They all ask respondents to report their own behavior with items such as "How many times did you exercise last week?"; "How many cigarettes have you smoked today?"; or "Record everything you eat over a two-week period." Self-report questionnaires are especially useful in evaluating the effects of a program in meeting its goals. Answers given confidentially or anonymously are more likely to be accurate. Unfortunately, students may not be totally honest if they can be identified, especially if the behavior is illegal.

The health behavior inventory relies on students' honesty in responding to the items, but can serve to help students become more aware of their own behaviors. The inventory contains a list of actions to which the student responds "yes" ("+") or "no" ("−"). This type of inventory is called a checklist. At the educator's option, choices such as "sometimes," "seldom," and "usually" can be added, making the inventory a rating scale. Positive answers indicate choices to practice skills that promote health literacy, maintain and improve health, prevent disease, and reduce health risk behaviors. Negative answers indicate choosing actions that may interfere with health literacy, harm health, and increase the risk of disease or injury and premature death (Meeks, Heit, & Page, 1996). Examples of items include the following:

1. I read food labels.

2. I get vigorous exercise at least three times per week.

3. I recycle.

The health behavior inventory is particularly useful with adult clients.

Individuals can be prompted to keep daily records, or diaries, of various activities. This can include recording things like exercise (time of day, how long, what activity, how you felt afterward), food selection, and perceptions and feelings related to the behavior. For example, a diary assignment might read, "For one month, record the date, time, and duration of each instance of physical exercise that lasted more than three minutes. Record how you felt, both emotionally and physically, after each exercise session." This type of measurement can be used to link the activity to attitude change.

Questionnaires can be constructed to elicit responses that indicate frequency of behavior. They can be crafted to produce detailed information much like that in a diary.

Self-reporting is a form of self-evaluation. In the school setting, student input is becoming more of an issue because a student who is part of the evaluation process cannot help getting involved. Such evaluation is also likely to be much more meaningful to the student (Bender et al., 1997). Students usually require some practice before becoming proficient at self-evaluation.

**Mastery**   An emerging trend in student evaluation is the mastery approach, which may have elements of observation and self-reporting. This can take many forms, but the central idea is that certain skills or competencies must be mastered to achieve an acceptable level of proficiency. The learner and educator often decide cooperatively what actions the learner must take to master the skills, what level of proficiency is acceptable, and the ways to demonstrate that proficiency. For instance, the student may be required to answer a certain number of questions on an examination, write a paper that expresses feelings about an issue satisfactorily, collect and analyze television advertisements for food products, and monitor his or her own diet for three weeks to demonstrate achievement of a certain minimal level of calories derived from fat. All materials showing actions taken to demonstrate mastery can be collected in a **portfolio**, which the teacher evaluates in light of the agreed-upon standards. In skill-based evaluations, the student/client may be required to perform a series of steps that culminate in demonstrating the skill. For instance, the first aid student may demonstrate mastery of CPR skills by performing a prescribed set of steps in the process of CPR on mannequins.

**Authentic Assessment**   In recent years, the **authentic assessment** approach (called "AA") to student evaluation has gained favor among educators, because it emphasizes meaning behind learning. It allows for students to participate actively in their own learning (Paris & Ayres, 1994; Terry & Pantle, 1994) in a constructive way. This approach allows teachers to examine students' basic skills, control of information, higher level of understanding, personal characteristics, and habits of mind. The designation "authentic" comes from the fact that these assessment strategies require the learners to demonstrate that they do certain things in real, out-of-school settings.

**portfolio**   a collection of student work and educator data from informal and performance assessments

**authentic assessment**   strategies that require learners to demonstrate that they do certain things in real, out-of-school settings

Assessments are authentic when they have meaning in themselves—when the learning they measure has value beyond the classroom and is meaningful to the learner (Kerka, 1995). For instance, knowing that a diet high in fat and low in fiber increases risk for cardiovascular disease and certain types of cancer can be assessed quite easily on a cognitive basis. If this knowledge is not translated into action, though (such as consuming a diet low in fat and high in fiber), it can be argued that health instruction has not been effective and the student has not truly internalized the information. AA has the potential for discovering if the skills, abilities, attitudes, and practices addressed in instructional objectives actually have been developed. Portfolios can be effective in authentic assessment.

Maksimowicz (1993) wrote that AA materials should do the following:

— reflect important themes and ideas

— be consistent with curriculum goals

— be rooted in real-world experiences and have application both inside and outside school

— be sensitive to students' developmental progress

— allow students to engage in critical thinking

Maksimowicz' statement is compelling because it provides criteria for authentic assessment as well as positive aspects of it.

AA techniques also

• allow students to demonstrate a rich array of what they know and can do;

• display products and processes of learning;

• are adaptable, flexible, ongoing, and cumulative; and

• allow multiple judgments of learning and achievement by providing multiple exhibits.

They can be more equitable in accommodating learning styles and acknowledging multiple ways of demonstrating competence. AA can engage worthy problems or tasks with real-life applicability. They can provide opportunities for learner self-evaluation and fairness in scoring procedures and their applications (Kerka, 1995). They also can increase learner interest, motivation, and independence (Grady, 1994).

The formats for AA can be lavishly multidimensional and varied. Darling-Hammond (1993) stated that examples and approaches fall into three categories, often overlapping: performance-based tasks and exhibitions, portfolios, and documentation over time.

**Performance-based tasks and exhibitions** includes activities such as simulations, product assessments, projects, checklists, and performance tasks. All of these methods have been used successfully in health education classes with children as young as grades 2–4 (Foucar-Szocki, 1994). Perhaps the key to success of these strategies is that they represent performance, evaluate against openly expressed standards, help students learn to evaluate themselves, and require public presentation and defense of their work—all critical aspects of AA (Darling-Hammond, 1994).

**Portfolios** are collections of student work. They are particularly popular tools in applying AA. They can provide an in-depth, personalized view of the student's progress and a rich array of what students know, do, and feel. Thus they can be used as a multidimensional tool to evaluate behavior, knowledge, attitudes, and critical thinking skills. When planning portfolio assessment, the teacher first must determine the purpose of the portfolio. If the purpose is to track student progress, the teacher must determine which learner goals will be assessed, what samples can demonstrate achievement of these goals, and what criteria will be used to evaluate the portfolio contents (Meeks, Heit, & Page, 1996). A real advantage of portfolios is that students can be involved in selecting their best work, which forces them to determine the strengths and weaknesses of their samples. This encourages self-reflection and self-evaluation.

Four classes of portfolio documentation have been identified (Collins, 1991):

1. Artifacts are actual samples of students' work. A health education artifact could be a student-designed brochure to educate others about a voluntary health agency, a student-produced video illustrating proper use of nutrition labels, a research paper on a health-related topic, or a copy of a completed test.

2. Reproductions are tangible evidence of student participation, such as photographs or a videotape of a student helping in a community recycling campaign or working at a school or community health fair.

3. Attestations are documents written about the student's work by someone other than the student. Examples include letters from the organizer of a health fair acknowledging the student's participation or letters describing the student's work with the elderly in a nursing home.

4. Productions are works the student prepares to document knowledge and skills. According to Cleary (1993), productions may include a student's written reflection of the portfolio's contents, with captions attached to each document describing the piece and what knowledge or skills the student gained while completing the piece.

**Documentation over time** is a form of self-reporting that can take numerous forms. One of the most useful is the student log or diary, in which the student records certain behaviors regularly. For instance, he or she may record the circumstances surrounding each cigarette smoked, efforts taken to reduce the number of cigarettes used, and a subjective appraisal of his or her success. Another example would entail recording snacks consumed over a month's time. These activities force the student to confront his or her own behavior and evaluate it. Anecdotal record keeping is another means of implementing documentation over time. Anecdotes could be recorded by the teacher, the parent, or the student.

Certainly, all categories of AA are more difficult to implement than more traditional methods of evaluation. Decisions about weight assigned to different examples of work and exactly how to evaluate each student's efforts are often difficult. AA has the added disadvantage of requiring much teacher time. In addition, in most classroom assessment, AA is only part of the student's evaluation; tests and other traditional methods are also used.

Any evaluation of behavior is questionable. This is unfortunate, because health behavior is an essential outcome of health instruction. Evaluating behaviors that occur outside the school setting is most difficult because certain kinds of behavior may not be evaluated for years after instruction, and the most significant impact on health behavior may never be evaluated at all. Measuring the amount of undesirable behavior that never happened because of effective instruction is virtually impossible.

## Grading

Most health educators who practice in a school setting are compelled to use grading to assign value to students' performance or change. Grades inform students, parents, administrators, and college admissions officers about the student's progress and work efficiency. Ideally, grades should not be an end in themselves. Instead, they should act as motivators for students to do their best and as guides for future courses of study (Anspaugh & Ezell, 1998). The following principles always should be paramount:

1. Make evaluations relevant to objectives.
2. Consider only the behaviors that reflect academic achievement to determine grades.
3. Consistently use only valid evidence as a basis for arriving at grades.
4. Evaluate fairly and consistently.
5. Take precautions to prevent cheating on tests and other measurement activities.
6. Make it clear to the students how they will be evaluated.
7. Allow students access to grade progress throughout the term.
8. Use more than one method of evaluation.
9. Never use grades as a tool for discipline; poor conduct, good attitude, or teacher frustration should not be a part of the grade.

Grades on test scores or evaluations of completed assignments or projects are impact evaluations at best. Final grades, although often assumed to constitute outcome evaluations because they become a part of a student's permanent record, are more often impact evaluations.

Students and parents expect classroom evaluation to result in grades. Student grades may have different meanings, depending upon the referencing framework within which they have has been assigned. Three referencing frameworks (Nitko, 1983) are common:

1. *Task-* or *criterion-referenced grades* are based upon absolute standards of achievement—for example, the requirement that a student answer 80 percent of the test questions correctly or do six pull-ups.

2. *Group-* or *norm-referenced grades* are based upon relative standards, in that the student's grade reflects his or her ranking compared with everyone else in the group. A common example of norm-referenced grades is the "curving" of test scores.

3. *Self-referenced grades* reflect a comparison between a pupil's performance and the teacher's perception of that individual's capability. For example, in classrooms with students who have a wide range of abilities, standards may be higher for some students than for others, allowing even students of low academic talent opportunities for positive feedback.

Although published over forty years ago, Diederich's (1964) words still ring clear and true:

> Teachers should not be in a position merely to declare that students are improving or not improving.... They should approach the task of evaluation not with the arrogance of a judge, but with the humility of an enquirer. The proper frame of mind for evaluation is fear and trembling. Then, if everything turns out all right, the relief of the teachers should be even more stupendous than that of the students!

## EVALUATION OF THE EDUCATOR

Although evaluation of students/clients commands most of the attention, any credible practitioner welcomes evaluation of his or her performance as a legitimate way of fostering improvement. In view of the current, often shrill rhetoric concerning teacher accountability, it becomes even more important. Retention, granting tenure for teachers, and upgrading of teacher skills are common uses of educator evaluation.

The task of evaluating teacher effectiveness is littered with faulty assumptions and uncontrollable sources of error. These problems seriously contaminate and threaten the reliability of conclusions that might be drawn from the obtained data, but should not preclude the teacher's careful and critical examination of his or her own performance and commitment to being a role model for students. In general, three approaches have been employed: (1) psychometric analysis of the relationship between measures of teacher behavior based on comparisons between pretest and post-test scores on standardized achievement tests; (2) systematic observations of teacher behavior, testing its consistency with specified criteria of acceptable performance; and (3) self-reports obtained by means of structured interviews or questions (Pollock & Middleton, 1994).

The practice of evaluating students at the beginning of the school year (pretest) and again at the end (post-test) and comparing the results is being considered in many states and districts *as a method to evaluate teachers.* This is a variation of the first approach. More common methods used in statewide assessments of teacher effectiveness involve students' mean scores on standardized achievement tests. Mean scores from school districts are compared with previous scores and those from other districts. They sometimes are even used to compare public school teaching with that in private schools. However, it is rather unusual for scientific analysis of teacher behavior to be studied in light of students' standardized achievement test scores; it is even more unusual for such scientific analysis to be used in individual teacher evaluation.

Many school districts and states are struggling with the issue of evaluating teacher performance, an issue that has become quite controversial. Obviously, variables—such as family education and structure and socioeconomic status of students, as well as curricular differences and education funding—can influence these comparisons, although they are seldom included in the assessment and evaluation. Teachers and parents often claim that scores on a single test (or even a series of tests) are insufficient to evaluate years of schooling, let alone the performance of teachers. Teachers may also have a tendency to "teach to the test" (Nickerson, 1989), turning the classroom into a laboratory for testing rather than an eclectic learning environment.

Evaluation of individual teachers often is based entirely on observations by administrators. In some cases, peers also observe the teacher and contribute to the evaluation. These observations usually are done in single visits, often consisting of less than a full class session. This hit-or-miss approach is sorely lacking in objectivity, thoroughness, validity, and reliability and seldom leads to professional growth on the teacher's part. Observations, when done uniformly by qualified evaluators, can be a valuable method of evaluating the program implementation skills of educators in a variety of settings.

Johnson and Orso (1986) conducted a broad study of teacher effectiveness standards that may lead to some useful criteria. They surveyed large school systems in all 50 states to identify consistencies among the states' evaluation instruments. Forty-eight systems—one each in 48 states—responded. The survey identified five categories of teacher behavior and criteria for their evaluation common to all of them. The five categories of behavior were (1) instruction, (2) classroom management, (3) professional responsibilities, (4) personal characteristics, and (5) interpersonal relations. The researchers concluded that teachers have difficulty in the first category—instructing—unless they have mastered the other four categories.

Interestingly, many states are providing rewards for teachers who acquire certification from the National Board for Professional Teaching Standards. Certification may further reduce the frequency and thoroughness with which teachers are evaluated on the local level.

Although evaluation of teachers can take many approaches, they should all produce opportunities to improve performance. Thorough analysis of one's evaluation coupled with conversations with supervisors and other educators can make evaluation a powerful tool of improvement. For teacher evaluation, one standard rises above the others. As Pollock and Middleton (1994) asserted, "Probably the most reliable gauge of a teacher's effectiveness is whether the instruction has enabled most, if not all, of the students to demonstrate successful achievement of the course objectives."

## KEY POINTS

1. Evaluation can serve many positive purposes, including improving individual and program performance and identifying students in need of special assistance.

2. Measurement, which determines quantity or quality of an object of interest, is a basic tool of evaluation. Evaluation compares the quantity or quality of the objective of interest to predetermined standards of acceptability.

3. Measurement instruments must be valid, reliable, sensitive, and objective. They must discriminate among those who possess the trait being measured, those who do not, and those who possess it in various degrees. They must have a sufficient level of administrability, or ease of use.

4. There are three levels of evaluation. Diagnostic evaluation is a component of needs assessment, yielding information about current status. Formative evaluation yields data on the program itself while it is being developed and implemented. In summative evaluation, we learn the degree to which the program has met predetermined goals and objectives.

5. Impact evaluation provides information about immediate, short-term effects. Outcome evaluation provides information about long-term or ultimate effects. Both are forms of summative evaluation.

6. Evaluating a learner is a somewhat different process from evaluating a program's effectiveness.

7. Many different types of tests and test items are available and useful to measure student knowledge. Educators should select the test items on the basis of applicability to the learners, content, objectives, and setting.

8. Measuring attitudes is not a simple process. However, a number of techniques—including the forced-choice format, Likert scale, semantic differential, and interview—can be applied effectively to assess attitudes.

9. Measuring behavior is often difficult and can be fraught with complications. Observations, self-report instruments, mastery, and authentic assessment are methods to assess behavior.

10. Evaluation of teachers is controversial and largely unscientific. Nevertheless, it has the potential to produce opportunities to improve teacher performance.

# REFERENCES

American Educational Research Association, American Psychological Association, & National Council on Measurement in Education. (1985). *Standards for educational and psychological testing.* Washington, DC: American Psychological Association.

Anspaugh, D.J., & Ezell, G. (1998). *Teaching today's health* (5th ed.). Boston: Allyn & Bacon.

Astin, A.W. (1992). *Principles of good practice for assessing student learning.* Washington, DC: American Association for Higher Education.

Bender, S.J., Neutens, J.J., Skonie-Hardin, S., & Sorochan, W.D. (1997). *Teaching health science: Elementary and middle school* (4th ed.). Boston: Jones and Bartlett.

Carmine, E.G., & Zeller, R.A. (1979). *Reliability and validity assessment.* Beverly Hills: Sage.

Cleary, M. (1993). Using portfolios to assess student performance in school health education. *Journal of School Health, 63*(9), 377–380.

Collins, A. (1991). Portfolios for biology teacher assessment. *Journal of School Personnel Evaluation Education, 5*(3), 147–167.

Creswell, Jr., W.H., & Newman, I.M. (1993). *School health practice* (10th ed.). St. Louis: Times Mirror/Mosby.

Darling-Hammond, L. (1993). *Authentic assessment in practice: A collection of portfolios, performance tasks, exhibitions, and documentation.* New York: National Center for Restructuring Education, Schools and Teaching, Columbia University.

Darling-Hammond, L. (1994, Fall). Setting standards for students: The case for authentic assessment. *Educational Forum, 59,* 14–21.

Diederich, P.B. (1964). The classroom teacher and the teacher-made test. *Education Horizons, 43*(3), 20.

Dignan, M.B., & Carr, P.A. (1992). *Program planning for health education and health promotion* (2nd ed.). Baltimore: Williams & Wilkins.

Ebel, R.L., & Frisbie, D.A. (1986). *Essentials of educational measurement* (4th ed.). Englewood Cliffs, NJ: Prentice-Hall.

Foucar-Szocki, D. (1994). *Becoming assessors: Authentic assessment for authentic instruction. A report of the Blue Ridge Assessment Project.* Charlottesville, VA: Albemarle County Schools.

Grady, J.B. (1994). Authentic assessment and tasks: Helping students demonstrate their abilities. *NASSP Bulletin, 78*(556), 92–98.

Green, L.W., & Kreuter, M.W. (1999). *Health promotion planning: An educational and ecological approach.* Mountain View, CA: Mayfield.

Hochbaum, G. (1982). Certain problems in evaluating and their implications for test development. *Health Values, 6*(1), 14–21.

Hopkins, C.D., & Antes, R.L. (1990). *Classroom measurement and evaluation* (3rd ed.). Itasca, IL: Peacock.

Johnson, N.C., & Orso, J.K. (1986). Teacher evaluation criteria. *ERS Spectrum, 4*(3), 33–36.

Kerka, S. (1995). *Techniques for authentic assessment* (ED381688). Columbus, OH: ERIC Clearinghouse on Adult, Career, and Vocational Education.

Kreuter, M.W., & Green, L.W. (1978). Evaluation of school health education: Identifying purpose, keeping perspective. *Journal of School Health, 48*(2), 228–235.

Lilienfeld, D.E., & Stolley, P.D. (1994). *Foundations of epidemiology* (4th ed.). New York: Oxford University Press.

Maksimowicz, M.L. (1993). *Focus on authentic learning and assessment in the middle school.* East Lansing: Michigan Association of Middle School Educators, Michigan State University.

McDermott, R.J., & Sarvela, P.D. (1999). *Health education evaluation and measurement: A practitioner's perspective* (2nd ed.). Boston: WCB/McGraw-Hill.

Meeks, L., Heit, P., & Page, R. (1996). *Comprehensive school health education: Totally awesome teaching strategies.* Blacklick, OH: Meeks Heit.

Miller, D.C. (1977). *Handbook of research design and social measurement* (3rd ed.). New York: Longman.

Mueller, D.J. (1986). *Measuring social attitudes.* New York: Teachers College Press.

National Council on Measurement in Education. (1990). *Standards for teacher competence in educational assessment of students.* Washington, DC.

National Task Force for the Preparation and Practice of Health Educators. (1985). *A guide for the development of competency-based curricula for entry-level health educators.* New York.

Nickerson, R.S. (1989). New directions in educational assessment. *Educational Researcher, 18*(9), 3–7.

Nitko, A. (1983). *Educational tests and measurements: An introduction.* New York: Harcourt Brace Jovanovich.

Oberteuffer, D., Harrelson, O.A., & Pollock, M.B. (1972). *School health education* (5th ed.). New York: Harper & Row.

Paris, S.G., & Ayres, L.R. (1994). *Becoming reflective students and teachers with portfolios and authentic assessment.* Washington, DC: American Psychological Association.

Patton, M.Q. (1980). *Qualitative evaluation.* Beverly Hills: Sage.

Patton, M.Q. (1982). *Practical evaluation.* Beverly Hills: Sage.

Payne, D.A. (1992). *Measuring and evaluating educational objectives.* New York: Merrill.

Pollock, M.B., & Middleton, K. (1994). *School health instruction: The elementary & middle school years* (3rd ed.). St. Louis: Mosby.

Rubinson, L., & Neutens, J.J. (1987). *Research techniques for the health sciences.* New York: Macmillan.

Smith, M., & Glass, G. (1987). *Research and evaluation in education and the social sciences.* Englewood Cliffs, NJ: Prentice-Hall.

Stake, R.E. (1975). *Evaluating the arts in education: A responsive approach.* Columbus, OH: Charles E. Merrill.

Terry, C.A., & Pantle, T.T. (1994). Authentic assessment: Reducing the fear and trembling. *Journal of Secondary Gifted Education, 6*(3), 44–51.

Veney, J.E., & Kaluzny, A.D. (1991). *Evaluation and decision making for health services* (2nd ed.). Ann Arbor, MI: Health Administration Press.

# Current and Future Issues in Health Promotion/Education

**H**ealth promotion, though evolving, will continue to face important issues in the future. Although health education has been part of children's educational experience for many years, the profession in many ways is still in its own adolescence. It must continue to mature, establishing its role in tomorrow's school systems, health care systems, worksites, and other venues. Technology, research, and world and national health problems will shape the development of health education and health promotion.

Although we have improved our ability to predict the health problems of tomorrow, we are still met with surprising challenges. The effects of AIDS on sexual attitudes and behavior as well as the health care and insurance industries would not have been predicted 25 years ago. The resurgence of tuberculosis is a surprise to most health authorities. Predicting the future is always difficult. Still, we can examine current issues and draw conclusions about approaching needs and coming events.

Health educators/promoters must be willing and prepared to take their place in the world of tomorrow. The social issues will change, forcing the content of courses, curricula, and programs to change. Clark (1994) made several cogent points regarding health education of the future:

- Our mission will be to develop more analytical thinkers who are more able to deal with an uncertain and complex environment.

- Community-based health education will be the focus of more health education interventions as it becomes more urgent to empower communities.

- More and more environmental activism will emerge, and it will cross age, economic, regional, cultural, and partisan lines.

- Health education will place more emphasis on values clarification, which will help us account for the different ways values are manifested in different cultures.

- The measure of successful health education in the future will be whether people judge the quality of their lives to be better because of it.

- Health educators can control the future to some extent and, to a larger extent, help individuals adjust to it. We must be prepared to act in both proactive and reactive ways.

## CREDENTIALING

**Credentialing** is a formal process applied to ensure that those practicing a profession meet acceptable standards. Efforts toward credentialing of educators

**credentialing**  a formal process applied to ensure that those practicing a profession meet acceptable standards; may apply to individuals, institutions, or programs

in America have historically been poor, inconsistent, and the least demanding of any profession. When compared with other professions (such as social work, medicine, nursing, and law), teaching has historically had the least demanding training requirements. Teachers can complete an unaccredited program, or no program at all, and still be licensed under emergency or alternative forms of certification. No state issues "emergency" or "alternative" licenses to people wishing to become social workers, physicians, nurses, or attorneys (Wise, 1994a). The nation cannot afford this type of laissez-faire approach to education.

Livingood et al. (1993) highlighted the importance of credentialing when they wrote, "Credentialing in some form is a dominant mechanism by which a division of expert labor convinces society that its practitioners capably provide the societal service." Individual credentialing may be through licensure, certification, or registration. Program or institutional credentialing may be through accreditation or approval. Credentialing has been applied at the state and national levels and is administered by state governments, independent organizations, and professional associations.

Credentialing of professionals has a number of benefits. If applied properly, it can (National Commission for Health Education Credentialing, 1989):

— attest to the individual's knowledge and skills deemed essential to the field of practice as delineated by the profession

— assist employers to identify qualified professionals

— assist the public in recognizing the basic competencies of those who are credentialed

— recognize a commitment to professional standards

— enhance the profession

— provide recognition to individual practitioners

— facilitate geographic mobility of qualified practitioners

— strengthen professional preparation

— promote an organized system of continuing education

Credentialing and standards of practice are means to control access to a profession. Certainly, they should not be seen as hidden justification for excluding other practitioners from the economic aggrandizement of health education (Clark, 1984; Green, 1985), but they should ensure that those practicing as health educators/promoters are competent to deliver the services offered by the profession.

## Credentialing of Teachers and Teacher Preparation Programs

"**Licensure** is the generic term referring to all forms of state control over the right to perform specific duties" (Gross, 1984). In occupational licensing, states determine that those licensed have a minimal degree of competency to ensure that the public health, safety, and welfare will be reasonably protected. Some professions require licensure under an occupational title, such as physician. This is not currently the case with health education or health promotion. However, a type of partial licensing referred to as **state teacher certification** (a few states use the term "teacher licensure") exists. Teacher certification is a process of legal recognition authorizing the individual holder of the certificate to perform specific services, usually teaching, in the public schools of the state. Some states require certification for administrative positions and some for teaching in colleges. The traditional method of attaining certification is to complete a college degree program of teacher education that meets the state certification requirements. Several states require applicants for certificates to pass all or part of the Praxis Series Assessments. A few states require other examinations as a requirement for certification. In most states, a structure is in place requiring continual professional development, including college courses, workshops, seminars, and inservice programs. In short, to maintain their certification, teachers must anticipate taking courses continually, earning inservice credits, and being observed and evaluated (Campbell, 1990).

**Registration** is a less-restrictive form of state control in which states merely maintain a list of individuals who perform certain tasks, without requiring qualification or passing an examination.

The person's name is simply entered on a list (Taub, 1993). Although this may be common in certain occupations, it seldom is utilized in education. In a few states, registries of health educators are maintained by professional associations at the local level. These registries are not necessarily under state control, but they can be made available to the state.

The credentialing of teachers is undergoing considerable reform. Alternative routes to certification or licensing is a recent trend. Rather than completing a traditional baccalaureate degree in a college or university teacher education program, alternative routes allow persons from other careers to obtain credentials. By 1998, 41 states and the District of Columbia had some type of alternative teacher certification program, and more than 80,000 people had been certified or licensed through these programs (Feistritzer, 1999). Alternative routes have become popular because of the threat of teacher shortages and the lack of ethnic diversity among teachers in many areas. The most effective alternative certification programs

— have a strong academic coursework component;

— are field-based, allowing individuals to get into classrooms early in their preparation;

— provide a qualified mentor to work with the candidates;

— allow candidates to go through their programs in cohorts rather than as isolated individuals; and

— are collaborative efforts involving state departments of education, institutions of higher education, and school districts.

Given the widespread acceptance of the alternative routes, they are likely to be the entry point for many more individuals in the future, including health educators.

Teacher credentialing will probably undergo change for many years into the future. Partners in this process include the National Council for the Accreditation of Teacher Education (NCATE), National Board for Professional Teaching Standards (NBPTS), the Council of Chief State School Officers (CCSSO), and the Interstate New Teacher Assessment and Support Consortium (INTASC). These organizations are working together to develop complementary standards, so that preparation standards reflect the skills and knowledge needed for state licensing examinations and so that both accreditation and individual credentialing help candidates and teachers build the skills needed for success on board certification assessments (Wise, 1996). The process involves a new philosophy of teacher preparation and recognition based primarily on demonstration of competencies.

INTASC, a program of the CCSSO, is a consortium of state education agencies, higher education institutions, and national education organizations. INTASC has produced model standards for licensing new teachers (see Box 13.1). The standards represent a common core of teaching knowledge and skills which will help all students acquire twenty-first century knowledge and skills. The standards were developed to be compatible with the advanced certification standards of NBPTS (INTASC, 1999). The core standards were designed to be performance-based—describing what teachers should know and be able to do—and they are connected to what students should know and be able to do in order to meet new K–12 standards.

INTASC is developing discipline-specific standards and performance assessments for credentialing teachers. A series of academies help teachers and teacher educators understand the design and function of an INTASC portfolio and how the portfolio assessment can be used for teacher licensing, individual professional development, and reform of teacher education programs (CCSSO, 1999). This approach to creating standards is based on a holistic conception of career development for teaching professionals. It describes rigorous expectations for beginning teachers and lays out elements of competent entry-level practice to ensure consistency with emerging visions of accomplished teaching. Through

**licensure**    all forms of state control over the right to perform specific duties

**state teacher certification**    legal recognition authorizing the individual holder of the certificate to perform specific services in public schools within the state

**registration**    placement of the individual's name on a list of those who perform certain tasks

## Box 13.1   INTASC Core Standards

- The teacher understands the central concepts, tools of inquiry, and structures of the discipline(s) he or she teaches and can create learning experiences that make these aspects of subject matter meaningful for students

- The teacher understands how children learn and develop, and can provide learning opportunities that support their intellectual, social and personal development.

- The teacher understands how students differ in their approaches to learning and creates instructional opportunities that are adapted to diverse learners.

- The teacher understands and uses a variety of instructional strategies to encourage students' development of critical thinking, problem solving, and performance skills.

- The teacher uses an understanding of individual and group motivation and behavior to create a learning environment that encourages positive social interaction, active engagement in learning, and self-motivation.

- The teacher uses knowledge of effective verbal, nonverbal, and media communication techniques to foster active inquiry, collaboration, and supportive interaction in the classroom.

- The teacher plans instruction based upon knowledge of subject matter, students, the community, and curriculum goals.

- The teacher understands and uses formal and informal assessment strategies to evaluate and ensure the continuous intellectual, social and physical development of the learner.

- The teacher is a reflective practitioner who continually evaluates the effects of his or her choices and actions on others (students, parents, and other professionals in the learning community) and who actively seeks out opportunities to grow professionally.

- The teacher fosters relationships with school colleagues, parents, and agencies in the larger community to support students' learning and well-being.

Source: Interstate New Teacher Assessment and Support Consortium (*INTASC*). *Model Standards for Beginning Teacher Licensing and Development*. Washington, D.C.: Council of Chief State School Officers, 1999. Available: http://www.ccsso.org/intascst.html. Reprinted with permission.

this process, it is hoped that licensing standards would describe the goals toward which teachers could work throughout their careers to achieve excellence in their profession (Ambach, 1996).

Adoption of a standards-based system for issuing teacher credentials has significant implications for teacher preparation. In order to produce teachers who can obtain state certification, teacher education programs must be designed so that their graduates have a strong foundation of content and pedagogical knowledge, can show their ability to apply this knowledge in the classroom, and have exhibited the professional behaviors specified by the standards. They should demonstrate required knowledge and skills with all students as a part of their teaching practice (Ambach, 1996).

The standards-based approach advocated by CCSSO and INTASC is being applied to teacher certification on the national level. The INTASC process addresses competencies for beginning teachers, and the National Board for Professional Teaching Standards applies standards for advanced teachers. NBPTS issues a voluntary national teaching certification. Note that licensure and certification are not the same. According to Gross (1984), "Certification, as distinct from licensure, is under the direct control of professions and professions do not have to deal with 51 separate jurisdictions." As defined by the U.S. Department of Health, Education, and Welfare in 1971, **certification** is

> the process by which a nongovernmental agency or association grants recognition to an individual who has met certain predetermined qualifications. Such qualifications may include: (a) graduation from an accredited or approved program; (b) acceptable performance on a qualifying examination or series of examinations; and/or (c) completion of a given amount of work experience.

In 1986, the Carnegie Forum on Education and the Economy recommended the formation of the National Board for Professional Teaching Standards. A year later, the board was founded with a mission to establish high and rigorous standards for what accomplished teachers should know and be able to do; to develop and operate a national, voluntary system to assess and certify teachers who meet these standards; and to advance related education reforms—all with the purpose of improving student learning. The 63-member board is comprised of teachers, school administrators, school board leaders, higher education officials, teacher union leaders, business and community leaders. The following propositions outline what the board values and believes should be honored in teaching (NBPTS, 1999):

- Teachers are committed to students and their learning.
- Teachers know the subjects they teach and how to teach those subjects to students.
- Teachers are responsible for managing and monitoring student learning.
- Teachers think systematically about their practice and learn from experience.
- Teachers are members of learning communities.

To be eligible for national certification, teachers must possess a baccalaureate degree from an accredited institution, have at least three years' teaching experience in a public or private school, and submit proof of a valid state teaching license.

The fee for assessment is $2,300. NBPTS is funded in part by grants from the U.S. Department of Education and the National Science Foundation.

The NBPTS certifies teachers based upon multiple assessments of teachers' professional skills, knowledge, and accomplishments. The NBPTS is setting advanced standards (as opposed to the entry-level standards required for state certification) in more than thirty certificate fields.

The NBPTS assessment system was developed to promote collegiality in teaching and to have an impact on teachers' role in education and on student learning and on the public perception of teaching and learning (Baratz-Snowden, Shapiro, & Streeter, 1993). The first standards assessment instruments were implemented in 1993.

Currently, assessment consists of two major elements:

- The first element is the structured portfolio, which consists of several classroom-based entries. Typically two entries are videotaped classroom interactions and two are collections of student work of particular kinds. Each entry must be accompanied by a detailed analysis of the teaching reflected in the work.

- The second element takes place at one of the 230 NBPTS assessment centers. The process consists of a full day of assessment exercises that are focused on pedagogical content knowledge. Candidates must respond to specific prompts, which may be simulations of situations to which teachers typically must respond or explorations of particular questions on pedagogical content topics and issues.

The professional development component requires continuing growth on the part of the certified teacher. This can be accomplished in institutions of higher education, at the schoolsite, or on a district-wide basis. It can go beyond these traditional growth opportunities to include independent study, working with a mentor, or working among independent peer groups (Baratz-Snowden, Shapiro, & Streeter, 1993). Certification renewal is required every ten years.

Among criticisms of the NBPTS plan, perhaps the most valid is that an undergraduate degree in education, or health education for that matter, is not a prerequisite for assessment or for certification. Thus, a person could gain national certification without completing an academic major in the discipline. Critics (e.g., Murphy, 1990; Cleary, 1991, 1992) also addressed problems with portfolio assessment, including fairness and consistency. Behind-the-scenes planning, coordination, and advocacy might never be evaluated. Development of an interdisciplinary health education curriculum would be difficult to evaluate in this way.

The voluntary nature of NBPTS certification is certainly debatable. There are advocates for using NBPTS as a piece of the licensure process for teachers. NBPTS is developing guidelines explaining how states and school districts may use certification (Wise, 1994a). The Vice President for Assessment and Research at the NBPTS wrote that the board "envisions that its system of certification would lead middle school administrators to encourage their

**voluntary certification**    the process by which a nongovernmental agency or association grants recognition to an individual who has met certain predetermined qualifications

teachers to acquire National Board Certification and to look for Board-certified teachers when hiring" and that "Board certification can assist administrators in making distinctions among faculty. . . ." (Baratz-Snowden, Shapiro, & Streeter, 1993).

The National Council on the Accreditation of Teacher Education, the Interstate New Teacher Assessment and Support Consortium, the National Education Association, and others are working with NBPTS to improve the profession of teaching. They envision a linked system of preservice preparation, extended clinical training, and continuing professional development in which board certification plays an important role. Both NCATE and INTASC are taking steps to see that their components of this process are aligned with the work of NBPTS (National Center for Research in Vocational Education, 1998). These links suggest an eventual revision of the voluntary nature of the certification.

National credentialing for teachers seems to be gaining appeal. It is possible that other national organizations also may offer national teacher certification. How national certification will be utilized remains to be seen but many feel that it will replace reciprocal certification between states. To predict that what has begun as voluntary will eventually become mandatory is logical.

It is in large part the responsibility of the NCATE to ensure that teacher preparation programs are preparing prospective teachers with the pedagogical knowledge and professional competencies necessary to meet practice standards. Through its continuing update of standards, NCATE is forcing the change in preparation to match rigorous licensing and board certification requirements.

The term **accreditation** applies only to institutions or programs within institutions, not to individuals. NCATE is a specialized accrediting body for teacher education programs. To be considered for NCATE accreditation, an institution must have regional accreditation and, if available, a state-approved teacher education program. NCATE may accredit any unit (college, school, or department) of higher education that prepares teachers (Taub, 1993). Application for accreditation is voluntary. To be accredited, an institution must (Wise, 1994b)

— establish specific criteria for admission to teacher education programs;

— have plans for monitoring a student's progress and criteria for graduating from the program;
— offer a curriculum that is based on what is currently known about sound professional practice;
— provide appropriate clinical and field experience; and
— incorporate national teaching standards into its curriculum.

NCATE is helping to shape modern teacher education curricula. Institutions applying for NCATE evaluation under the revised standards have reported a good deal of change in their elementary and secondary programs. NCATE clearly is flexing its muscles and exerting considerable leverage over individual institutions. Many states have pressured institutions within their borders to acquire accreditation. The universal applications of NCATE standards, although no doubt improving the quality of professional preparation programs, is also reducing much of the autonomy that programs and institutions enjoyed in the past. It is widely believed that students seeking to major in a teacher education program, including that for school health education, may be more attracted to an institution that has NCATE accreditation.

NCATE accredits teacher education programs in school health education, exerting substantial influence directly on professional preparation. In the absence of specific standards for health education performance, NCATE contracts with the American Association for Health Education (AAHE)—a division of the American Alliance for Health, Physical Education, Recreation and Dance (AAHPERD)—to review the portfolios of institutional departments of health education. The review, composed largely of examining syllabi of required courses, is based on the Role Delineation Curriculum Project Framework (National Commission for Health Education Credentialing, 1996). Therefore, NCATE program approval and subject content accreditation are based on the responsibilities and competencies identified by the Role Delineation Project, implemented by the NCHEC, and evaluated for the CHES (Certified Health Education Specialist) designation.

As the credentialing of teachers evolves, the collaboration of CCSSO, INTASC, NBPTS, and

NCATE will lead to the general adoption of standards of good teaching and teacher preparation. These standards will be used to credential beginning and advanced teachers and teacher preparation programs.

# Certified Health Education Specialist (CHES)

The purposes of the National Commission for Health Education Credentialing are to certify health education specialists, promote professional development, and strengthen professional preparation. NCHEC's voluntary professional certification, the Certified Health Education Specialist (CHES), purports to establish a national standard for health education practice. Additional benefits appear in Box 13.2.

The certificate is awarded to those who pass an examination composed of 150 multiple choice items, which are revised from time to time. Beginning in 1992, only individuals who have a degree with a health education emphasis from an accredited institution of higher education are eligible for certification. The test assesses mastery of the responsibilities and competencies listed in Appendix

---

**Box 13.2  Benefits of the CHES Credential**

1. It affords professional recognition and professional status.
2. It provides a sense of confidence of one's abilities to meet the competencies required of the profession.
3. It helps define the practice of health education to others by standardizing competencies.
4. It recognizes that health education is a developing profession moving closer to recognition by others.
5. It may make the holder more employable.
6. It may make the individual's job more secure.
7. It may affect salary determination.
8. It requires the individual to stay current in his/her profession.

---

B. Recertification, required every five years, is based upon continuing education criteria developed by the commission.

NCHEC evolved from the work of the National Task Force on the Preparation and Practice of Health Educators. The task force, initiated in 1978, was charged with developing a credentialing system. During the charter certification phase, 1,558 CHES certificates were awarded without testing. In 1990, the first certification examination was given, and 644 more health education specialists were certified. The number of CHESs has continued to grow rapidly. By 1999, approximately 5,500 individuals had been certified by NCHEC (1999).

The NCHEC's credentialing process has not avoided debate and controversy (Cortese, 1990; Livingood, 1989; O'Rourke, 1990; Orrebo & Williamson, 1990; Butler, 1997). Gold (1989) questioned the voluntary nature of the process:

> What began as voluntary is now often touted as mandatory. Even if the words on paper say "voluntary," the message being given by some of the proselytizers is that certification is a must. They are told if they do not become credentialed, it demonstrates lack of support for the profession. Students and employers alike are led to believe that they must acquire and hire only these professionals. How is that voluntary? More importantly, how do we know that the certified health education specialist is better than a health educator who is not?

Gold's final point is absorbing in light of the fact that no objective data have been presented to demonstrate that CHESs perform more effectively than "non-CHESs." No published empirical studies have supported or dispelled the argument that individual credentialing has directly affected the quality of health education practice (Doyle & Cissell, 1998). We will examine some of the criticisms and some of the positive results of the certification.

Pahz (1998), in describing reasons that students may not apply for CHES certification, pointed out weaknesses in the credentialing process. First, the

---

**accreditation**  a voluntary process of recognizing institutions and programs that meet certain criteria, the goals they have set for themselves, and that they have the personnel and financial resources to accomplish their objectives

cost of the exam and of obtaining continuing education credits may be too high for people just entering the profession. Although the costs may seem comparable to those required of professions like medicine and law, those professions typically afford higher income early in the career. Nonetheless, the costs are not staggering and may be outweighed by the potential advantages of certification.

Critics are also concerned that the testing instrument fails to discriminate between those who possess the required competencies and those who do not. The very high pass rate, little changed by instituting a requirement of a degree in the field, may lend credence to this argument. This should be a worrisome issue for the profession. The test has also been criticized for measuring generic competencies in a multiple choice format, and some observers question whether standardized criteria and testing can measure the capabilities of a profession characterized by diverse work settings and skill applications (Gold, Gilbert, & Greenberg, 1989; Orrebo & Williamson, 1990).

Another issue is the perception of the generic, homogeneous health educator. The Role Delineation Project concluded that health educators, regardless of setting, have responsibilities in common and, therefore, competencies in common. This tends to produce the perception that health educators—whether teaching in an elementary school, conducting a program at a YMCA or a senior citizens' center, directing worksite health promotion programs, or planning and supervising educational programs for a state public health department—are all the same, performing the same functions. The CHES credential perpetuates this idea. Even though many health educators agree with this perception, many others see a diverse profession with variation in the roles, competencies, and functions of professionals in different settings.

The concept of the generic health educator carries significant ramifications for professional preparation. The CHES credential indicates acquisition of competencies and skills without testing for possession of health content knowledge. This practice is somewhat in conflict with many of the textbooks written for content areas such as human sexuality, substance abuse, and consumer health, as well as some of the methods texts that contain chapters or sections on the teaching of various content areas. It also conflicts with the philosophies of many institutions that provide courses in health content and begs the question: Shouldn't a competent educator possess a foundation of knowledge about the subject he or she teaches?

The question of whether the full competencies should be applied in school health at the undergraduate level has been raised (McMahon, Bruess, & Lohrmann, 1987; Butler, 1997). Gilbert and Sawyer (1995) accurately pointed out that for an individual to believe he or she can function well as a health educator without training in educational principles is ludicrous. Further, many school health educators consider themselves content specialists, whereas the responsibilities and competencies refer only to accessing information and require no foundation of knowledge about health-related topics.

The voluntary nature of CHES may soon be obsolete. In 1997, NCHEC celebrated Arkansas legislation requiring most people who function as health educators to be CHES. Similar legislation in other states soon followed. For practical purposes, credentialing as a health educator may have little meaning for classroom health teachers because they receive professional certification from their states. Indeed, those practicing in schools appear to be least likely to apply for CHES. Lohrmann, Gold, & Jubb (1987) stated that two things should occur for the role delineation competencies to have full application to school health instruction:

> First, states must move to a certification standard that requires a major in health education for a teacher to be certified to teach health. Second, a career path must be established in school health instruction for those who aspire to the master health teacher level or health education coordinator. The states then could require these individuals meet standards of a credentialed professional health educator.

Schwartz and associates (1999), however, suggested that

> If a state were to require that all health educators certified to teach in public schools or work in their community health agencies were CHESs, this would greatly increase the prestige and market demand for health educators.

However, if only a CHES is allowed to implement school health education, such programs may be eliminated from the budget when money is scarce

(Girvan & Kearnes, 1993; Luebke & Bohnenblust, 1994).

Proponents of the CHES credential and the framework upon which it is based make convincing arguments for its advancement. The framework itself provides an excellent self-study instrument for those planning to become health educators and for those who teach them (Pollock & Carlyon, 1996). There is also reason to believe that the credential has enhanced professional identity (Girvan, Hamburg, & Miner, 1993; Livingood, 1996). In addition, with a more clearly defined profession, greater job satisfaction and skill-based confidence among practicing health educators may result, contributing to numerical stability and growth (Doyle & Cissell, 1998).

There is good reason to believe that certified individuals will be at an employment advantage in community and public health settings (Alperin & Miner, 1993). They may also be perceived as more capable to participate in joint school-community health education programs (Cleary & Birch, 1995; Luebke & Bohnenblust, 1994).

Linked to employment advantage is the prospect of staking claim to our professional identity. Already other professions, including social work, nursing, and psychology have begun competing for health education practice roles. The Pew Health Professions Commission (1995) stated that "clinicians of the future will be required to . . . sharpen their skills in areas ranging from clinical prevention to health education" and proposed to revitalize the health professions and "regulate the health education and practice environment," a clear signal that health education must claim its place among other health professions or lose the power to regulate its own practice and training. CHES supporters believe that certification may contribute to recognition from other health-related professions. The framework and certification is a step in the direction of protecting the integrity of the profession.

## Community and Public Health Program Credentialing

The Society for Public Health Education and the American Association for Health Education sponsor a voluntary credential of undergraduate programs that prepare health educators for work in all settings. However, programs in community or public health are most likely to apply for this credential. Approval is granted through the SOPHE/AAHE Baccalaureate Program Approval Committee (SABPAC) and is recognized by the profession as a standard for entry-level health education preparation programs.

The Council on Education for Public Health (CEPH) is an independent agency recognized by the U.S. Department of Education to accredit schools of public health and certain graduate public health programs, such as community health education and preventive medicine programs offered in settings other than schools of public health. The primary professional degree in the field is the Master of Public Health, but other masters and doctoral degree programs are accredited as well (CEPH, 1999). Accreditation by CEPH is a voluntary process.

Although NCATE, SABPAC, and CEPH accreditation and approval are technically "voluntary," the prestige of a teacher education program or public/community health program is enhanced greatly by this recognition. In the future, the influence of the accreditation and approval process and the organizations that implement it will continue to grow. All three organizations rely on the areas of responsibility and related competencies published by the National Commission for Health Education Credentialing, Inc. (see Appendix B). Reliance on one set of standards will help ensure that entry-level health educators meet minimum requirements and, at the same time, will enforce a sense of similarity and conformity in colleges and departments of teacher education and public health.

## Institutional Accreditation

Institutional accreditation is a voluntary process that functions in the private sector. Begun by individual professional associations as a way of achieving collective status, accreditation has evolved over the years into an organized process.

In 1975, the Council on Postsecondary Accreditation (COPA) was developed as an umbrella organization to recognize, review, and coordinate existing accrediting bodies of all types. COPA was dissolved in 1993 and replaced by the Council on

Higher Education Accreditation (CHEA) in 1996. CHEA is a nonprofit membership organization of higher education institutions and regional, national, and specialized professional accrediting bodies (National Teaching and Learning Forum, 1999). It is also a national policy center and clearinghouse on accreditation for the entire higher education community. To maximize its benefits to educational establishment, CHEA (CHEA, 1999)

— coordinates research, analysis, debate, meetings, and other activities and processes that improve accreditation;

— collects and disseminates data and information about accreditation, its "best practices" and quality assurance;

— fosters communication and exchange on accreditation issues within the higher education community;

— mediates disputes between institutions of higher learning and accreditors as necessary; and

— works, through accreditation, to maintain institutional quality and diversity.

CHEA represents 8 regional accreditors, 42 specialized and professional accrediting associations, and 5 national accrediting organizations that accredit mostly seminaries, distance learning institutions, and independent colleges and schools. For purposes of college and university institutional accreditation, the nation is divided into eight regions: Middle States, New England (higher education; vocational, technical and career institutions), North Central, Northwest, Southern, and Western (community and junior colleges; senior colleges and universities). The regional accrediting associations ascertain whether an institution meets certain basic criteria, meets the goals it has set for itself, and has the personnel and financial resources to accomplish its objectives now and in the future (Greenberg, 1994).

The power vested in CHEA is illustrated by the fact that the U.S. Department of Education officially recognizes accrediting agencies and associations for determining institutions' eligibility for federal assistance. This recognition has been translated into fiscal and administrative support for educational programs that meet accreditation standards, thus making accreditation an important issue to institutions of higher education. It also affects students' choice of institutions because institutions that are not accredited are not eligible for most federal assistance programs for students.

The process of accreditation usually takes the following steps (U.S. Society & Values, 1997):

1. The establishment of standards

2. An institutional self-study, in which performance is measured against established standards

3. On-site evaluation by a team of outside educators selected by the accrediting agency

4. Publication of the fact that the institution met the standards

5. Periodic re-evaluation of the institution's programs

Although it is only beginning to evaluate actual teaching and learning, institutional accreditation has been a useful tool in assessing important aspects of an institution's performance, maintaining standards of quality, and giving additional meaning to a professional license or degree. Institutional accreditation of a college or university does not mean that each specific curriculum or department is accredited.

In 1992, Congress passed the Higher Education Amendments, which authorized the DOE to impose standards for academic progress and accreditation that are likely to increase federal involvement in higher education. These standards concern length of educational programs, tuition, student achievement, and graduation rates. Although these standards address important issues, the historic independence of higher education from the federal government may be threatened.

# ACCOUNTABILITY AND PROFESSIONAL PREPARATION

The age of accountability has arrived in public education. Other programs funded by governments always evidence the intent to hold funding recipients accountable. It appears that all education programs, regardless of setting, will be finally forced to document that they are achieving goals set for them. Increasing competition for resources will require teachers to demonstrate program effectiveness more accurately. Serious observers of the political scene in education recognize that all who practice in educational settings will have to justify their programs. In education, accountability is interpreted to mean that educators and institutions are to be answerable for what their clients learn (Browder, 1973). In health education and health promotion, this includes learner behavior. Evaluative strategies will become more critical to program continuation. Sophisticated assessment tools must be designed and implemented to monitor program success.

Schools of the future will have to state their objectives in behavioral terms, develop their curricula to match educational standards and objectives, and be evaluated based on competencies or performance of learners. The internal structure and management of schools may undergo serious alterations, and school administrators may lose much of the autonomy they have enjoyed in the past. We may see situations in which local and state governments take over the day-to-day operation of public schools, possibly assisted by members of the business community.

The issue of accountability will also affect institutions of higher education much more intensely. As we have seen, accrediting agencies such as NCATE and SABPAC are becoming more dominant in the planning and evaluation of programs in the nation's colleges and universities. State departments of education are very willing to become partners with NCATE in accreditation of teacher preparation programs, leading to close approximation of state teacher certification standards with NCATE standards. College and university programs that prepare teachers will be characterized by their similarity. In addition, because accreditation of both teacher preparation programs in health education and community health education programs are based on the same standards, the academic preparation of practitioners in various settings (and for various audiences) is likely to become parallel.

Those practicing in certain settings have already experienced the force of the accountability movement. Worksite and managed care settings often continue health promotion programs based on the program managers' ability to demonstrate that objectives are met. Unfortunately, these evaluations are often done on the short term and are based on fiscal, rather than health-enhancement, objectives.

Public and community health organizations will be forced to demonstrate their progress toward goals with more clarity. Funding organizations are becoming more concerned with results of these agencies' efforts and will probably force clear demonstration of improvement of health status.

The number of students pursuing health education graduate training is increasing and is expected to do so for the foreseeable future. This interest is attributed to the increasing U.S. population, growing public and corporate interest in health and wellness, recognition of health education as means to help control escalating health care costs, shift in health services delivery to managed care organizations, and other societal trends. There also is an influx of other health professionals—from, for example, nursing, social work, and business—into graduate health education. Many of these professionals seeking advanced health education degrees may lack the requisite entry-level competencies (Merrill et al., 1998). Therefore, college and university offerings and faculty may need to expand to provide graduate programs that include both undergraduate and graduate health education/promotion competencies.

Health educators are likely to find many opportunities for employment in managed care organizations. Thus, health educators must be able to adapt to differing methods of health care delivery and changing concepts in health education. The communications industry and corporate health environment may be future employment settings as well. Each will require professional preparation programs to match their individual requirements to coursework.

Graduate health education programs should provide basic education in the behavioral and social sciences as well as training in program planning, implementation, and evaluation. They should also emphasize competencies in budgeting and management of health education programs, information management and technology, communications and interpersonal skills training, media advocacy, and linguistically and culturally appropriate care (Merrill et al., 1998).

Ethical issues will continue to place pressure on health educators/promoters and those who train them. It is likely that ethical considerations related to assisted suicide, DNA registries, health insurance and rationing health care, surrogate parenthood, genetic engineering, alternative health care, chemical abortion, and other issues will place professionals in the forefront of policy determination, research, and public education. In addition, interdisciplinary training that illustrates and clarifies the many ethical considerations facing the profession and the society will be needed.

The profession will be called upon to address issues such as violence, especially among youths; sexually explicit language and behavior portrayed in movies, television, the Internet and other media; increase in child abuse and child pornography; changes in family structure; breakdown of parent-child and grandparent-grandchild bonds; as well as problems as yet unforeseen. Professional preparation programs, schools, and communities must adjust to these changes and design creative ways to reverse some of their negative effects.

Professionals will be under more pressure to be on the "cutting edge" of educational technology. Professional preparation programs must train practitioners to be comfortable and competent with changing technology. Unfortunately, education has not kept up with the pace of advancing technology, perhaps due to lack of technological training of faculty, financial constraints, or poor understanding of changes occurring in K–12 classrooms (NCATE, 1997).

# CHANGING TECHNOLOGY IN EDUCATION

"Changing technology" refers to the rapidly changing media that are used to conduct education. Just as today's technology was yesterday's dream, tomorrow's educational technology is today's dream. The dreams will continue to unfold.

Leaders in education, governmental entities, and business expect teachers and their graduates to possess minimum technology skills. At least 35 states have established "standards for technological fluency, with most currently working toward integrating them into the academic standards" (Milken Family Foundation, 1998).

Most institutions of higher education have implemented a computer literacy policy. However, technology is improving so rapidly that, by the time students graduate from college, their technological skill is usually obsolete. Therefore, we should teach the flexibility to see beyond today and not be overcome by new and even revolutionary methodology. Programs that are truly current recognize that currency is only momentary. Professional preparation programs will be required to produce professionals who develop new media as technology advances, assess technology and software, and are flexible enough to experiment with new modalities constantly and make them central rather than supplementary to teaching. The ability to tailor programs to individual needs also will be a major requirement of future educational programs, calling for more technological proficiency among health educators.

Multiple sources predict that technological competence will become a central component in professional preparation of teachers, including school health educators (Corbett-Perez, 2000). Accrediting agencies will exert considerable influence on improving the skills of educators in the use of educational technology. In 1997 NCATE recommended an emphasis on technology as "central to the teacher preparation process" and is introducing accreditation standards that will "undoubtedly raise the bar for the use of technology in teaching and learning" (NCATE, 1997). Teacher preparation standards in the components of Content Studies for Initial Teacher Preparation, Professional and Pedagogical Studies, and Professional Education Faculty Qualifications make reference to the use of and skills in computers and technology. The International Society for Technology in Education has proposed basic standards for educational computing and literacy. The Association for Educational Communications and Technology has assisted NCATE in developing technology standards for teacher preparation. The International Technology Education Association, with the full support of NCATE, is developing standards for technology education through the *Technology for All Americans* project. In the future, no area of education will be without standards for technology and computer competence.

It is now possible to conduct college courses with a great deal of interaction among students and faculty, although they never actually sit in the same room. Professors and students communicate through electronic mail and the Internet. Through fiber optics, satellite communication, interactive television, and the World Wide Web, classes can be conducted across the campus, across the country, or around the globe. Some institutions award degrees through satellite-delivered courses to students who never set foot on the campus. The college of tomorrow will be more open and less centralized, with less institutional control over the where, when, and how of learning. Educators will prepare lessons and courses to be delivered to students in their homes thousands of miles away. The implications for rural and other underserved populations is enormous. The skills required for these environments will not come about intuitively; they must be developed by colleges and universities, many of which are far behind in current technology.

It is not inconceivable that, given the uniformity imposed by accrediting bodies and the ability to offer coursework technologically, universities will begin to merge. As more courses are taught via the Internet and satellite transmission, the size of university faculties may shrink dramatically.

The implications are vast and extend even to the elementary classroom. Worksite wellness centers, the community health agencies, and other practice settings may offer health promotion services to recipients who are away from the site.

A report (Macy Research Associates, 1995) prepared for the American Heart Association found that

- Installation of technology in American schools is rapidly moving forward.
- Distance learning likely will be a growth area within the next few years.
- Telecommunications and use of on-line services will be areas of growth in education.
- There is consensus that educational technology and electronic media will continue to grow, probably at high rates.
- Continued growth in the home computer market will influence the educational technology market.

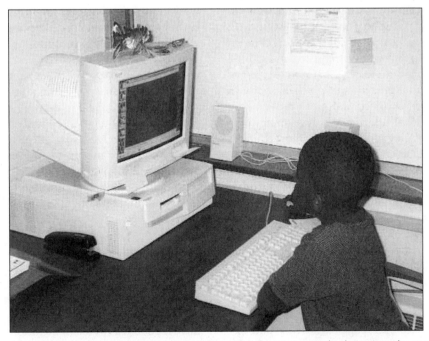

Computer-assisted and web-based learning are becoming the norm, even in elementary classrooms.

The study found a paucity of computer-driven software available in health education. As health educators develop educational technologies, they should try to ensure that the systems and methods are convenient to outside resources, focus on transferring and exchanging data, are easy to use, and facilitate learning while luring the learner to accomplish other challenging tasks. There is no doubt that technology can contribute to a richer learning environment.

A good example of the use of advanced technology is the hypertext/hypermedia learning module. It is self-contained and transportable and allows interdisciplinary team training and content to be introduced throughout and among discipline-specific program curricula. Hypermedia programs are software applications that enable users to create and choose links between disparate materials—such as video, graphic, textual, and audio materials—and to choose links among the related concepts. These multiple uses of material reinforces interdisciplinary perspectives and sets up a structure for communicative learning, critical thinking, and self-reflection (Kovacich et al., 1997).

Applications of the Internet and on-line services are being developed at a rapid pace. Who can predict what the state of the art will be in fifteen years? All we can say is that it will be advanced. Many of today's educators have not kept up with technological innovations. Those who remain in this rut will find themselves antiquated and of little real service to their students. Classroom teachers of the future will not be evaluated on their ability to prepare and deliver a lecture but, instead, on how effective they are at utilizing and developing computer programs and applications to allow students to progress at their own pace.

The "methods and materials" courses of tomorrow will be much different from those of today. Professors, teachers, and students should have the spirit of adventurers where educational technology is concerned. The more they experiment, the more skills they develop. The more they explore, the more they learn. An important part of health educators' role in the future will be helping people learn how to learn. The future holds an explosion of new information, which will be delivered in thousands of scientific papers and new and expanded journals, many of them electronic. We must train people to select and use data, be analytical, make decisions, and tailor their own solutions to their own needs. This will require the capacity to correlate and cross-index information to reveal interrelationships that are more difficult to establish today.

# CHANGING CONSUMER POPULATIONS

The relative risks for different groups will vary as a function of the resources associated with their demographic and related social-structural characteristics (age, gender, race, or ethnicity); the nature of the ties between and among them (family members, friends, neighbors); and the schools, jobs, incomes, and housing that characterize the neighborhoods in which they live. The corresponding rewards and resources associated with these individual and social arrangements include social status (prestige and power), social capital (social support), and human capital (productive potential) (Aday, 1993). Future and current demographic changes will shift the balance of these resources, producing vulnerable and underserved populations. Faced with economic, cultural, linguistic, and physical barriers, underserved people are disproportionately affected by certain illnesses and conditions, including injuries, alcoholism, and heart disease (Marin et al., 1995). This will require communities to design programs and policies to confront uncertainties to health in these populations.

The Children's Defense Fund identifies risks to children. These risks are often concentrated in minority groups and in low-income populations. Box 13.3 presents some alarming facts that not only apply to the changing consumer populations in America but also affect the overall wellness of society.

## The Very Young

The first national education goal for the year 2000 is guaranteeing that all children enter school ready to learn. Although this objective has not been met, there is good reason for its inclusion and its continued pursuit. To get a true opportunity for success in school and after, children must enter kindergarten prepared. Early childhood education is just a part of the broader intellectual, social, emotional, and physical development children need to succeed in the crucial elementary grades. Family and community supports play vital roles in ensuring that young children grow up in healthy environments that nurture continuous development (Annie E. Casey Foundation, 1999).

Millions of young children are at risk for failure at school and health problems. For example, some 32 percent of children are not living with two parents, and 19 percent live in homes where the head

---

### Box 13.3   Every Day in America for all Children

- 2 children under age 5 are murdered
- 6 children and youth under age 20 commit suicide
- 10 children and youth under age 20 are homicide victims
- 12 children and youth under age 20 die from firearms
- 35 children and youth under age 20 die from accidents
- 77 babies die
- 151 babies are born at very low birth weight
- 218 children are arrested for violent crimes
- 399 children are arrested for drug abuse
- 406 babies are born to mothers who received late or no prenatal care
- 798 babies are born at low birth weight
- 1,352 babies are born to teen mothers
- 1,540 babies are born without health insurance
- 2,140 babies are living in poverty
- 2,316 babies are born to mothers who are not high school graduates
- 2,806 students drop out of school
- 3,445 babies are born to unmarried mothers
- 5,044 children are arrested
- 17,297 public school students are suspended

Source: Children's Defense Fund. (2000). *The State of America's Children–Yearbook 2000*, Washington, DC. Reprinted by permission.

---

of the household is a high school dropout (U.S. Bureau of the Census, 1998a). Both factors that affect the time families spend together—an attribute of strong families (Moore, 1993)—and the child's learning pace, especially in the early years (Duncan & Brooks-Gunn, 1997). We must, as a society, attend to the basic needs of young children. If we do not concern ourselves with the nutrition, health care, emotional development, and family life of infants and preschoolers, it may be too late for many children before they reach school age.

Improving the health of American children requires a wide range of interventions. Many of these already are in place and functioning. Head Start is an example of a successful program that provides many services—health screening, nutrition education, and healthy diet are examples—to young children. Head Start has a wonderful record of assisting at-risk children to develop readiness for school. Currently, access to Head Start services is limited primarily to those in low-income families. In the future, similar programs may be available to all children. Even though this program has demonstrated the practicality and cost-effectiveness of early health services and health education, less than half of eligible children are enrolled.

Other programs have proven that they can make a difference in young children's lives. Physicians participating in the national Reach Out and Read program provide reading material to children aged 6 months to 5 years and their parents at each office visit. Volunteers read to young children in doctors' waiting rooms to demonstrate the fun and closeness reading can bring to families. The Smart Start program in North Carolina provides children under age 6 access to high-quality and affordable child care, health care, and other critical family services. Both of these programs help children arrive at school healthy, motivated, and ready to learn. American families need help from programs such as these as well as from schools, health care facilities, public welfare institutions, businesses, and religious organizations.

As has been pointed out repeatedly in this book, health and education are interrelated. Children whose lives are impeded by depression, physical abuse, substance abuse, obesity, or hunger are not healthy children. Children who are not healthy are

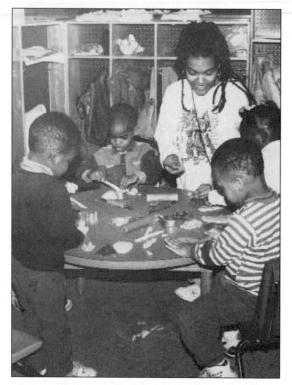

Creative preschool education programs can do much to enhance children's self-esteem, social skills, and overall well-being.

impaired as learners. Lack of health and misdiagnosed or untreated conditions can interfere with a child's ability to attend school regularly or to participate in recreational and other social activities that enhance development (Zuckerman & Norton, 1999). To improve the academic achievement of children, schools and other institutions must devote more attention to health concerns through health services and health education. Health care services must be made available to the nation's 10 million children who are not covered by any health insurance (U.S. Bureau of the Census, 2000). We are likely to see a continuing growth in the number of school-based clinics and partnerships between schools, including preschools, and health care providers.

Traditionally, society's responsibility for educating children began as they entered school. However, in 1995, 59 percent of preschool children were in some type of nonparental arrangements on a regular basis and 28 percent were in full-time nonparental care. Children at greater risk of school failure spent more time per week in nonparental care, on average, than did other children (National Center for Education Statistics, 1998). However, children from higher income families are more likely to attend early childhood programs (National Center for Health Statistics, 1998). Because it is widely documented that children from higher income families are generally healthier and do better academically, it becomes obvious that the amount of time spent in day care, the quality of the nonparental care, and the health and educational opportunities afforded there are critical. In the future, more emphasis will be placed on the welfare of preschool children. Day care facilities offer a tremendous opportunity to provide health education and to help young children develop the skills of coping, decision making, and valuing. High-quality early childhood care and preschool education can stimulate cognitive development, increase school readiness, and advance academic achievement in early elementary grades (Annie E. Casey Foundation, 1999). Licensed day care centers soon may be compelled to prove that they provide a range of educational experiences that meet criteria for skill development and health education. This may necessitate links with early childhood education centers and the formal education system.

## The Elderly

The aging of the American population creates an increased need for health-related programs and services for older adults. According to the U.S. Bureau of the Census (1996), persons 65 years of age or older represent 12.6 percent of the U.S. population. About half of all the people who have ever lived to be 65 or older are alive today (Center for the Advancement of Health, 1998). From 2000 to 2010, the population 65 years of age and older is expected to increase by 13.5 percent and the population 85 years of age or older will increase by 33 percent. This population shift illustrates both a need for health-related programs for the elderly and an opportunity for professional health educators and health promoters to establish themselves as serious contributors to the welfare of the older population.

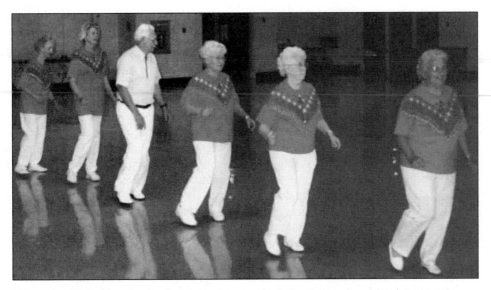

This senior citizens' line dancing troupe encourages physical activity and social maintenance.

When thinking of aging, we should recognize that it is a series of political, economic, social, religious, physiological, and behavioral events. The dependency that is often equated with aging is socially created and may be diminished through increasing economic capabilities, enhancing opportunities for productive work, enriching social responsibilities, and decreasing the degree of deterioration experienced by older people (Sheinfeld Gorin, 1998). Programs that maintain functional independence rather than simply lengthening life will be needed, along with policies designed to encourage health promotion in older people.

Health promotion programs of the future should focus on positive changes in health behavior such as exercise and smoking cessation that are beneficial and may even slow the disease process (Hermanson et al., 1988; Donahue et al., 1988). They must also provide education and services relating to immunizations for pneumococcal pneumonia and influenza and about compliance with medication regimens. Demonstrating prevention of further health decline and maximizing functional capacities would be enough to justify health education for the elderly, but benefits go far beyond that point. Improving the quality of life of elders has been associated with reduced medical costs and greater independence (Boult et al., 1994; Stewart, King, &

Haskell, 1993). Evidence exists that even modest health promotion interventions can increase quality of life, including physical functioning, freedom from fatigue and pain, and perceptions of one's health (Stewart & King, 1991).

The future will bring increased use of screening tools in primary care for assessment of depression and early cognitive deficits, such as deterioration of memory, orientation, general intellect, specific cognitive functioning, and social functioning. Health educators will play a crucial role in encouraging patients to undergo these assessments and interpreting their results and implications.

Although the treatment of chronic diseases of the elderly is advancing rapidly, much of what can be done for the elderly population is tied to educating the rest of society about the aged. Many frequently held misconceptions about the elderly can prejudice others toward them. Stereotyping of the elderly leads to approaches that treat them as an entirely different and discrete segment of the population at the very time of their lives when the elderly themselves are striving to retain an integrated place in society (Stewart, 1993). Reducing these mistaken notions can be of great service to seniors. For instance, psychological and medical studies indicate that aging is not associated with physical and mental failing (Rodeheffer et al., 1984; Schaie, 1983,

1989; Williams & Katzman, 1988). Instead, any decline seems to be attributable to the presence of disease (Williams, 1991).

Most older Americans live in their own homes and are healthy despite chronic illnesses (Schuster, 1995). Many are in excellent health. Services will be needed to keep elderly people in their homes rather than in nursing homes. However, some elders cannot live and manage their own personal care needs independently and require community resources and family aid to help them maintain a sense of autonomy. This may require educating the elder or the family about the availability of services and about the skills necessary to meet individuals' needs. In many cases, establishing a social network that encourages both giving and receiving affection and respect is valuable in raising self-esteem and ameliorating loneliness (Heckheimer, 1989).

The health education professional should recognize the importance of influencing the kin and significant others of the elderly about ways of providing affective support to the elderly. Elderly people who are isolated and lonely tend to present the gravest health and welfare problems and the most formidable behavior change problems as well. We should endorse roles that help them feel useful and wanted, shelter them from the economic hazards to which they may be subject, tend to needs they may be unable to meet by their own efforts, and, where necessary, ease the transition to institutional care (Stewart, 1993). Innovative and varied interventions must focus not only upon existing support systems but also upon facilitating formation of new ones so the elderly will be less isolated.

Many of the aged population were raised in a period when the religious group was of primary importance. They also tend to have much time to think of spiritual matters. Health educators can help promote the spiritual health of elderly people by assisting them in altruistic activities; arranging access to religious services or ceremonies; encouraging them to share their love and wisdom through "grandparenting"; and facilitating sharing through organ donation agreements, teaching others, or discussing memories with others.

We are only beginning to explore the opportunities for health promotion of elderly people. Nursing homes, senior citizen centers, schools, recreation centers, clubs, health maintenance organizations, and hospitals have a chance to offer much needed education about issues such as safe exercise, changing nutritional needs, compliance with medical advice, proper use of medications, and availability of services. Health educators/promoters can be a vital part of programming of services and education for the elderly population.

Older adults will become more and more active politically. The membership of the AARP already has influenced a great deal of legislation and program development. Health promoters should bear in mind that providing services for elderly can forge a political bond that can strengthen both profession and constituency.

## The Changing Family

The structure of the family has changed dramatically in the past few decades. Beyond the obvious reality of more women working outside the home, other significant changes suggest that we need to reconsider our concept of family. In the future, families are expected to be smaller, more nontraditional, and to operate with a new set of norms.

The number of female householders is over 12.6 million in the United States. This situation is most evident in African-American households, where about half of families are married couples and half are female head-of-house (U.S. Bureau of the Census, 1998b). Childbirth to unmarried women, especially teens, increased at an alarming pace through 1990. However, the rate began to decrease in the early 1990s and has gone down for several years, a trend that has great potential to improve the lives of children. The decrease in teen birth rates was 7 percent overall, but 20 percent in African Americans. However, the out-of-wedlock birth rate still approaches 70 percent among African Americans and 25 percent among whites. Single-parent households face a unique set of health and social problems, most of which are linked to poverty. Schools, public health departments, voluntary health agencies, and the worship community must find creative ways to deal with these problems.

Changes in family composition and structure have already contributed to unfavorable outcomes for children. Many parents seem to lack the commitment necessary to the development of their children. Uhlenberg and Eggebeen (1986) wrote, "We suggest that it is an erosion of the bond between parent and child—one characterized by parental commitment and willingness to sacrifice self-interest—that is the significant cause of declining well-being of American adolescents after 1960." Still, we cannot expect to reinvent the family. We can, however, help families function in more effective and supportive ways.

Nontraditional families such as homosexual couples with children, cohabiting couples, single parents, and older people with children can pose considerable pressure for the society in the form of challenges to traditional values and need for fiscal and social services. In addition, lack of affordable child care, divorce, and the need to change jobs because of downsizing, layoffs, and transfers may produce much family stress. New policies, laws, and procedures will be necessary to address these changes. New modalities and messages in health education will be needed in recognition of these families' needs.

## Cultural and Ethnic Diversity

We are undergoing a massive change in culture in our society. We are literally looking different as a nation and the conventional majority values and norms are being challenged as we become a more diverse, more ethnic, more integrated culture. Health educators have long prided themselves with working across cultures. . . . These cultural changes are . . . greater than we have experienced previously (Clark, 1994).

As Clark's words imply, we as a nation are undergoing a massive change in ethnic makeup. Minorities have higher birth rates than whites. In addition, more immigrants are arriving from South America, Asia, and Mexico than from Europe. This cultural transmutation presents awesome opportunities and challenges for health promoters. It also is a clarion call to recruit students from diverse racial, ethnic, and cultural backgrounds into the profession; so far, efforts have been inadequate (Merrill et al., 1998).

The U.S. Census Bureau reported (1999a) that, in mid-1990, whites constituted 83.9 percent of the total U.S. population; by mid-1999, whites constituted 82.3 percent. During the same period, the African-American population increased from 12.3 percent to 12.8 percent; the Asian/Pacific Islander population increased from 3 percent to 4 percent; Hispanic population increased from 9 percent to 11.5 percent; and the Native American/Native Alaskan population increased from 0.7 percent to 0.9 percent. Some states are more affected by increases in minority populations than others. For instance between 1990 and 1998, 15 states recorded increases of over 25 percent in their African-American populations and 22 states saw increases of 50 percent or more in their Hispanic populations.

Already, in some cities, the majority of public school children are nonwhite. America is undergoing mammoth changes in culture. We look different, think differently, and hold different values than before. The majority values and norms will continue to change as our society becomes more diverse. Helping students accept and value diversity will become an increasingly important function of health educators. We must continue serving the various ethnic minorities in effective ways because they bring unique health problems and because these groups can reciprocate with support for our profession.

At one time, many held the perception that the United States was a "melting pot" where each individual would share similar language, values, and beliefs. Clearly, as English and Videto (1997) pointed out, this is not the case. Society expects each of us to acknowledge and respect the cultural norms of the diverse sub-populations that reflect contemporary society. Diversity and multicultural emphases are not new to health educators, who have long been accomplished at working across cultures and being sensitive to individual differences.

The health status of ethnic/racial minority populations in the United States has been influenced by the aftermath of past racial restrictions in educational, employment, housing, political, and other institutional systems. Despite much progress, continued inequities can be seen in disproportionate numbers who are poor, homeless, living in substandard housing, in prisons, unemployed, and/or school dropouts (Ho, 1992).

Minority groups, particularly people who are foreign-born, are more likely to be without health insurance. In 1998, 16.3 percent of the population was without health insurance coverage for the entire year. The uninsured rate among Hispanic populations was 35.3 percent compared with 11.9 percent of non-Hispanic whites. Foreign-born populations had a 34.1 percent uninsured rate compared with 14.4 percent of natives. Poor immigrants were even worse off: 53.3 percent were without health insurance (U.S. Bureau of the Census, 1999b).

Members of ethnic/racial minorities face many health problems and exhibit some behaviors that put them at greater risk than whites in the United States. For instance, age-adjusted death rates are about 58 percent higher for the African-American population compared with the white population, and the infant mortality rate for African-American infants is more than twice that of whites (National Center for Health Statistics, 1998). Nearly twice as many African-American persons than white persons report they are in fair or poor health (CDC, 1998a). African-Americans also have higher rates of homicide, stroke, cirrhosis, and diabetes (Nakamura, 1999). Non-Hispanic African Americans and Hispanic Americans accounted for 47 percent and 20 percent, respectively, of persons diagnosed with AIDS in 1997 (CDC, 1998b), far exceeding their percentages of the population at large. Among those considered to be more likely to be exposed to or infected with tuberculosis are Asian Americans and Pacific Islanders, African Americans, Hispanic Americans, and Native Americans (CDC, 1999). Native Americans and Alaska Natives have very high prevalence of tobacco use, although they smoke fewer cigarettes per day than whites (CDC, 1998c). When compared with the majority population, Hispanic Americans have higher infant mortality rates, shorter life expectancies, and higher rates of sexually transmissible diseases, but lower rates of some chronic disorders (Nakamura, 1999). These few examples, coupled with the growth of ethnic minorities in the United States, are clear indications that the work of health promoters/educators should be in great demand in the very near future. They also indicate that professionals must develop skills to deal with minority populations. Some helpful techniques to accomplish this are shown in Box 13.4.

---

**Box 13.4    Working Effectively with Minority Group Members**

- Become aware of differences within the group by asking questions and getting involved in small-group discussions.
- Seek involvement and input and listen to people of different backgrounds without bias; avoid being defensive.
- Learn the beliefs and feelings of specific groups about particular issues.
- Read about current and emerging issues that concern different groups and read literature that is popular among different groups.
- Learn about the language, humor, gestures, norms, expectations, and values of different groups.
- Attend events that appeal to members of specific groups.
- Become attuned to cultural clichés, stereotypes, and distortions you may encounter in the media.
- Use examples to which people of different cultures and backgrounds can relate.
- Learn the facts before you make statements or form opinions about different groups.

Source: *Planned Approach to Community Health: Guide for the Local Coordinator*, National Center for Chronic Disease Prevention and Health Promotion, Centers for Disease Control and Prevention, USDHHS, 1992, Washington, DC: USDHHS.

---

Health promoters must learn to deal not only with the changing demographics and the unique risks that each vulnerable group carries, but also with those who would exploit them. There is evidence, for example, that some industries (such as suppliers of tobacco and alcoholic beverages) view the niches occupied by youths, minorities, and women as ones they most want to penetrate (White, 1988) through targeted advertisements and product placement. Health promotion specialists will have to develop an arsenal of weapons to counter the tactics of those who would exploit the vulnerable.

# RESPONSIBILITY FOR HEALTH

The responsibility for health once lay predominately with the family and the community. Then the Industrial Revolution, growth of urban areas, and expansion of the health care delivery system shifted responsibility for health primarily to the medical community. With the publication of the Lalonde Report, (see Chapter 2) and the acceptance of the Health Field concept (Chapter 1), the responsibility for health moved to the individual with assistance from the political and health care systems and from health promotion professionals. Later, the Canadian approach shifted farther in the direction of social reform.

The future will see a shift in the focus of responsibility from the individual to a more shared view. It is very important to recognize the inequities between upper and lower socioeconomic levels. Overemphasizing the individual's personal responsibility may have led to a "victim-blaming" mentality. Such a practice stigmatizes people who are unhealthy or disabled. The responsibility for health should, and most likely will be, shared by all segments of society, not just the health care industry and the individual. Responsibility will rest more in schools, our places of employment, and especially in our communities. This multisectoral approach, which looks at the social, economic, and environmental issues that affect health, can and should include public health and health education. The role of government will include leadership in the development and coordination of programs at the local and regional levels.

Specific issues such as quality of housing, education, poverty, workplace hazards, environmental threats, and exposure to carcinogens may be tomorrow's frontier for health educators/promoters to explore. Macro-level interventions, such as high taxes on tobacco and speed limit reduction (Minkler, 1999) as well as mandatory seat belt use have been shown to be effective.

Community organization may bear an unprecedented burden in the future. Community organization is defined as the process by which community groups are helped to identify common problems or goals, mobilize resources, and in other ways, develop and implement strategies for reaching the goals they have set collectively (Minkler & Wallerstein, 1997). Inherent to this approach are **empowerment**, participation, and coalition building. The resources of the community, both human and

material, can be harnessed and channeled into collective action to solve its own problems. These efforts will build ownership in the community and generate continued responsibility for the program among those residing in the community. Social involvement and participation can be significant factors in improving perceived control, individual coping capacity, health behaviors, and health status (Cohen & Syme, 1985; Eng, Briscoe, & Cunningham, 1990). The health educator, working with community members, can be an important change agent, empowering people to make a difference in their own lives and improving their quality of life (International Union for Health Education, 1991; Fincham, 1992). Implicit in this effort will be the advocacy for legislation to limit the effects of poverty and programs to help people move out of poverty to become self-sufficient.

## POLITICAL ACTIVISM AND ADVOCACY

Many of the issues mentioned previously are political in nature. Others, such as physician-assisted suicide, medical use of fetal stem cells, government support for the tobacco industry, preservation of environmental resources, provision of medical treatment and health insurance, media exploitation of violence and sex, and reduction in firearm deaths have distinctly political implications. Certainly, as citizens, health promoters should be involved in the process by which these issues are addressed.

O'Rourke (1989) foresaw a climate of shifting emphasis. He predicted that health educators will be involved less with changing individual behavior and more with alleviating the causes of social and health problems and with creating "public understanding of the political issues involved in public health programs." He believes our arsenal of health-promoting strategies should contain not only those directed toward self-help and self-care but also

**empowerment**    an enabling process through which individuals or communities take control over their lives and their environment

those directed toward promoting a healthful environment, a safer workplace, and a caring medical system; promoting public participation; developing healthful public policy, a community approach to health status improvement, a caring and sharing philosophy, and a focus that is not overly reliant on individual effort. This approach requires that we advocate for the role of health promotion with elected officials so that they become our allies.

This macro level of activity, which recognizes health education as a political function as well as an education activity, seeks to create public understanding of the political issues involved in public health problems. It adopts a broadened perspective incorporating the simple realization that individuals, communities, and societies are related to one another.

As professionals, health educators will need to become even more politically active at the local and state levels. Calls for less government and regulation may result in shifting some federal powers to the states, causing declines in funding. State and local functions such as the development of health education curricula, especially elements addressing human sexuality, are already political. The relatively recent development of 'school-based health clinics has faced extensive political debate. Supporters for these and other health services must become involved in the political process. They must energize their supporters to become advocates in the political and social arenas.

The debate on health care reform continues. We must ensure that health educators are included as reimbursable health professionals—that is, designated as appropriate providers. Professional certification and credentialing will greatly enhance our standing in this area. We must look for every avenue to obtain the status of designated provider in the future health care system, whether it be by state authorization, legislation, or from approval by state alliances.

Our profession is relatively new to these processes. "Becoming involved" does not necessarily mean running for public office, although that is one effective way. Forming coalitions, authoring legislation, writing letters, and lobbying by professional organizations are effective ways to affect public policy through the political system. Innovative practicum experiences designed to examine the politics of health and education is an idea that designers of future college requirements should consider.

# ENTREPRENEURSHIP, VENDORSHIP, AND REIMBURSEMENT

More health promoters/educators of the future will opt for self-employment. Worksite health promotion has provided an opportunity that will continue to grow. Software development, textbook writing, grant writing, evaluation contracting, program development, training, and professional speaking are a few of the routes to successful entrepreneuring. Health educators will offer consultation, program planning, and evaluation to businesses and health care facilities. An individual might be under contract with several businesses at one time, leading to considerable financial opportunity.

## Entrepreneurship

Many health educators already are selling their services as consultants, a practice that will continue and expand. Technological innovations implemented by college professors will free them to do more consulting. This could become a part of the faculty member's workload, providing significant income to the institution.

Entrepreneurs must be clever enough to spot future trends and watch the political scene. A number of trends will continue to demand attention, including AIDS education, new contraception methods, geriatrics, environmental issues, bioethics, genetic testing and counseling, varied family styles, minorities becoming majorities, preventive medicine, alternative therapies, and poverty. By being well positioned, savvy, and willing to work hard, health educators can increase their personal incomes by providing valuable educational and consultative services. Changes in insurance coverage and the insurance/health care partnership will open this marketplace to health educators with a penchant for consulting.

## Vendorship

Similarly, the role of vendor seems to be on the horizon for our profession—specifically, the ability to secure financial reimbursement for services from insurance companies and other third-party payers via formal recognition as suppliers of services. This would provide health education/promotion as an alternative point for the patient/client to enter the health care system. The likelihood of this happening has been greatly enhanced by the creation of a classification for the occupation of health educator by the U.S. Department of Labor's Standard Occupational Classification Policy Review Committee. It could also cultivate growth in health-related partnerships linking academic and community practice settings with managed care and public health. To acquire vendorship privileges, professions must acquire recognition by society that, in addition to formal training, national licensing, or certification requirements, are sufficiently rigorous to protect the public from incompetent practitioners (Cleary, 1993). The CHES credential, coupled with accreditation of professional preparation programs, is a good start in this direction. Cleary (1993) stated that access to third-party-payment reimbursement will depend upon professional preparation programs becoming more aligned with the CHES exam. Eligibility to take the exam may be contingent upon graduation from a SABPAC, CEPH, or NCATE-accredited program.

## Reimbursement

Another force working in favor of vendorship is the increasingly favorable political climate toward third-party reimbursement for non–health care practitioners who can establish effectiveness. Cost reduction is a key to this effectiveness for the political and insurance interests. As the health care system undergoes change, medicine will become a partner with health education (Clark, 1994). Health educators have developed growing abilities to conduct increasingly sophisticated behavioral change programs and to employ more rigorous quantitative and qualitative evaluation methods to document both short- and long-term results (Cleary, 1990; Steckler et al., 1992). This message that

prevention is less costly than treatment has reached the medical community (although not necessarily the insurance industry) and will inevitably lead to a stronger link between health promotion and medicine. The knowledge that the decrease in death rates and improvements in health status have been a result of better nutrition, improved behaviors, control of infectious diseases through immunizations, and better sanitation and environmental conditions—not new developments in medical technology—will offer opportunities to establish stronger footholds and eventually power in the health care delivery system.

Health educators can assist patients by helping them understand their options regarding physician choice, health care insurance, type of care, and intensity of services. They can also assist medical organizations by contributing to more one-on-one contact, improving patterns of communication between patient and provider, and enhancing patient compliance with treatment regimens (Lorig, Manzonson, & Holman, 1993). These services can increase patient satisfaction.

# SOCIAL MARKETING AND ADVOCACY

Social marketing has come of age in the field of public health and will likely be employed by practitioners with increased frequency and expertise in other settings. It provides a framework within which program specialists can effect population-based change in health behavior (Lefebvre & Rochlin, 1997). Andreasen (1995) defined social marketing as

> the application of commercial marketing technologies to the analysis, planning, execution, and evaluation of programs designed to influence the voluntary behavior of target audiences in order to improve their personal welfare and that of their society.

Social marketing is

— a key benefit to individuals and society, (as opposed to commercial marketing practices that focus on profit and organizational benefits);

— a focus on behavior, not on awareness or attitude change; and

— centered on the target audience's having a primary role in the process.

The utility and effectiveness of social marketing is dependent upon how well the target audience is heard and understood, how well barriers and benefits to new behaviors are strategically and tactically addressed, and how well program components are integrated and managed. The practice of social marketing lies in developing and implementing integrated elements whose objective is a specific change in behavior. Strategies are developed to guide planners in developing specific tactics to meet this objective. These strategies dictate which tactics are appropriate (Lefebvre & Rochlin, 1997).

The theoretical base of social marketing lies in economics, where the concept of exchange is paramount. Kotler and Armstrong (1997) defined marketing as

> A social and managerial process by which individuals and groups obtain what they need and want through creating and exchanging products and value with others.

Exchange is the act of obtaining something desired by offering something in return. Health promoters, in social marketing, offer the recipient something of value—such as feeling better, living longer, and having more energy—as a result of behavior change. Although the health promoter may not receive anything tangible, the client must be convinced that what he or she is giving in return (e.g., suffering through nicotine withdrawal and relinquishing the pleasure of smoking) for the behavior change results in a positive exchange. Bonaguro and Miaoulis (1983) pointed out several similarities between health promotion and marketing. Both disciplines

— strive to motivate the consumer to behaviors

— identify target populations

— attract and hold the attention of consumers if they are to be successful

— convey information and possess something of value to the consumer

— involve an exchange of some sort

— give the consumer the choice of accepting or rejecting the action

Social marketing efforts are characterized by their devotion to being consumer-driven. As Ling and associates (1992) noted,

> Social marketing has had a beneficial impact on how the public health sector educates the public and persuades

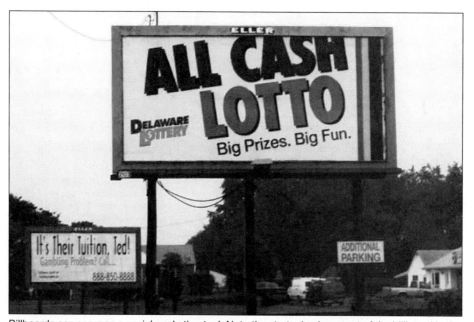

Billboards can serve as a social marketing tool. Note the strategic placement of the billboard in the background.

communities and individuals to adopt healthy practices. With its emphasis on clients, social marketing has sharpened the focus on the public. It has brought more precision to audience analysis and segmentation. . . . These data provide critical information for the formulation of better targeted and more effective messages, thus leading to more appropriate message design, more effective delivery, and, above all, better reception by the public.

Social marketing strategies can take many forms. Media form an important group of options for social marketers. Media practically frame social reality and shape the public consciousness about science (Nelkin, 1989). The better health promoters become at utilizing the media, the more effective they will be at changing individual behaviors and effecting social and political changes relating to health. Media—television; journals, magazines, newspapers, both electronic and print; radio; the Internet—have huge power to shape public thinking. They have a unique ability to provoke reflection, to create issues for debate, and to offer plans for positive action (Bogart, 1989). They literally tell

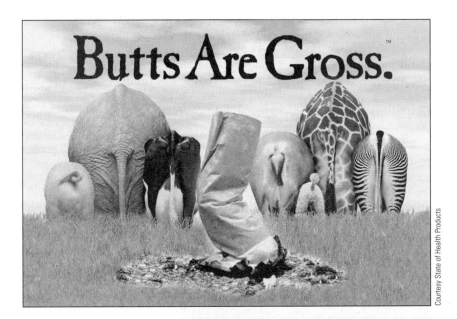

Courtesy State of Health Products

Courtesy State of Health Products

Nonprofit organizations, such as the American Cancer Society, are adept at marketing their messages. Clever themes can be placed on posters, tee-shirts, placemats, or other commonly seen items.

people what to think about. Health promotion specialists can use the media to awaken community interest and foster the development of interest groups. In the future, health educators will become more accomplished at using media to raise aspirations, encourage discussions, shape policy, market programs, and improve the overall quality of life.

Health promoters/educators need to attract and hold the consumers' attention just as the purveyor of products utilizes advertisements to attract and hold attention. However, this presents a major problem for educators, who, while trying to present their product in a positive, and attractive way, cannot use the misleading and exploitative tactics sometimes seen in commercial advertising.

We also must recognize that a change in behavior requires an exchange. In buying and selling merchandise, money is exchanged for the product. In health promotion, consumers are asked to exchange certain behaviors for intangible effects such as confidence and self-efficacy, feelings of satisfaction, value for health, or a feeling of well-being, as well as more measurable effects such as fewer illnesses and longer lifespan. The challenge to the health educator/promoter is to advocate the exchange of lifestyle for intangible benefits.

The issue in the consumer's mind is whether the cost of the action is equal to the benefits and, in the end, the consumer must make the decision. Perhaps it would be more palatable for many educators to accept Kotler's (1982) definition of social marketing as "the design, implementation, and control of programs seeking to increase the acceptability of a social idea or practice."

Many avenues of communication are available to health educators as tactics to market their messages and services. Examples include public service announcements, billboards, announcements in church bulletins, audiovisual self-help materials, worksite efforts to develop peer support systems, spokespeople on television and radio talk shows, special events such as health screenings, community coalitions to advocate for safe exercise areas, and bits of information in local professional newsletters.

Health educators and health promoters function in a marketplace culture. People will not come pounding on our doors begging for our services. Successful practitioners will adapt their skills to this environment.

## KEY POINTS

1. Credentialing is a process applied to ensure that those practicing a profession meet acceptable standards. Teacher credentialing takes several forms and is administered by state governments and professional organizations created for that purpose.

2. The Certified Health Education Specialist credential has the potential to advance the profession and contribute to recognition among other health related professions.

3. Educators and educational institutions must become more efficient at demonstrating that they meet their objectives. Evidence of effectiveness will be required at all levels and in all settings.

4. The rapid change in technology will alter methods, skills, and the look of education.

5. Health promoters must become more adept at addressing the needs of diverse populations. Changes in the family and society will force professionals into different paradigms of practice.

6. Opportunities for increased income through various models and modes of practice will confront health educators/promoters. They will become entrepreneurs and vendors of services subject to third-party reimbursement.

7. Health promoters will need to become better at advocating for health-related behaviors and programs through political action and social marketing.

# REFERENCES

Aday, L.A. (1993). *At risk in America: The health and health care needs of vulnerable populations in the United States.* San Francisco: Jossey-Bass.

Alperin, M., & Miner, K.R. (1993). Professional relevance: Meeting the contemporary public health agenda. *Journal of Health Education, 24*(5), 299–304.

Ambach, G. (1996). Standards for teachers: Potential for improving practice. *Phi Delta Kappan, 78*(3), 207–210.

Andreasen, A.R. (1995). *Marketing social change: Changing behavior to promote health, social development, and the environment.* San Francisco: Jossey-Bass.

Annie E. Casey Foundation. (1999). *Success in school: Education ideas that count* [On-line]. Available: http://www.aecf.org/initiatives/success/school.htm

Baratz-Snowden, J., Shapiro, B.C., & Streeter, K.R. (1993). National board for professional teaching standards: Making a profession. *Middle School Journal, 83*(2), 68–71.

Bogart, L. (1989). *Press and public: Who reads what, when, where, and why in American newspapers.* Hillsdale, NJ: Lawrence Erlbaum.

Bonaguro, J.A., & Miaoulis, G. (1983). Marketing: A tool for health education planning. *Health Education, 14*(1), 6–11.

Boult, C., Kane, R., Louis, T., Boult, L., & McCaffrey, D. (1994) Chronic conditions that lead to functional limitations in the elderly. *Journal of Gerontology: Medical Sciences, 49*(1), m28–m36.

Browder, L.H. (1973). *An administrator's handbook on educational accountability.* Arlington, VA: American Association of School Administrators.

Butler, J.T. (1997). NCHEC and its responsibilities and competencies require reexamination. *American Journal of Health Studies, 13*(4), 169–173.

Campbell, D. (1990). Theory into practice. In J.W. Butzow (Ed.), *Toward a model of post-baccalaureate teacher education.* Harrisburg, PA: Pennsylvania Academy for the Profession of Teaching.

Center for the Advancement of Health. (1998). Getting old: A lot of it is in your head. *Facts of Life: Issue Briefings for Health Reporters, 3*(2). [On-line] Available: http://www.cfah.org/website2/fol3-2.htm

Centers for Disease Control and Prevention. (1998a). *Health status* [On-line]. Available: http://www.cdc.gov/nchswww/fastats/hstatus.htm

Centers for Disease Control and Prevention. (1998b). *The HIV/AIDS epidemic in the United States, 1997–1998* [On-line]. Available: http://www.ced.gov/nchstp/hiv_aids/pubs/facts/hivrepfs.htm

Centers for Disease Control and Prevention. (1998c). *Tobacco use among U.S. racial/ethnic minority groups* [On-line]. Available: http://www.cdc.gov/nccdphp/osh/sgr-min-fs-nat.htm

Centers for Disease Control and Prevention. (1999). *Core curriculum on tuberculosis: What the clinician should know* [On-line]. Available: http://www.cdc.gov/nchstp/tb/pubs/corecurr.htm#RTFToC09

Clark, K. (1984). The implications of developing a professionwide code of ethics. *Health Education Quarterly, 10*(2), 120–125.

Clark, N. (1994). Health educators and the future: Lead, follow, or get out of the way. *Journal of Health Education, 25*(3), 136–141.

Cleary, M.J. (1990). Evaluating the supportive disciplines of health education: A conceptual model and example. *Health Education, 21*(6), 18–22.

Cleary, M.J. (1991). Restructured schools: Challenges and opportunity for school health education. *Journal of School Health, 61*(4), 172–175.

Cleary, M.J. (1992). Is board certification necessary for school health educators? *Journal of School Health, 62*(4), 121–125.

Cleary, M.J. (1993). Credentialing and vendorship: Are we ready? *Journal of Health Education, 24*(5), 285–287.

Cleary, M.J., & Birch, D.A. (1995). Monitoring trends in education: Implications for professional preparation in school health education. *Journal of Wellness Perspectives, 12*(1), 7–13.

Cohen, S., & Syme, S.L. (Eds.). (1985). *Social support and health.* Orlando, FL: Academic Press.

Corbett-Perez, S. (2000). Implications for mandatory national technology competencies for professional preparation in health education. *Journal of Health Education, 31*(2), 74–78.

Cortese, P. (1990). Health education credentialing: An idea whose time has come. *Health Education Quarterly, 17*(3), 247–251.

Council for Higher Education Accreditation. (1999). *About CHEA* [On-line]. Available: http://www.chea.org/About/index.html

Council of Chief State School Officers. (1999). *Interstate New Teacher Assessment and Support Consortium* [On-line]. Available: http://ccsso.org/intasc.html

Council on Education for Public Health. (1999). *About CEPH* [On-line]. Available: http://www.ceph.org/about.htm

Donahue, R., Abbott, R., Reed, D., & Yano, K. (1988). Physical activity and coronary heart disease in middle-aged and elderly men: The Honolulu heart program. *American Journal of Public Health, 78*(6), 683–685.

Doyle, E.I., & Cissell, W.B. (1998). A critical analysis of the CHES credentialing issue: Bridging the gap between vision and outcomes. *Journal of Health Education, 29*(4), 213–220.

Duncan, G.J., & Brooks-Gunn, J. (1997). *Consequences of growing up.* New York: Russell Sage Foundation.

Eng, E., Briscoe, J., & Cunningham, A. (1990). The effect of participation in state projects on immunization. *Social Science and Medicine, 30*(12), 1349–1358.

English, G.M., & Videto, D.M. (1997). The future of health education: The knowledge to practice paradox. *Journal of Health Education, 28*(1), 4–8.

Feistritzer, C.E. (1999). *Teacher quality and alternative certification programs: Testimony before the House Committee on Education and the Workforce, May 13, 1999* [On-line]. Available: http://www.ncei.com/Testimony051399.htm

Fincham, S. (1992). Community health promotion program. *Social Science and Medicine, 35*(8), 239–249.

Gilbert, G.G., & Sawyer, R.G. (1995). *Health education: Creating strategies for school and community health.* Boston: Jones and Bartlett.

Girvan, J.T., Hamburg, M.V., & Miner, K. (1993). Credentialing the health education profession. *Journal of Health Education, 40*(5), 260.

Girvan, J.T., & Kearns, R.O. (1993) The case for school health educators becoming certified health education specialists. *Journal of Health Education, 24*(5), 296–298.

Gold, R.S. (1989). Credentialing and the future of health education. *Wellness Perspectives: Research, Theory, and Practice, 6*(1), 49–54.

Gold, R.S., Gilbert, G.G., & Greenberg, J. (1989). Credentialing movement and the future of health education. *Wellness Perspectives: Research, Theory and Practice, 6*(1), 46–55.

Green, L.W. (1985). What is the society for public health education if not an open society? SOPHE presidential address, 1984. *Health Education Quarterly, 12*(4), 285–292.

Greenberg, M. (1994). A fresh look at accreditation. *The Chronicle of Higher Education, 41*(2), B1–B2.

Gross, S.J. (1984). *Of foxes and hen houses: Licensing and the health professions.* Westport, CT: Quorum Books.

Heckheimer, E.F. (1989). *Health promotion of the elderly in the community.* Philadelphia: W. B. Saunders.

Hermanson, B., Omenn, G., Kronmal, R., & Gersh, B. (1988) Beneficial six-year survival outcomes from smoking cessation in older men and women with coronary artery disease: Results from the CASS registry. *New England Journal of Medicine, 319*(21), 1365–1369.

Ho, M. (1992). *Minority children and adolescents in therapy.* Newbury Park, CA: Sage.

International Union for Health Education, World Health Organization. (1991). Meeting global health challenges: A position paper on health education. *Hygiea,* Special Supplement.

Interstate New Teacher Assessment and Support Consortium. (1999). *Model standards for beginning teachers licensing and development* [On-line]. Available: http://isu.indstate.edu/dickinson/cimt200/intascin.htm

Kotler, P. (1982). *Marketing for nonprofit organizations.* Englewood Cliffs, NJ: Prentice-Hall.

Kotler, P. & Armstrong, G. (1997). *Marketing: An introduction* (4th ed.). Upper Saddle River, NJ: Prentice-Hall.

Kovacich, J., Cook, C., Pelletier, V., & Weaver, S. (1997). Building interdisciplinary teams on-line in rural health care. In P. Knight (Ed.), *Masterclass: Curriculum, learning and teaching at master's level:* London, UK: Cassell.

Lefebvre, R.C., & Rochlin, L. (1997). Social marketing. In K. Glanz, F.M. Lewis, & B.K. Rimer (Eds.), *Health behavior and health education: Theory, research, and practice* (2nd ed.). San Francisco: Jossey-Bass.

Ling, J.C., Franklin, B.A., Lindsteadt, J.F., & Gearon, A.N. (1992). Social marketing: Its place in public health. *Annual Review of Public Health, 13,* 341–362.

Livingood, W. (1989). Health education certification: Professional foundation for the 21st century. *Wellness Perspectives: Research, Theory, and Practice, 6*(1), 37–45.

Livingood, W.C. (1996). Becoming a health education profession: Key to societal influence. *Health Education Quarterly, 23*(4), 421–430.

Livingood, W., Woodhouse, L.D., Godin, S., Eickmeier, J., Cosgrove, W., & Howard, M. (1993). Credentialing and competition for social jurisdiction. *Journal of Health Education, 24*(5), 282–284.

Lohrmann, D.K., Gold, R.S., & Jubb, W.H. (1987). School heath education: A foundation for school health programs. *Journal of School Health, 57*(10), 420–425.

Lorig, K.R., Manzonson, D.P., & Holman, H.R. (1993). Evidence suggesting that health education for self-management in patients with chronic arthritis has sustained benefits while reducing health care costs. *Arthritis and Rheumatism, 36*(4), 439–446.

Luebke, J.K., & Bohnenblust, S.E. (1994). Responsibilities and competencies: Implications for health education professional preparation programs. *Journal of Health Education, 25*(4), 227–229.

Macy Research Associates. (1995). *AHA's youth market technology application study: Technology trends.* Dallas: American Heart Association.

Marin, G., Burhansstipanov, L., Connell, C.M., Gielen, A.C., Helitzer-Allen, D., Lorig, K., Morisky, D.E., Tenney, M., & Thomas, S. (1995). A research agenda for health education among underserved populations. *Health Education Quarterly, 22*(3), 346–363.

McMahon, J.D., Bruess, C.E., & Lohrmann, D.K. (1987). Three applications of the role delineation project 1985 curriculum framework. *Journal of School Health, 57*(7), 272–279.

Merrill, R., Chen, D.W., Gielen, A., McDonald, E., Auld, E., Mulrooney, S.J., & Sampson, N.H. (1998). The future health education workforce. *Journal of Health Education, 29*(5), S59–S64.

Milken Family Foundation. (1998). *Technological fluency.* [On-line]. Available: http://www.milkenexchange.org/teaching/learning-tf.html

Minkler, M. (1999). Personal responsibility for health? A review of the arguments and the evidence at century's end. *Health Education and Behavior, 26*(1), 121–140.

Minkler, M., & Wallerstein, N. (1997). Improving health through community organization and community building. In K. Glanz, F.M. Lewis, & B.K. Rimer (Eds.), *Health behavior and health education: Theory, research, and practice* (2nd ed.). San Francisco: Jossey-Bass.

Moore, K.A. (1993). *Family strengths and youth behavior problems: Analysis of three national survey databases.* Washington, DC: Child Trends.

Murphy, J. (1990). Helping teachers prepare to work in restructured schools. *Journal of Teacher Education, 41*(4), 50–56.

Nakamura, R.M. (1999). *Health in America: A multicultural perspective.* Boston: Allyn & Bacon.

National Board for Professional Teaching Standards. (1999). *About the NBPTS* [On-line]. Available: http://www.nbpts.org

National Center for Education Statistics. (1998). *Statistical analysis report: Characteristics of early care and education programs: Data from the 1995 National Household Education Survey* [On-line]. Available: http://www.nces.ed.gov/pubs98/98128.html

National Center for Health Statistics. (1998). *Final mortality data for 1996 sets new records—highest life expectancy and lowest infant mortality rate* [On-line]. Available: http://www.cdc.gov/nchswww/releases/98facts/98shets/finmort.htm

National Center for Research in Vocational Education. (1998). *National Board for Professional Teaching Standards certification program* [On-line]. Available: http://ncrve.berkeley.edu

National Commission for Health Education Credentialing. (1989). *Information about the NCHEC.* New York: NCHEC.

National Commission for Health Education Credentialing. (1996). *A competency-based framework for professional development for certified health education specialists.* Allentown, PA.

National Commission for Health Education Credentialing. (1999). *NCHEC* [On-line]. Available: http://www.nchec.org

National Council for the Accreditation of Teacher Education. (1997). *Technology and the new professional teacher: Preparing for the 21st century classroom.* [On-line]. Available: http://www.ncate.org/projects/tech/TECH.HTM

National Teaching and Learning Forum. (1999). *Higher education associations* [On-line]. Available: www.ntlf.com/html/lib/assoc/chea.htm

Nelkin, D. (1989). Journalism and science: The creative tension. In M. Moore (Ed.), *Health risks and the press: Perspectives on media coverage of risk assessment and health.* Washington, DC: The Media Institute.

O'Rourke, T. (1989). Reflections on directions in health education: Implications for policy and practice (AAHE Scholar Presentation). *Health Education, 20*(6), 4–14.

O'Rourke, T. (1990). Credentialing and the future of health education: A rebuttal. *Wellness Perspectives: Research, Theory, and Practice, 6*(3), 55–63.

Orrebo, B., & Williamson, J. (1990). Certification and its discontents: A history of the moratorium. *Health Education Quarterly, 17*(3), 243–247.

Pahz, J.A. (1998). Debating CHES. *The CHES Bulletin, 9*(2), 20–22.

Pew Health Professions Commission (1995). *Critical issues: Revitalizing the health professions for the twenty-first century.* San Francisco.

Pollock, M.B., & Carlyon, W. (1996). Seven responsibilities and how they grew: The story of a curriculum framework. *Journal of Health Education, 27*(2), 81–87.

Rodeheffer, R., Gerstenblith, G., Becker, L., Fleg, J., Weisfeldt, M., & Lakatta, E. (1984). Exercise cardiac output is maintained with advancing age in healthy human subjects: Cardiac dilation and increased stroke volume compensate for a diminished heart rate. *Circulation, 69*(2), 203–213.

Schaie, K. (1983). The Seattle longitudinal study: A 21-year exploration of psychometric intelligence in adulthood. In K. Schaie (Ed.), *Longitudinal Studies of Adults' Psychological Development.* New York: Guilford Press.

Schaie, K. (1989). Perceptual speed in adulthood: Cross sectional and longitudinal studies. *Psychology and Aging, 4*(4), 443–453.

Schuster, C. (1995). Have we forgotten the older adults? An argument in support of more health promotion programs for and research directed toward people 65 years and older. *Journal of Health Education, 26* (6), 338–344.

Schwartz, L.W., O'Rourke, T.W., Eddy, J.M., Auld, E., & Smith, B. (1999). Use and impact of the competencies for entry-level health educators on professional preparation programs. *Journal of Health Education, 30*(4), 209–214.

Sheinfeld Gorin. S. (1998). Future directions for health promotion. In S. Sheinfeld Gorin & J. Arnold, *Health promotion handbook.* St. Louis: Mosby.

Steckler, A., McLeroy, K.R., Goodman, R.M., Bird, S.T., & McCormick, L. (1992). Toward integrating qualitative and quantitative methods: An introduction. *Health Education Quarterly, 19*(1), 1–8.

Stewart, A., & King, A. (1991). Evaluating the efficacy of physical activity for influencing quality of life outcomes in older adults. *Annals of Behavioral Medicine, 13*(2), 108–116.

Stewart, A., King, A., & Haskell, W. (1993). Endurance exercise and health-related quality of life in 50 to 65 year-old adults. *Gerontologist, 33*(6), 782–789.

Stewart, G.W. (1993). Social and behavioral change strategies. *Health Education Quarterly.* Supplement 1, S113–S135.

Taub, A. (1993). Credentialing: The basics. *Journal of Health Education, 24*(5), 261–262.

Uhlenberg, P., & Eggebeen, D. (1986, Winter). The declining well-being of American adolescents. *The Public Interest, 82,* 25–38.

U.S. Bureau of the Census. (1996). *Population projections of the United States by age, sex, race and Hispanic origin: 1995–2050.* Washington, DC.

U.S. Bureau of the Census. (1998a). *Current population survey.* Washington, DC: U.S. Government Printing Office.

U.S. Bureau of the Census. (1998b). *Families by type, race, and Hispanic origin* [On-line]. Available: http://www.census.gov/population/socdemo/hh-fam/98pplb.txt

U.S. Bureau of the Census. (1999a). *Population estimates* [On-line]. Available: www.census.gov/population/estimates/state/rank/strnktb5.txt and www.census.gov/population/estimates/nation/intfile3-1.txt

U.S. Bureau of the Census. (1999b). *Health insurance coverage: 1998* [On-line]. Available: http:www.census.gov/hhes/hlthins/hlthin98/hlt98/hlt98asc.html

U.S. Bureau of the Census. (2000). Children without health insuance coverage: 1998 and 1999 [Online]. Available: http://www.census.gove/hhes/hlthins/hlthin99/fig02.gif

U.S. Department of Health, Education and Welfare. (1971). *Report on licensure and related health personnel credentialing.* (DHEW Publication No. (HSM) 72–11). Washington, DC: Government Printing Office.

U.S. Society & Values. (1997). *The accreditation process* [On-line]. Available: http://194.90.114.5/publish/journals/society/december97/accred.html

White, L.C. (1988). *Merchants of death: The American tobacco industry.* New York: Beech Tree Books.

Williams, T. (1991). Health care trends for older people. *Biofeedback and Self-Regulation, 16*(4), 337–347.

Williams, T., & Katzman, B. (1988). Public policy issues. In L. Jarvik & C. Winograd (Eds.), *Treatment for the Alzheimer patient.* New York: Springer.

Wise, A.E. (1994a). Teaching the teachers. *American School Board Journal, 181*(6), 22–25.

Wise, A.E. (1994b). The NCATE seal of approval. *American School Board Journal, 181*(6), 25.

Wise, A.E. (1996). Building a system of quality assurance for the teaching profession: Moving into the 21st century. *Phi Delta Kappan, 78*(3), 191–192.

Young, I.M. (1990). *Justice and the politics of difference.* Princeton, NJ: Princeton University Press.

Zuckerman, S., & Norton, S. (1999). *Snapshots of America's families: Health status of nonelderly adults and children.* Washington, DC: The Urban Institute.

# Code of Ethics for the Health Education Profession

## PREAMBLE

The Health Education profession is dedicated to excellence in the practice of promoting individual, family, organizational, and community health. Guided by common ideals, Health Educators are responsible for upholding the integrity and ethics of the profession as they face the daily challenges of making decisions. By acknowledging the value of diversity in society and embracing a cross-cultural approach, Health Educators support the worth, dignity, potential, and uniqueness of all people.

The Code of Ethics provides a framework of shared values within which Health Education is practiced. The Code of Ethics is grounded in fundamental ethical principles that underlie all health care services: respect for autonomy, promotion of social justice, active promotion of good, and avoidance of harm. The responsibility of each Health Educator is to aspire to the highest possible standards of conduct and to encourage the ethical behavior of all those with whom they work.

Regardless of job title, professional affiliation, work setting, or population served, Health Educators abide by these guidelines when making professional decisions.

## ARTICLE I: RESPONSIBILITY TO THE PUBLIC

A Health Educator's ultimate responsibility is to educate people for the purpose of promoting, maintaining, and improving individual, family, and community health. When a conflict of issues arises among individuals, groups, organizations, agencies, or institutions, Health Educators must consider all issues and give priority to those that promote wellness and quality of living through principles of self-determination and freedom of choice for the individual.

**Section 1:** Health Educators support the right of individuals to make informed decisions regarding health, as long as such decisions pose no threat to the health of others.

**Section 2:** Health Educators encourage actions and social policies that support and facilitate the best balance of benefits over harm for the affected parties.

**Section 3:** Health Educators accurately communicate the potential benefits and consequences of the services and programs with which they are associated.

**Section 4:** Health Educators accept the responsibility to act on issues that can adversely affect the health of individuals, families, and communities.

**Section 5:** Health Educators are truthful about their qualifications and the limitations of their expertise and provide services consistent with their competencies.

**Section 6:** Health Educators protect the privacy and dignity of individuals.

**Section 7:** Health Educators actively involve individuals, groups, and communities in the entire educational process so that all aspects of the process are clearly understood by those who may be affected.

**Section 8:** Health Educators respect and acknowledge the rights of others to hold diverse values, attitudes, and opinions.

**Section 9:** Health Educators provide services equitably to all people.

# ARTICLE II: RESPONSIBILITY TO THE PROFESSION

Health Educators are responsible for their professional behavior, for the reputation of their profession, and for promoting ethical conduct among their colleagues.

**Section 1:** Health Educators maintain, improve, and expand their professional competence through continued study and education; membership, participation, and leadership in professional organizations; and involvement in issues related to the health of the public.

**Section 2:** Health Educators model and encourage nondiscriminatory standards of behavior in their interactions with others.

**Section 3:** Health Educators encourage and accept responsible critical discourse to protect and enhance the profession.

**Section 4:** Health Educators contribute to the development of the profession by sharing the processes and outcomes of their work.

**Section 5:** Health Educators are aware of possible professional conflicts of interest, exercise integrity in conflict situations, and do not manipulate or violate the rights of others.

**Section 6:** Health Educators give appropriate recognition to others for their professional contributions and achievements.

# ARTICLE III: RESPONSIBILITY TO EMPLOYERS

Health Educators recognize the boundaries of their professional competence and are accountable for their professional activities and actions.

**Section 1:** Health Educators accurately represent their qualifications and the qualifications of others whom they recommend.

**Section 2:** Health Educators use appropriate standards, theories, and guidelines as criteria when carrying out their professional responsibilities.

**Section 3:** Health Educators accurately represent potential service and program outcomes to employers.

**Section 4:** Health Educators anticipate and disclose competing commitments, conflicts of interest, and endorsement of products.

**Section 5:** Health Educators openly communicate to employers expectations of job-related assignments that conflict with their professional ethics.

**Section 6:** Health Educators maintain competence in their areas of professional practice.

# ARTICLE IV: RESPONSIBILITY IN THE DELIVERY OF HEALTH EDUCATION

Health Educators promote integrity in the delivery of health education. They respect the rights, dignity, confidentiality, and worth of all people by adapting strategies and methods to the needs of diverse populations and communities.

**Section 1:** Health Educators are sensitive to social and cultural diversity and are in accord with the law when planning and implementing programs.

**Section 2:** Health Educators are informed of the latest advances in theory, research, and practice, and use strategies and methods that are grounded in and contribute to development of professional standards, theories, guidelines, statistics, and experience.

**Section 3:** Health Educators are committed to rigorous evaluation of both program effectiveness and methods used to achieve results.

**Section 4:** Health Educators empower individuals to adopt healthy lifestyles through informed choice rather than by coercion or intimidation.

**Section 5:** Health Educators communicate the potential outcomes of proposed services, strategies, and pending decisions to all individuals who will be affected.

# ARTICLE V: RESPONSIBILITY IN RESEARCH AND EVALUATION

Health Educators contribute to the health of the population and to the profession through research and evaluation activities. When planning and conducting research or evaluation, Health Educators do so in accordance with federal and state laws and regulations, organizational and institutional policies, and professional standards.

**Section 1:** Health Educators support principles and practices of research and evaluation that do no harm to individuals, groups, society, or the environment.

**Section 2:** Health Educators ensure that participation in research is voluntary and is based upon the informed consent of the participants.

**Section 3:** Health Educators respect the privacy, rights, and dignity of research participants, and honor commitments made to those participants.

**Section 4:** Health Educators treat all information obtained from participants as confidential unless otherwise required by law.

**Section 5:** Health Educators take credit, including authorship, only for work they have actually performed and give credit to the contributions of others.

**Section 6:** Health Educators who serve as research or evaluation consultants discuss their results only with those to whom they are providing service, unless maintaining such confidentiality would jeopardize the health or safety of others.

**Section 7:** Health Educators report the results of their research and evaluation objectively, accurately, and in a timely fashion.

# ARTICLE VI: RESPONSIBILITY IN PROFESSIONAL PREPARATION

Those involved in the preparation and training of Health Educators have an obligation to accord learners the same respect and treatment given other groups by providing quality education that benefits the profession and the public.

**Section 1:** Health Educators select students for professional preparation programs based upon equal opportunity for all and the individual's academic performance, abilities, and potential contribution to the profession and the public's health.

**Section 2:** Health Educators strive to make the educational environment and culture conducive to the health of all involved and free from sexual harassment and all forms of discrimination.

**Section 3:** Health Educators involved in professional preparation and professional development engage in careful preparation; present material that is accurate, up-to-date, and timely; provide reasonable and timely feedback; state clear and reasonable expectations; and conduct fair assessments and evaluation of learners.

**Section 4:** Health Educators provide objective and accurate counseling to learners about career opportunities, development, and advancement, and assist learners secure professional employment.

**Section 5:** Health Educators provide adequate supervision and meaningful opportunities for the professional development of learners.

# Responsibilities and Competencies for Health Educators

Responsibilities, competencies, and subcompetencies for graduate level health educators are in italics. All others are for entry-level health educators.

## Responsibility I: Assessing Individual and Community Needs for Health Education

### Competency A:

Obtain health-related data about social and cultural environments, growth and development factors, needs, and interests.

#### Subcompetencies:

1. Select valid sources of information about health needs and interests.
2. Utilize computerized sources of health-related information.
3. Employ or develop appropriate data-gathering instruments.
4. Apply survey techniques to acquire health data.
5. *Conduct health-related assessment in communities.*

### Competency B:

Distinguish between behaviors that foster and those that hinder well-being.

#### Subcompetencies:

1. Investigate physical, social, emotional, and intellectual factors influencing health behaviors.
2. Identify behaviors that tend to promote or compromise health.
3. Recognize the role of learning and affective experience in shaping patterns of health behavior.
4. *Analyze social, cultural, economic, and political factors that influence health.*

### Competency C:

Infer needs for health education on the basis of obtained data.

#### Subcompetencies:

1. Analyze needs assessment data.
2. Determine priority areas of need for health education

### Competency D:

*Determine factors that influence learning and development.*

#### Subcompetencies:

1. *Assess individual learning styles.*
2. *Assess individual learning literacy.*
3. *Assess the learning environment.*

# Responsibility II: Planning Effective Health Education Programs

## Competency A:

Recruit community organizations, resource people, and potential participants for support and assistance in program planning.

**Subcompetencies:**

1. Communicate the need for the program to those who will be involved.
2. Obtain commitments from personnel and decision makers who will be involved in the program.
3. Seek ideas and opinions of those who will affect or be affected by the program.
4. Incorporate feasible ideas and recommendations into the planning process.
5. *Apply principles of community organization in planning programs.*

## Competency B:

Develop a logical scope and sequence plan for a health education program.

**Subcompetencies:**

1. Determine the range of health information requisite to a given program of instruction.
2. Organize the subject areas comprising the scope of a program in logical sequence.
3. *Review philosophical and theory-based foundations in planning health education programs.*
4. *Analyze the process for integrating health education as part of a broader health care or education program.*
5. *Develop a theory-based framework for health education programs.*

## Competency C:

Formulate appropriate and measurable program objectives.

**Subcompetencies:**

1. Infer educational objectives that facilitate achievement of specified competencies.

2. Develop a framework of broadly stated, operational objectives relevant to a proposed health education program.

## Competency D:

Design educational programs consistent with specified program objectives.

**Subcompetencies:**

1. Match proposed learning activities with those implicit in the stated objectives.
2. Formulate a wide variety of alternative educational methods.
3. Select strategies best suited to implementation of educational objectives in a given setting.
4. Plan a sequence of learning opportunities building upon, and reinforcing mastery of, preceding objectives.
5. *Select appropriate theory-based strategies in health program planning.*
6. *Plan training and instructional programs for health professionals.*

## *Competency E:*

*Develop health education programs using social marketing principles.*

**Subcompetencies:**

1. *Identify populations for health education programs.*
2. *Involve participants in planning health education programs.*
3. *Design a marketing plan to promote health education.*

# Responsibility III: Implementing Health Education Programs

## Competency A:

Exhibit competence in carrying out planned educational programs.

**Subcompetencies:**

1. Employ a wide range of educational methods and techniques.

2. Apply individual or group process methods as appropriate to given learning situations.

3. Utilize instructional equipment and other instructional media effectively.

4. Select methods that best facilitate practice of program objectives.

5. *Assess, select, and apply technologies that will contribute to program objectives.*

6. *Develop, demonstrate, and model implementation strategies.*

7. *Deliver educational programs for health professionals.*

8. *Use community organization principles to guide and facilitate community organization.*

## Competency B:

Infer enabling objectives as needed to implement instructional programs in specified settings.

**Subcompetencies:**

1. Pretest learners to ascertain present abilities and knowledge relative to proposed program objectives.

2. Develop subordinate measurable objectives as needed for instruction.

## Competency C:

Select methods and media best suited to implement program plans for specific learners.

**Subcompetencies:**

1. Analyze learner characteristics, legal aspects, feasibility, and other considerations influencing choices among methods.

2. Evaluate the efficacy of alternative methods and techniques capable of facilitating program objectives.

3. Determine the availability of information, personnel, time, and equipment needed to implement the program for a given audience.

4. *Critically analyze technologies, methods, and media for their acceptability to diverse groups.*

5. *Apply theoretical and conceptual models from health education and related disciplines to improve program delivery.*

## Competency D:

Monitor educational programs, adjusting objectives and activities as necessary.

**Subcompetencies:**

1. Compare actual program activities with the stated objectives.

2. Assess the relevance of existing program objectives to current needs.

3. Revise program activities and objectives as necessitated by changes in learner needs.

4. Appraise applicability of resources and materials relative to given educational objectives.

# Responsibility IV:
# Evaluating Effectiveness of Health Education Programs

## Competency A:

Develop plans to assess achievement of program objectives.

**Subcompetencies:**

1. Determine standards of performance to be applied as criteria of effectiveness.

2. Establish a realistic scope of evaluation efforts.

3. Develop an inventory of existing valid and reliable tests and survey instruments.

4. Select appropriate methods for evaluating program effectiveness.

5. *Identify existing sources of health related databases.*

6. *Evaluate existing data gathering instruments and processes.*

7. *Select appropriate qualitative and/or quantitative evaluation design.*

8. *Develop valid and reliable evaluation instruments.*

## Competency B:

Carry out evaluation plans.

**Subcompetencies:**

1. Facilitate administration of the tests and activities specified in the plan.

2. Utilize data collecting methods appropriate to the objectives.

3. Analyze resulting evaluation data.

4. Implement appropriate qualitative and quantitative evaluation techniques.

5. Apply evaluation technology as appropriate.

## Competency C:

Interpret results of program evaluation.

### Subcompetencies:

1. Apply criteria of effectiveness to results obtained from a program.

2. Translate evaluation results into terms easily understood by others.

3. Report effectiveness of educational programs in achieving proposed objectives.

4. *Implement strategies to analyze data from evaluation assessments.*

5. *Compare evaluation results to other findings.*

6. *Make recommendations from evaluation results.*

## Competency D:

Infer implications from findings for future program planning.

### Subcompetencies:

1. Explore possible explanations for important evaluation findings.

2. Recommend strategies for implementing results of evaluation.

3. *Apply findings to refine and maintain programs.*

4. *Use evaluation findings in policy analysis and development.*

# Responsibility V: Coordinating Provision of Health Education Services

## Competency A:

Develop a plan for coordinating health education services.

### Subcompetencies:

1. Determine the extent of available health education services.

2. Match health education services to proposed program activities.

3. Identify gaps and overlaps in the provision of collaborative health services.

## Competency B:

Facilitate cooperation between and among levels of program personnel.

### Subcompetencies:

1. Promote cooperation and feedback among personnel related to the program.

2. Apply various methods of conflict reduction as needed.

3. Analyze the role of health educator as liaison between program staff and outside groups and organizations.

## Competency C:

Formulate practical modes of collaboration among health agencies and organizations.

### Subcompetencies:

1. Stimulate cooperation among personnel responsible for community health education programs.

2. Suggest approaches for integrating health education within existing health programs.

3. Develop plans for promoting collaborative efforts among health agencies and organizations with mutual interests.

4. *Organize and facilitate groups, coalitions, and partnerships.*

## Competency D:

Organize the in-service training programs for teachers, volunteers, and other interested personnel.

### Subcompetencies:

1. Plan an operational, competency-oriented training program.

2. Utilize instructional resources that meet a variety of in-service training needs.

3. Demonstrate a wide range of strategies for conducting in-service programs.

4. *Facilitate collaborative training efforts among health agencies and organizations.*

# Responsibility VI: Acting as Resource Person in Health Education

## Competency A:

Utilize computerized health information retrieval systems effectively.

**Subcompetencies:**

1. Match an information need with the appropriate retrieval system.
2. Access principal on-line and other database health information resources.
3. *Select a data system commensurate with program needs.*
4. *Determine relevance of various computerized health information resources.*
5. *Assist in establishing and monitoring policies for use of data gathering practices.*

## Competency B:

Establish effective consultative relationships with those requesting assistance in solving health-related problems.

**Subcompetencies:**

1. Analyze parameters of effective consultative relationships.
2. Describe special skills and abilities health educators need for consultation activities.
3. Formulate a plan for providing consultation to other health professionals.
4. Explain the process of marketing health education consultative services.
5. *Apply networking skills to develop and maintain consultative relationships.*

## Competency C:

Interpret and respond to requests for health information.

**Subcompetencies:**

1. Analyze general processes for identifying the information needed to satisfy a request.

2. Employ a wide range of approaches in referring requesters to valid sources of health information.

## Competency D:

Select effective educational resource materials for dissemination.

**Subcompetencies:**

1. Assemble educational material of value to the health of individuals and community groups.
2. Evaluate the worth and applicability of resource materials for given audiences.
3. Apply various processes in the acquisition of resource materials.
4. Compare different methods for distributing educational materials.
5. *Apply communication theory and principles in the development of health education materials.*

# Responsibility VII: Communicating Health and Health Education Needs, Concerns, and Resources

## Competency A:

Interpret concepts, purposes, and theories of health education.

**Subcompetencies:**

1. Evaluate the state of the art of health education.
2. Analyze the foundations of the discipline of health education.
3. Describe major responsibilities of the health educator in the practice of health education.
4. *Articulate the historical and philosophical bases of health education.*

## Competency B:

Predict the impact of societal value systems on health education programs.

**Subcompetencies:**

1. Investigate social forces causing opposing viewpoints regarding health education needs and concerns.

2. Employ a wide range of strategies for dealing with controversial health issues.

3. *Analyze social, cultural, demographic and political factors that influence decision makers.*

4. *Predict the future health education needs based upon societal changes.*

5. *Respond to challenges to health education programs.*

## Competency C:

Select a variety of communication methods and techniques in providing health information.

### Subcompetencies:

1. Utilize a wide range of techniques for communicating health and health education information and education.

2. Demonstrate proficiency in communicating health information and health education needs.

3. *Demonstrate both proficiency and accuracy in oral and written presentations.*

4. *Use culturally sensitive communication methods and techniques.*

## Competency D:

Foster communication between health care providers and consumers.

### Subcompetencies:

1. Interpret the significance and implications of health care providers' messages to consumers.

2. Act as liaison between consumer groups and individuals and health care provider organizations.

## *Responsibility VIII: Apply Appropriate Research Principles and Methods in Health Education*

### *Competency A:*

*Conduct thorough reviews of literature.*

#### *Subcompetencies:*

1. *Employ electronic technology for retrieving references.*

2. *Analyze references to identify those pertinent to selected health education issues or programs.*

3. *Select and critique sources of health information.*

4. *Evaluate the research design, methodology and findings from the literature.*

5. *Synthesize key information from the literature.*

### *Competency B:*

*Use appropriate qualitative and quantitative research methods.*

#### *Subcompetencies:*

1. *Assess the merits and limitations of qualitative and quantitative research methods.*

2. *Apply qualitative and/or quantitative research methods in research designs.*

### *Competency C:*

*Apply research to health education practice.*

#### *Subcompetencies:*

1. *Use appropriate research methods and design in assessing needs.*

2. *Use information derived from research for program planning.*

3. *Select implementation strategies based upon research results.*

4. *Employ research design, methods and analysis in program evaluation.*

5. *Describe how research results inform health policy development.*

6. *Use research results to inform health policy development.*

7. *Use protocol for dissemination of research findings.*

## *Responsibility IX: Administering Health Education Programs*

### *Competency A:*

*Develop and manage fiscal resources.*

#### *Subcompetencies:*

1. *Prepare proposals to obtain resources through grants, contract, and other internal and external sources.*

2. *Develop and manage realistic budgets to support program requirements.*

## Competency B:

*Develop and manage human resources.*

### Subcompetencies:

1. *Assess and communicate qualifications of personnel needed for programs.*
2. *Recruit, employ, and evaluate staff members.*
3. *Provide staff development.*
4. *Demonstrate leadership in managing human resources.*
5. *Apply human resource policies consistent with relevant laws and regulations.*

## Competency C:

*Exercise organizational leadership.*

### Subcompetencies:

1. *Analyze the organization's culture in relationship to program goals.*
2. *Assess the political climate of the organization, community, state and nation regarding conditions that advance or inhibit the goals of the program.*
3. *Conduct long-range and strategic planning.*
4. *Develop strategies to reinforce or change organizational culture to achieve program goals.*
5. *Develop strategies to influence public policy.*

## Competency D:

*Obtain acceptance and support for programs.*

### Subcompetencies:

1. *Apply social marketing principles and techniques to achieve program goals.*
2. *Employ concepts and theories of public relations and communications to obtain program support.*
3. *Incorporate demographically and culturally sensitive techniques to promote programs.*
4. *Use needs assessment information to advocate for health education programs.*

## Responsibility X: Advancing the Profession of Health Education

## Competency A:

*Provide a critical analysis of current and future needs in health education.*

### Subcompetencies:

1. *Relate health education issues to larger social issues.*
2. *Articulate health education's role in policy formation at various organizational and community levels.*

## Competency B:

*Assume responsibility for advancing the profession.*

### Subcompetencies:

1. *Analyze the role of the health education associations in advancing the profession.*
2. *Participate in professional organizations.*
3. *Develop a personal plan for professional growth.*

## Competency C:

*Apply ethical principles as they relate to the practice of health education.*

1. *Analyze the interrelationships among ethics, values, and behavior.*
2. *Relate the importance of a code of ethics to professional practice.*
3. *Subscribe to a professionally recognized health education code of ethics.*

Source: *A Competency-Based Framework for Graduate-Level Health Educators,* The National Commission for Health Education Credentialing, Inc., 1999. Allentown, PA: The National Commission for Health Education Credentialing, Inc. Reprinted by permission of The National Commission for Health Education Credentialing, Inc., Society for Public Health Education, and American Alliance for Health, Physical Education, Recreation and Dance/American Association for Health Education.

# National Health Education Standards For Students Organized by Grade

## GRADES K–4

### Health Education Standard 1:

Students will comprehend concepts related to health promotion and disease prevention.

**Performance Indicators**: As a result of health instruction in Grades K–4, students will:

1. describe relationships between personal health behaviors and individual well being.
2. identify indicators of mental, emotional, social, and physical health during childhood.
3. describe the basic structure and functions of the human body systems.
4. describe how the family influences personal health.
5. describe how physical, social, and emotional environments influence personal health.
6. identify common health problems of children.
7. identify health problems that should be detected and treated early.
8. explain how childhood injuries and illnesses can be prevented.

### Health Education Standard 2:

Students will demonstrate the ability to access valid health information and health-promoting products and services.

**Performance Indicators**: As a result of health instruction in Grades K–4, students will:

1. identify characteristics of valid health information and health-promoting products and services.
2. demonstrate the ability to locate resources from home, school, and community that provide valid health information.
3. explain how media influences the selection of health information, products, and services.
4. demonstrate the ability to locate school and community health helpers.

### Health Education Standard 3:

Students will demonstrate the ability to practice health-enhancing behaviors and reduce health risks.

**Performance Indicators**: As a result of health instruction in Grades K–4, students will:

1. identify responsible health behaviors.
2. identify personal health needs.
3. compare behaviors that are safe to those that are risky or harmful.
4. demonstrate strategies to improve or maintain personal health.

5. develop injury prevention and management strategies for personal health.

6. demonstrate ways to avoid and reduce threatening situations.

7. apply skills to manage stress.

## Health Education Standard 4:

Students will analyze the influence of culture, media, technology, and other factors on health.

**Performance Indicators**: As a result of health instruction in Grades K–4, students will:

1. describe how culture influences personal health behaviors.

2. explain how media influences thoughts, feelings, and health behaviors.

3. describe ways technology can influence personal health.

4. explain how information from school and family influences health.

## Health Education Standard 5:

Students will demonstrate the ability to use interpersonal communication skills to enhance skills.

**Performance Indicators**: As a result of health instruction in Grades K–4, students will:

1. distinguish between verbal and non-verbal communication.

2. describe characteristics needed to be a responsible friend and family member.

3. demonstrate healthy ways to express needs, wants, and feelings.

4. demonstrate ways to communicate care, consideration, and respect of self and others.

5. demonstrate attentive listening skills to build and maintain healthy relationships.

6. demonstrate refusal skills to enhance health.

7. differentiate between negative and positive behaviors used in conflict situations.

8. demonstrate non-violent strategies to resolve conflicts.

## Health Education Standard 6:

Students will demonstrate the ability to use goal setting and decision-making skills to enhance health.

**Performance Indicators:** As a result of health instruction in Grades K–4, students will:

1. demonstrate the ability to apply a decision-making process to health issues and problems.

2. explain when to ask for assistance in making health-related decisions and setting health goals.

3. predict outcomes of positive health decisions.

4. set a personal health goal and track progress toward its achievement.

## Health Education Standard 7:

Students will demonstrate the ability to advocate for personal, family, and community health.

**Performance Indicators:** As a result of health instruction in Grades K–4, students will:

1. describe a variety of methods to convey accurate health information and ideas.

2. express information and opinions about health issues.

3. identify community agencies that advocate for healthy individuals, families, and communities.

4. demonstrate the ability to influence and support others in making positive health choices.

# GRADES 5–8

## Health Education Standard 1:

Students will comprehend concepts related to health promotion and disease prevention.

**Performance Indicators:** As a result of health instruction in Grades 5–8, students will:

1. explain the relationship between positive health behaviors and the prevention of injury, illness, disease, and premature death.

2. describe the interrelationship of mental, emotional, social, and physical health during adolescence.

3. explain how health is influenced by the interaction of body systems.

4. describe how family and peers influence the health of adolescents.

5. analyze how environment and personal health are interrelated.

6. describe ways to reduce risks related to adolescent health problems.

7. explain how appropriate health care can prevent premature death and disability.

8. describe how lifestyle, pathogens, family history, and other risk factors are related to the cause or prevention of disease and other health problems.

## Health Education Standard 2:

Students will demonstrate the ability to access valid health information and health-promoting products and services.

**Performance Indicators:** As a result of health instruction in Grades 5–8, students will:

1. analyze the validity of health information, products, and services.

2. demonstrate the ability to utilize resources from home, school, and community that provide valid health information.

3. analyze how media influences the selection of health information and products.

4. demonstrate the ability to locate health products and services.

5. compare the costs and validity of health products.

6. describe situations requiring professional health services.

## Health Education Standard 3:

Students will demonstrate the ability to practice health-enhancing behaviors and reduce health risks.

**Performance Indicators:** As a result of health instruction in Grades 5–8, students will:

1. explain the importance of assuming responsibility for personal health behaviors.

2. analyze a personal health assessment to determine health strengths and risks.

3. distinguish between safe and risky or harmful behaviors in relationships.

4. demonstrate strategies to improve or maintain personal and family health.

5. develop injury prevention and management strategies for personal and family health.

6. demonstrate ways to avoid and reduce threatening situations.

7. demonstrate strategies to manage stress.

## Health Education Standard 4:

Students will analyze the influence of culture, media, technology, and other factors on health.

**Performance Indicators:** As a result of health instruction in Grades 5–8, students will:

1. describe the influence of cultural beliefs on health behaviors and the use of health services.

2. analyze how messages from media and other sources influence health behaviors.

3. analyze the influence of technology on personal and family health.

4. analyze how information from peers influences health.

## Health Education Standard 5:

Students will demonstrate the ability to use interpersonal communication skills to enhance health.

**Performance Indicators:** As a result of health instruction in Grades 5–8, students will:

1. demonstrate effective verbal and non-verbal communication skills to enhance health.

2. describe how the behavior of family and peers affects interpersonal communication.

3. demonstrate healthy ways to express needs, wants, and feelings.

4. demonstrate ways to communicate care, consideration, and respect of self and others.

5. demonstrate communication skills to build and maintain healthy relationships.

6. demonstrate refusal and negotiation skills to enhance health.

7. analyze the possible causes of conflict among youth in schools and communities.

8. demonstrate strategies to manage conflict in healthy ways.

## Health Education Standard 6:

Students will demonstrate the ability to use goal setting and decision-making skills to enhance health.

**Performance Indicators:** As a result of health instruction in Grades 5–8, students will:

1. demonstrate the ability to apply a decision-making process to health issues and problems individually and collaboratively.

2. analyze how health-related decisions are influenced by individuals, family, and community values.

3. predict how decisions regarding health behaviors have consequences for self and others.

4. apply strategies and skills needed to attain personal health goals.

5. describe how personal health goals are influenced by changing information, abilities, priorities, and responsibilities.

6. develop a plan that addresses personal strengths, needs, and health risks.

## Health Education Standard 7:

Students will demonstrate the ability to advocate for personal, family, and community health.

**Performance Indicators:** As a result of health instruction in Grades 5–8, students will:

1. analyze various communication methods to accurately express health information and ideas.

2. express information and opinions about health issues.

3. identify barriers to effective communication of information, ideas, feelings, and opinions about health issues.

4. demonstrate the ability to influence and support others in making positive health choices.

5. demonstrate the ability to work cooperatively when advocating for healthy individuals, families, and schools.

# GRADES 9–11

## Health Education Standard 1:

Students will comprehend concepts related to health promotion and disease prevention.

**Performance Indicators:** As a result of health instruction in Grades 9–11, students will:

1. analyze how behavior can impact health maintenance and disease prevention.

2. describe the interrelationships of mental, emotional, social, and physical health throughout adulthood.

3. explain the impact of personal health behaviors on the functioning of the body systems.

4. analyze how the family, peers, and community influence the health of individuals.

5. analyze how the environment influences the health of the community.

6. describe how to delay onset and reduce risks of potential health problems during adulthood.

7. analyze how public health policies and government regulations influence health promotion and disease prevention.

8. analyze how the prevention and control of health problems are influenced by research and medical advances.

## Health Education Standard 2:

Students will demonstrate the ability to access valid health information and health-promoting products and services.

**Performance Indicators:** As a result of health instruction in Grades 9–11, students will:

1. evaluate the validity of health information, products, and services.

2. demonstrate the ability to evaluate resources from home, school, and community that provide valid health information.

3. evaluate factors that influence personal selection of health products and services.

4. demonstrate the ability to access school and community health services for self and others.

5. analyze the cost and accessibility of health care services.

6. analyze situations requiring professional health services.

## Health Education Standard 3:

Students will demonstrate the ability to practice health-enhancing behaviors and reduce health risks.

**Performance Indicators:** As a result of health instruction in Grades 9–11, students will:

1. analyze the role of individual responsibility for enhancing health.

2. evaluate a personal health assessment to determine strategies for health enhancement and risk reduction.

3. analyze the short-term and long-term consequences of safe, and risky or harmful behaviors.

4. develop strategies to improve or maintain personal, family, and community health.

5. develop injury prevention and management strategies for personal, family, and community health.

6. demonstrate ways to avoid and reduce threatening situations.

7. evaluate strategies to manage stress.

## Health Education Standard 4:

Students will analyze the influence of culture, media, technology, and other factors on health.

**Performance Indicators:** As a result of health instruction in Grades 9–11, students will:

1. analyze how cultural diversity enriches and challenges health behaviors.

2. evaluate the effect of media and other factors on personal, family, and community health.

3. evaluate the impact of technology on personal, family, and community health.

4. analyze how information from the community influences health.

## Health Education Standard 5:

Students will demonstrate the ability to use interpersonal communication skills to enhance health.

**Performance Indicators:** As a result of health instruction in Grades 9–11, students will:

1. demonstrate skills for communicating effectively with family, peers, and others.

2. analyze how interpersonal communication affects relationships.

3. demonstrate healthy ways to express needs, wants, and feelings.

4. demonstrate ways to communicate care, consideration, and respect of self and others.

5. demonstrate strategies for solving interpersonal conflicts without harming self or others.

6. demonstrate refusal, negotiation, and collaboration skills to avoid potentially harmful situations.

7. analyze the possible causes of conflict in schools, families, and communities.

8. demonstrate strategies used to prevent conflict.

## Health Education Standard 6:

Students will demonstrate the ability to use goal setting and decision-making skills to enhance health.

**Performance Indicators:** As a result of health instruction in Grades 9–11, students will:

1. demonstrate the ability to utilize various strategies when making decisions related to health needs and risks of young adults.

2. analyze health concerns that require collaborative decision making.

3. predict immediate and long-term impact of health decisions on the individual, family, and community.

4. implement a plan for attaining a personal health goal.

5. evaluate progress toward achieving personal health goals.

6. formulate an effective plan for lifelong health.

## Health Education Standard 7:

Students will demonstrate the ability to advocate for personal, family, and community health.

**Performance Indicators:** As a result of health instruction in Grades 9–11, students will:

1. evaluate the effectiveness of communication methods for accurately expressing health information and ideas.

2. express information and opinions about health issues.

3. utilize strategies to overcome barriers when communicating information, ideas, feelings, and opinions about health issues.

4. demonstrate the ability to influence and support others in making positive health choices.

5. demonstrate the ability to work cooperatively when advocating for healthy communities.

6. demonstrate the ability to adapt health message and communication techniques to characteristics of a particular audience.

Source: This represents the work of the Joint Committee on National Health Education Standards. Copies can be obtained through the American School Health Association, American Association for Health Education, or the American Cancer Society.

# Leading Health Indicators
# from *Healthy People 2010*

| Indicator | Focus Area-Objective Number | Objectives |
|---|---|---|
| Physical Activity | 22-2 | Increase the proportion of adults who engage regularly, preferably daily, in moderate physical activity for at least 30 minutes per day. |
| | 22-7 | Increase the proportion of adolescents who engage in vigorous physical activity that promotes cardiorespiratory fitness 3 or more days per week for 20 or more minutes per occasion. |
| Obesity and Overweight | 19-2 | Reduce the proportion of adults who are obese. |
| | 19-3 | Reduce the proportion of children and adolescents who are overweight or obese. |
| Tobacco Use | 27-1a | Reduce cigarette smoking by adults. |
| | 27-3ba | Reduce cigarette smoking by adolescents. |
| Substance Abuse | 26-10a | Increase the proportion of adolescents not using alcohol or any illicit drugs during the past 30 days. |
| | 26-10c | Reduce the proportion of adults using any illicit drugs during the past 30 days. |
| | 26-11c | Reduce the proportion of adults engaging in binge drinking of alcoholic beverages during the past month. |
| Responsible Sexual Behavior | 13-6 | Increase the proportion of sexually active persons who use condoms. |
| | 25-11 | Increase the proportion of adolescents who abstain from sexual intercourse or use condoms if currently sexually active. |
| Mental Health | 18-9b | Increase the proportion of adults with recognized depression who receive treatment. |

| Indicator | Focus Area-<br>Objective Number | Objectives |
|---|---|---|
| Injury and Violence | 15-15 | Reduce deaths caused by motor vehicle crashes. |
| | 15-32 | Reduce homicides. |
| Environmental Quality | 8-1a | Reduce the proportion of persons exposed to air that does not meet the U.S. Environmental Protection Agency's health-based standards for ozone. |
| | 27-10 | Reduce the proportion of nonsmokers exposed to environmental tobacco smoke. |
| Immunization | 14-24 | Increase the proportion of young children who receive all vaccines that have been recommended for universal administration for at least 5 years. |
| | 14-29 | Increase the proportion of noninstitutionalized adults who are vaccinated annually against influenza and ever vaccinated against pneumococcal disease. |
| Access to Health Care | 1-1 | Increase the proportion of persons with health insurance. |
| | 1-4a | Increase the proportion of persons who have a specific source of ongoing care. |
| | 16-6a | Increase the proportion of pregnant women who begin prenatal care in the first trimester of pregnancy. |

Source: Healthy People 2010 (Conference ed. in two vols.), U.S. Department of Health and Human Services, 2000, Washington, DC: U.S. Government Printing Office.

# Resources for Health Promotion

## PROFESSIONAL ORGANIZATIONS AND ASSOCIATIONS

**American Academy of Pediatrics**
141 Northwest Point Blvd.
Elk Grove Village, IL 60007-1098
847-228-5005
http://www.aap.org

**American Alliance for Health, Physical Education, Recreation and Dance**
1900 Association Drive
Reston, VA 22091
800-213-7193
http://www.aahperd.org

**American Association for Health Education**
1900 Association Drive
Reston, VA 20191
800-213-7193
http://www.aahperd.org/aahe/aahe-main.html

**American Association of School Administrators**
1801 North Moore Street
Arlington, VA 22209
703-528-0700
http://www.aasa.org

**American Association of Sex Educators, Counselors and Therapists**
435 N. Michigan Avenue, Suite 1717
Chicago, IL 60611-4067
312-664-0828
http://www.aasect.org

**American College Health Association**
P.O. Box 28937
Baltimore, MD 21240-8937
410-859-1500
http://www.acha.org

**American College of Sports Medicine**
401 West Michigan Street
Indianapolis, IN 46206-3233
317-637-9200
http://www.acsm.org

**American Dental Association**
211 East Chicago Avenue
Chicago, IL 60611
312-621-8099
http://www.ada.org

**American Dietetic Association**
216 West Jackson Blvd.
Chicago, IL 60606-6995
800-877-1600
http://www.eatright.org

**American Federation of Teachers**
555 New Jersey Avenue, NW
Washington, DC 20001
202-879-4400
http://www.aft.org

**American Medical Association**
515 North State Street
Chicago, IL 60610
312-464-4500
http://www.ama-assn.org

**American Nurses Association**
600 Maryland Avenue, SW, Suite 100 West
Washington, DC 20020
800-274-4ANA (-4262)
http://www.ana.org

**American Optometric Association**
243 North Lindbergh Blvd.
St. Louis, MO 63141
314-991-4100
http://www.aoanet.org

**American Osteopathic Association**
142 East Ontario Street
Chicago, IL 60611
800-621-1773
http://www.am-osteo-assn.org

**American Psychiatric Association**
1400 K Street
Washington, DC 20005
202-682-6000
http://www.psych.org

**American Psychological Association**
750 First Street, NE
Washington, DC 20002-4242
202-336-5500
http://www.apa.org

**American Public Health Association**
800 I Street, NW
Washington, DC 20001-3710
202-777-APHA (-2742)
http://www.apha.org

**American School Counselor Association**
801 North Fairfax Street, Suite 310
Alexandria, VA 22314
800-306-4722
http://www.schoolcounselor.org

**American School Food Service Association**
700 South Washington Street, Suite 300
Alexandria, VA 22314
703-739-3900
http://www.asfsa.org

**American Social Health Association**
P.O. Box 13827
Research Triangle Park, NC 27709
800-342-2437
http://www.ashatd.org

**Association for Worksite Health Promotion**
60 Revere Drive, Suite 500
Northbrook, IL 60002
847-480-9574
http://www.awhp.org

**Association of State and Territorial Directors of Health Promotion and Public Health Education**
750 First Street, NE, Suite 1050
Washington, DC 20002
202-312-6460
http://www.astdhpphe.org

**Association of State and Territorial Health Officials**
1275 K Street, NW, Suite 800
Washington, DC 20005-4006
202-371-9090
http://www.astho.org

**Canadian Association for Health, Physical Education, and Recreation**
333 River Road
Ottawa, Ontario, Canada KIL 8H9

**Canadian Public Health Association**
1565 Carling Avenue, Suite 400
Ottawa Ontario, Canada K1Z 8R1
613-725-3769
FAX 613-725-9826
http://www.cpha.ca

**Coalition of National
Health Education Organizations**
University of South Florida,
    College of Public Health
13201 Bruce B. Downs Blvd.
Tampa, FL 33612-3805
http://www.med.usf.edu/~kmbrown/NCHEO.htm

**Coalition on Sexuality and Disability, Inc.**
122 East 23rd Street
New York, NY 10010
212-242-3900

**Council of Chief State School Officers**
1 Massachusetts, NW, Suite 700
Washington, DC 20001
202-408-5505
http://www.ccsso.org

**Eta Sigma Gamma**
200 University Avenue
Muncie, IN 47306
800-715-2559
http://www.cast.ilstu.edu/temple/esg.htm

**International Union
for Health Promotion and Education**
North American Regional Office/IUHPE
c/o APHA
800 I Street, NW
Washington, DC 20001-3710

**National Association of School Psychologists**
4340 East West Highway, Suite 402
Bethesda, MD 20814
301-657-0270
http://www.naspweb.org

**National Association of School Nurses**
P.O. Box 1300
Scarborough, ME 04070-1300
207-883-2117
http://www.nasn.org

**National Association of Social Workers**
750 First Street, NE, Suite 700
Washington, DC 20002-4241
202-408-8600
http://www.naswdc.org

**National Association
of State Boards of Education**
1012 Cameron Street
Alexandria, VA 22314
703-684-4000
http://www.nasbe.org

**National Commission
for Health Education Credentialing, Inc.**
944 Marcon Blvd., Suite 310
Allentown, PA 18103
888-624-3248
http://www.nchec.org

**National Education Association**
1201 16th Street, NW
Washington, DC 20036
202-822-4000
http://www.nea.org

**National Environmental Health Association**
720 S. Colorado Blvd.
South Tower, Suite 970
Denver, CO 80246-1925
303-756-9090
http://www.neha.org

**National School Boards Association**
1680 Duke Street
Alexandria, VA 22314
703-683-7590
http://www.nsba.org

**National Wellness Association**
1300 College Court
Box 827
Stevens Point, WI 54481-0827
715-342-2969
http://www.wellnessnwi.org/nwa/

**National Wellness Institute**
South Hall, 1319 Fremont Street
Stevens Point, WI 54481
800-244-8922
http://www.nationalwellness.org

**Society for Public Health Education**
750 First Ave., NE, Suite 910
Washington, DC 20002-4242
202-408-9804
http://www.sophe.org

**Wellness Councils of America**
9802 Nicholas Street, Suite 315
Omaha, NE 68114
402-827-3590
http://www.welcoa.org

# NONPROFIT ORGANIZATIONS

**Alcoholics Anonymous**
General Service Office
475 Riverside Drive
New York, NY 10015
212-870-3400
http://www.alcoholics-anonymous.org

**Alzheimer's Association**
919 North Michigan Avenue, Suite 1000
Chicago, IL 60611-1676
800-272-3900
http://www.alz.org

**American Anorexia Bulimia Association, Inc.**
165 West 46th Street, Suite 1108
New York, NY 10036
212-575-6200
http://www.aabainc.org

**American Cancer Society**
1599 Clifton Road, NE
Atlanta, GA 30329-4251
800-ACS-2345 (227-)
http://www.cancer.org

**American Diabetes Association**
1701 N. Beauregard Street
Alexandria, VA 22311
800-DIABETES (342-2383)
http://www.diabetes.org

**American Foundation for the Blind, Inc.**
11 Penn Plaza, Suite 300
New York, NY 10001
212-502-7600
http://www.afb.org/afb

**American Heart Association**
National Center
7272 Greenville Avenue
Dallas, TX 75231
800-AHA-USA1 (242-8721)
http://amhrt.org

**American Institute of Stress**
120 Park Avenue
Yonkers, NY 10703
http://www.stress.org

**American Lung Association**
1740 Broadway
New York, NY 10019-4374
800-LUNG-USA (586-4872)
http://www.lungusa.org

**American Lupus Society**
260 Maple Court, Suite 123
Ventura, CA 93003
800-331-1802

**American National Red Cross**
1621 North Kent Street, 11th Floor
Arlington, VA 22209
703-248-4222
http://www.redcross.org

**Arthritis Foundation**
1330 West Peachtree Street
Atlanta, GA 30309
404-872-7100
http://www.arthritis.org

**Action for Smoking or Health**
2013 H Street, NW
Washington, DC 20006
202-659-4310
http://www.ash.org

**BEST Foundation for a Drug-Free Tomorrow**
725 South Figueroa, Suite 1615
Los Angeles, CA 90017
800-ALERT10 (253-7810)
http://www.projectalert.best.org

**Canadian Cancer Society**
10 Alcorn Avenue, Suite 200
Toronto, Ontario M4V 3B1
416-961-7223
http://www.cancer.ca

**Cystic Fibrosis Foundation**
6931 Arlington Road
Bethesda, MD 20814
800-344-4823
http://www.cff.org

**Epilepsy Foundation of America**
4351 Garden City Drive
Landover, MD 20785
800-EFA-1000 (332-)
http://www.efa.org

**Girls Incorporated**
120 Wall Street, 3rd Floor
New York, NY 10005
212-509-2000
www.girlsinc.org

**Greenpeace International**
Keizersgracht 176
1016 DW
Amsterdam, The Netherlands
31 20 523 62 22
http://www.greenpeace.org

**Juvenile Diabetes Foundation**
120 Wall Street
New York, NY 10005
800-JDF-CURE (533-2873)
http://www.jdfcure.org

**Leukemia Society of America**
600 Third Avenue
New York, NY 10016
212-573-8484
http://www.leukemia.org

**The Lung Association (Canada)**
1900 City Park Drive, Suite 508
Blair Business Park
Gloucester, Ontario, Canada K1J 1A3
613-747-6776
http://www.lung.ca

**Lupus Foundation of America**
1300 Piccard Drive, Suite 200
Rockville, MD 20850-5303
800-558-0121
http://www.lupus.org

**March of Dimes Birth Defects Foundation**
1275 Mamaroneck Avenue
White Plains, NY 10605
888-MODIMES (663-4637)
http://www.modimes.org

**Mothers Against Drunk Driving**
P.O. Box 541688
Dallas, TX 75354-1688
800-GET-MADD (438-6233)
http://www.madd.org

**Muscular Dystrophy Association**
National Headquarters
3300 East Sunrise Drive
Tucson, AZ 85718
800-572-1717
http://www.mdausa.org

**National Association on HIV Over Fifty**
Midwest AIDS Training & Education Center
University of Illinois at Chicago
808 South Wood Street, m/c 779
Chicago, IL 60612
312-996-1426
http://www.uic.edu/depts/matec/nahof_
resources.html

**National Association for Sickle-Cell Disease, Inc.**
3345 Wilshire Boulevard
Los Angeles, CA 90010-1880
800-421-8453

**National Center for Health Education**
72 Spring Street, Suite 208
New York, NY 10012
212-334-9470
http://www.nche.org

**National Child Safety Council**
P.O. Box 1368
Jackson, MI 49204
800-222-1464

**National Children's Center for Rural and Agricultural Health and Safety**
1000 North Oak Avenue
Marshfield, WI 54449
888-924-SAFE (-7233)
http://www.research.marshfieldclinics.org/
children/action/support.htm

**National Council
for Reliable Health Information**
P.O. Box 1276
Loma Linda, CA 92354
909-824-4690
http://www.ncrhi.org

**National Council on Aging**
409 Third Avenue SW, 2nd Floor
Washington, DC 20024
202-479-1200
http://www.ncoa.org

**National Council on Alcoholism
and Drug Dependence**
12 West 21st Street
New York, NY 10010
212-206-6770
http://www.ncadd.org

**National Easter Seals Society**
70 East Lake Street
Chicago, IL 60601-5907
312-726-6200
http://www.friend-partners.org

**National Kidney Foundation**
30 East 33rd Street, Suite 1100
New York, NY 10016
800-622-9010
http://www.kidney.org

**National Multiple Sclerosis Society**
733 Third Avenue
New York, NY 10017
800-344-4867
http://www.nmss.org

**National Mental Health Association**
1021 Prince Street
Alexandria, VA 22314-2971
703-684-7722
http://nmha.org

**National Osteoporosis Foundation**
1233 22nd Street, NW
Washington, DC 20037-1292
202-223-2226
http://www.nof.org

**National Safety Council**
1121 Spring Lake Drive
Itasca, IL 60143-3201
630-285-1121
http://www.nsc.org

**National Stroke Association**
96 Inverness Drive, E, Suite I
Englewood, CO 80112-5112
800-STROKES (787-6537)
http://www.stroke.org

**National Youth Sports Safety Foundation**
333 Longwood Avenue, Suite 200
Boston, MA 02145
617-277-1171
http://www.nyssf.org

**Planned Parenthood Federation of America**
810 Seventh Avenue
New York, NY 10019
212-541-7800
http://www.plannedparenthood.org

**Sexuality Information and
Education Council of America**
130 West 42nd Street, Suite 350
New York, NY 10036-7801
212-819-9770
http://www.siecus.org

**Sierra Club**
85 Second Street, 2nd Floor
San Francisco, CA 94105-3441
415-977-5500
http://www.sierraclub.org

**United Cerebral Palsy**
1660 L Street, NW, Suite 700
Washington, DC 20036
800-872-5827
http://www.ucpa.org

# GOVERNMENT WEBSITES

**Administration for Children and Families**
http://www.acf.dhhs.gov

**Behavioral Risk Factor
Surveillance System (BRFSS)**
http://www.cdc.gov/nccdphp/brfss

**American Health Foundation**
http://www.ahf.org

**Centers for Disease Control and Prevention**
http://www.cdc.gov

**CDC National AIDS Clearinghouse**
http://www.cdcnac.org

**CDC Prevention Guidelines Database**
http://aepo.xdv.www.epo.cdc.gov/wonder/
prevguid/prevguid.htm

**Combined Health Information Database**
http://chid.nih.gov

**Consumer Information Center**
http://www.pueblo.gsa.gov

**Consumer Product Safety Commission**
http://www.cpsc.gov

**Division of Adolescent and School Health**
http://www.cdc.gov.nccdphp/dash

**Environmental Protection Agency**
http://www.epa.gov

**Federal Government—Statistical Data**
http://www.fedstats.gov

**FedWorld**
http://www.fedworld.gov

**Food and Drug Administration**
http://www.fda.gov

**Library of Congress**
http://www.lcweb.loc.gov

**Morbidity & Mortality Weekly Report**
http://www2.cdc.gov/mmwr

**National Agricultural Library**
www.nalusda.gov

**National Center for Health Statistics**
http://www.cdc.gov/nchswww

**National Center for Injury
Prevention and Control**
http://www.cdc.gov/ncipc/pub-res/prevguide.htm

**National Health Information Clearinghouse**
http://nhic-nt.gov/medlineplus

**National Highway Traffic Safety Administration**
http://www.nhtsa.dot.gov

**National Institute
for Occupational Safety and Health**
http://www.cdc.gov/niosh/homepage.html

**National Institutes of Health**
http://www.nih.gov

**National Library of Medicine**
http://www.nlm.nih.gov

**National Prevention Information Network**
http://www.cdcnpin.org

**Occupational Health and Safety Administration**
http://www.osha.gov

**Office of Disease Prevention
and Health Promotion**
http://www.odphp.osophs.dhhs.gov

**U.S. Department of Agriculture**
http://www.usda.gov

**U.S. Department of Education**
http://www.ed.gov

**U.S. Department of Health and Human Services**
http://www.dhhs.gov

**Youth Risk Behavior Survey**
http://www.cdc.gov/nccdphp/dash/yrbs

**WONDER on the Web (MMWR articles and CDC Prevention Guidelines)**
http://wonder.cdc.gov

# VENDORS

**Adventure North, Inc.**
P.O. Box 128
Pillager, MN 56473

**Advocate Fitness**
205 Touhy, Suite 122
Park Ridge, IL 60068

**Aerobics and Fitness Association**
15250 Ventura Blvd., Suite 200
Sherman Oaks, CA 91403
http://www.aerobics.com

**American Corporate Health Programs & American Institute for Preventive Medicine**
30445 Northwestern Hwy., #350
Farmington Hills, MI 48334

**American Health Foundation**
675 Third Avenue, 11th Floor
New York, NY 10017
212-551-2509

**Aquatic Access, Inc.**
417 Nolan Way
Louisville, KY 40223
800-325-LIFT (-5438)

**Biedna and Company**
499 Flora Place
Fremont, CA 94536-4408

**BIOSIG Instrument, Inc.**
P.O. Box 860
Champlain, NY 12919
800-463-5470

**Body Profile, Inc.**
16800 South Woodland Road
Shaker Heights, OH 44120
216-752-5970

**Cardio Theater**
12 Piedmont Center, Suite 105
Atlanta, GA 30305

**Corporate Fitness Works**
18558 Office Park Drive
Gaithersburg, MD 20879

**Denice Ferko-Adams & Associates**
Wellness Resources
Coopersburg, PA 18036-1514

**DINE Systems, Inc**
586 North French Road
Amherst, NY 14228
800-688-1848
http://www.dinesystems.com

**ETR Associates**
P.O. Box 1830
Santa Cruz, CA 95061-1830
800-321-4407
http://www.etr.org

**Futrex, Inc.**
6 Montgomery Village Ave., Suite 620
Gaithersburg, MD 20879

**Gatorade Sport Science Institute**
617 West Main Sreet
Barrington, IL 60010
847-304-2314
http://www.gssiweb.com

**Great Performances**
14964 NW Greenbrier Parkway
Beaverton, OR 97006

**HealthCare Education Associates**
1729 East Palm Canyon, Suite A
Palm Springs, CA 92264
619-323-4032

**Health Awareness, Inc.**
53426 Hunters Crossing
Utica, MI 48315

**Healthy Achievers**
22 Hayes Road
Madbury, NH 03820

**Hope Publications**
350 East Michigan Avenue, Suite 301
Kalamazoo, MI 49007

**Krames Communications**
1100 Grundy Lane
San Bruno, CA 94066-3030

**LifeCare Resources, Inc.**
540 North Golden Circle Five, #300
Santa Ana, CA 92705

**Mayo Health Information**
200 First Street, SW
Rochester, MN 55905

**Office Workouts, Inc.**
29399 Agoura Road, Suite 113
Agoura Hills, CA 91301

**Pro Source Fitness**
3500 West 80th Street, Suite 130
Bloomington, MN 55431

**State of Health Products**
800 Washington Avenue North, Suite 513
Minneapolis, MN 55401
800-428-8868
http://www.buttout.com

**Tanita Corporation of America**
2625 South Clearbrook Drive
Arlington Heights, IL 60005

**Welltech International**
P.O. Box 411183-251
St. Louis, MO 63141

# ADDITIONAL WEBSITES

**Academy Curriculum Exchange**
http://ofcn.org/cyber.serv/academy/ace

**AIDS Research Information Center**
http://www.critpath.org/aric

**Alan Guttmacher Institute**
http://www.agi-usa.org

**Alcohol, Tobacco, and Drug Abuse**
http://www.healthtouch/com/level1/leaflets/
    102504/102601.htm
http://www.edc.org/hec
http://wcovesoft.com/csap.html
http://www.csa.ca/atod/orgsinfo.htm
http://www.nida.nih.gov
http://www.drugfreekids.com
http://boots.co.uk/main.html
http://www.lindesmith.org
http://www.health.org
http://www.cdc.gov/nccdphp/osh/tobacco
http://www.stic.neu.edu
http://www.scarcnet.org
http://www.no-smoke.org
http://www.quittobacco.com

**Alternative Medicine**
http://www.quackwatch.com
http://www.altmed.od.nih.gov/nccam

**AskERIC Lesson Plan Collection**
http://ericir.syr.edu/Virtual/Lessons

**Awesome Library (lesson plans)**
www.neat-schoolhouse.org/awesome.html

**C. Everett Koop's Shapeup America**
http://www.shapeup.org/sua

**Canadian Consumer Health Information**
http://www.hwc.ca/links/english.html

**Canadian Institute for Health Information**
http://www.cihi.ca

**Columbia Education Center**
http://www.col-ed.org/cur

**Connections+ (Lesson plans)**
http://www.mcrel.org/resources/plus

**Consumer Issues**
http://www.ConsumerResearch.com
http://www.consumerreports.org
http://www.cpsc.gov
http://www.fraud.org

**Dietary Guidelines for Americans**
http://www.usda.gov/cnpp/DietGd.pdf

**DrKoop.com**
http://www.drkoop.com

**Duke University's Healthy Devil On-Line**
http://h-devil-www.mc.duke.edu/h-devil

**Emory University Resources**
http://www.cc.emory.edu/WHSCL/medweb.html

**Encarta**
http://encarta.msn.com/schoolhouse/default.asp

**Epidemiology: The World Wide
Web Virtual Library**
http://www.epibiostat.ucsf.edu/epidem/
    epidem.html

**Families USA Foundation**
http://www.familiesusa.org

**Fitness Link**
http://www.fitnesslink.com

**Fun with Food Science**
http://www.aces.uiuc.edu/~Whitesid/
    4-H/index.html

**The Global Health Network**
http://www.pitt.edu/HOME/GHNet/GHNet.html

**Go Ask Alice**
http://alice.columbia.edu

**Hall of Health**
http://www.hallofhealth.org

**Harvard Medical Web**
http://www.med.harvard.edu

**Health Education Electronic Mail
Directory (HEDIR)**
http://www.siu.edu/~kittle/HEDIR/Menu.html

**Health Education Professional Resources**
http://www.nyu.edu/education/hepr

**Health Education Program of the American
Academy of Family Physicians Foundation**
http://www.healthanswers.com/health_
    answers/aafpf

**Health Finder**
http://www.healthfinder.gov/libraries.htm

**HealthGate**
http://www.healthgate.com

**Health Information Center**
http://nhic-nt.health.org

**HealthLine**
http://www.health-line.com

**Health and Medical Libraries**
http://arcade.uiowa.edu/hardin-www/hslibs.html

**Health Promotion on the Internet**
http://www.monash.edu.au/health/index.htm

**Health Promotion Online**
http://www.hc-sc.ca/health-promotion-sante

**Health Teacher with Web MD**
http://www.healthteacher.com

**Infoseek Health Channel**
http://www.infoseek.com/Topic?tid=1207

**Institute for Health Promotion Research**
http://www.ihpr.ubc.ca

**Intelihealth**
http://www.intelihealth.com/IH/ihtIH

**The International Institute for Health Promotion**
http://www.healthy.american.edu/iihp.html

**Job Stress Network,
Center for Social Epidemiology**
http://www.workhealth.org

**KidsHealth**
http://kidshealth.org

**Leafy Greens Council**
http://www.leafy-greens.org/default.htm

**Mayo Clinic Health Oasis**
http://www.mayohealth.org

**Medscape**
http://www.medscape.com

**Mind over Matter**
http://www.nida.hih.gov/MOM/MOMIndex.html

**National Center for Education
in Maternal and Child Health**
http://www.ncemch.georgetown.edu

**The New England Journal of Medicine**
http://www.nejm.org

**New York Online Access to Health**
http://noah.cuny.edu

**Nutrition Expedition**
http://fsci.umn.edu/nutrexp

**The Ottawa Charter on Health Promotion**
http://www.who.dk/policy/ottawa.htm

**Quackwatch**
http://www.quackwatch.com

**Reducing Occupational Stress**
http://www.workhealth.org/prevent/prred.htm

**Safer Sex**
http://www.safersex.org

**Sexually Transmissible Diseases,
including HIV/AIDS**
http://www.ams.quensu.ca/sexcntr/links.htm
http://www.indiana.edu/~aids/index.html
http://www.unspeakable.com/truth.html

**Shape Up America!**
http://www.shapeup.org

**Stress Free Net**
http://www.stressfree.com

**Teacher.net (lesson plans
under keyword "health")**
http://teachers.net/lessons

**Teacher's Desk**
http://www.teachersdesk.com

**Tobacco Documents (previously secret)**
http://www.house.gov/commerce/TobaccoDocs
http://www.gate.net/%7Ejcannon/tobacco.html
http://www.tobaccoresolution.com
http://www.house.gov/commerce/TobaccoDocs/
   documents.html
http://www.tobaccodocuments.org
http://tobacco.org
http://www.gate.net/~jcannon/liggett

**Virtual Library of Public Health**
http://www.ldb.org/vl/index.htm

**WellTech**
http://com/workplacehealth

**West Healthed**
http://ww.tiac.net/users/rwest

**World Health Organization**
http://www.who.int

**Worldwatch Institute**
http://www.worldwatch.org

# Glossary

**accountability**   the concept that educators and institutions are answerable for what their clients learn

**accreditation**   a voluntary process of recognizing institutions and programs that meet certain criteria, the goals they have set for themselves, and that they have the personnel and financial resources to accomplish their objectives

**administrability**   the ease with which a measurement instrument can be utilized in appropriate ways

**administrative assessment**   an analysis of the policies, resources, and circumstances prevailing in an organization that facilitate or hinder the development of the health promotion program

**affective domain**   emotions, feelings, and attitudes

**attitudes**   people's perceptions of or feelings about their environment and the things in it

**authentic assessment**   strategies that require learners to demonstrate that they do certain things in real, out-of-school settings

**autonomy**   the ethical principle that people should be free to decide their own course of action as long as they do no harm to others

**bacteriology phase**   the period of time between 1880 and 1910, when means to counteract specific diseases were made possible by the discovery that specific microorganisms cause specific diseases

**behavioral assessment**   a systematic analysis of the behavioral links to the goals or problems identified in the epidemiological and social assessments

**behavioral objective**   a statement of desired outcome that indicates who is to demonstrate how much of what action by when

**beliefs**   acceptance of or confidence in an alleged fact or body of facts as true or right without positive knowledge or proof; perceived truth

**beneficence**   the ethical principle that people, especially professionals, should contribute to the health and welfare of others; not doing harm is not enough

**code of ethics**   a statement of principles prescribing the responsibilities of a profession in general terms

**cognitive domain**   learning, consisting of acquiring knowledge and information on an intellectual level

373

**community health education**
The application of a variety of methods that result in the education and mobilization of community members in actions for resolving health issues and problems which affect the community. These methods include, but are not limited to, group process, mass media, communication, community organization, organization development, strategic planning, skills training, legislation, policy making and advocacy (1990 Joint Committee on Health Education Terminology, 1991).

**community organization**    the process by which community groups identify common problems or goals, mobilize resources, and develop and implement strategies for reaching the goals they collectively have set

**competency**    an acceptable level of skill proficiency required to carry out an activity

**comprehensive school health instruction**    the development, delivery, and evaluation of a planned, sequential preschool–12 curriculum (with goals, objectives, content sequence, and specific classroom lessons) that includes, but is not limited to, the following major content areas: community health, consumer health, environmental health, family life, mental and emotional health, injury prevention and safety, nutrition, personal health, prevention and control of disease, substance use and abuse

**concepts**    major components of a theory

**constructs**    concepts developed or adopted for use in a particular theory

**credentialing**    a formal process applied to ensure that those

practicing a profession meet acceptable standards; may apply to individuals, institutions, or programs

**criterion-referenced tests**    tests that have an absolute pass or fail score

**cues to action**    stimuli that provoke a health-related event

**determinants of health**    critical influences that determine the health of individuals and communities

**developmental objectives**    in the context of *Healthy People 2010*, objectives for which current surveillance systems do not provide sufficiently valid and reliable data to establish a baseline

**diagnostic evaluation**    evaluation to determine the needs of an individual or group prior to planning the program activities

**discrimination**    the ability of a measurement instrument to provide different scores between respondents who possess the quality being measured and those who do not

**disease**    the underlying defect or malfunction within the organism

**distributive justice**    the theory advancing the ideal of just distribution of goods, needs, punishment, and reward to all

**duplication**    submitting a manuscript or its essence to more than one journal simultaneously

**educational assessment**    the delineation of factors that predispose, enable, and reinforce a specific behavior or that, through behavior, affect environmental changes

**educational goals**    broad statements of the program's

effect on the agency or on the learner/client

**educator objectives**    objectives that address the methodology, techniques, informational content, and other aspects the instructor determines to be necessary to achieve the behavioral objectives

**emotional health**    the ability to feel and express the full range of human emotions, give and receive love, achieve a sense of fulfillment and purpose in life, and develop psychological hardiness

**employee assistance program**    initiative for the purpose of helping employees cope with health problems that affect work

**empowerment**    an enabling process through which individuals or communities take control over their lives and their environment

**enabling factor**    factors that are present before a behavior occurs that allow the behavior to be carried out by providing the necessary ability, skills, opportunity, or resources

**environmental assessment**    (also called ecological assessment) a systematic analysis of factors in the social and physical environment that interact with behavior to produce health effects or quality-of-life outcomes (adapted from Green & Kreuter, 1999)

**environmental factors**    determinants outside the person that can be modified to support behavior, health, or quality of life

**epidemiological assessment**    the delineation of the extent, distribution, and causes of a health problem in a defined population

**ethics**    a branch of philosophy that deals with systematic approaches to understanding morality

**evaluation**   comparison of an object of interest against a standard of acceptability

**expectancies**   values placed by the individual on what is expected to occur

**expectations**   certain events that the individual expects to occur in a particular situation

**formative evaluation**   the ongoing process of evaluation while the program is being developed and implemented; also called process evaluation

**fragmentation**   breaking down data from a study into several parts (the "least publishable unit") for the purpose of increasing the number of publications in which the study results can appear

**hardiness**   an optimistic and committed approach to life, viewing problems as challenges that can be handled

**health literacy**   the capacity of individuals to obtain, interpret, and understand basic health information and services, and the competence to use the information and services in ways that enhance health

**health promotion phase**   the period of time beginning in 1975 and continuing into the present, when educational, political, social, and economic interventions are employed to promote adaptations that will improve or protect individuals' health

**health protection**   legal or fiscal controls, other regulations and policies, and voluntary codes of practice, aimed at the enhancement of health and the prevention of illness

**health resources phase**   the period of time between 1910 and 1960, characterized by enormous financial investments in hospitals, health personnel, and biomedical research

**health risk appraisal** questionnaires used to estimate individuals' health risks by comparing behaviors and current health status to those of a cross section of healthy people who are the same age and gender as the user

**heredity**   genetic background that programs each of us in some ways

**illness**   the presentation of visible symptoms

**impact evaluation**   evaluation of a program or curriculum in terms of its immediate, short-term effects

**incidence**   number of new cases of a disease in a certain period of time

**justice**   the ethical principle that every person should be treated fairly and similarly

**knowledge**   the intellectual acquaintance with facts, truth, or principles

**learning**   change of behavior brought about by experience, insight, perception, or a combination of the three, that causes the individual to approach future situations differently

**licensure**   all forms of state control over the right to perform specific duties

**maturation**   a developmental process during which a person manifests traits, the blueprint of which is carried on the genes

**measurable objectives**   in the context of *Healthy People 2010*, objectives for which there are valid and reliable data from currently established, nationally representative data systems

**measurement**   determination of quantity or quality of an object of interest

**mediators**   factors that facilitate or help bring about a change in personal behavior

**mental (or intellectual) health** ability to make sound decisions and think critically

**miasma phase**   the period of time from 1850 to 1880, when disease was thought to be caused by noxious vapors

**model**   a subclass of theory used to represent processes and relationships among variables

**multiphasic screening**   the use of various tests, conducted separately or in a single session, to identify health problems or deviations from the average

**natural law**   the theory that individuals have the right to select their personal health behavior or lifestyle

**needs assessment**   a planned process that identifies the reported needs of an individual or a group

**nonmalificence**   the ethical principle that a professional should do no harm or impose unreasonable intentional risk of harm

**norm-referenced tests**   tests where an individual's score is compared to a group score

**objectives**   precise statements that map out the tasks necessary to reach a goal

**objectivity**   the ability of a measurement instrument to yield similar results on successive occasions and to yield similar results when administered by different people

**optimal health**   the highest level of health possible under the current set of environmental conditions and the individual's capacity

**outcome evaluation**   evaluation of a program or curriculum in terms of its long-term or ultimate effects

**paternalism**   the theory that the government may intervene into personal lives and liberties by invoking *parens patriae* power of the state

**patient education**   health education in health care delivery settings to patients and their families

**philosophy**   statement summarizing an individual's or group's attitudes, beliefs, values, principles, and state of mind

**physical health**   the absence of disease and disability; functioning adequately from the perspective of physical and physiological abilities; the biological integrity of the individual

**plagiarism**   the unauthorized use of the works or ideas of others without proper credit or permission

**planning**   the process of making decisions as to what topic to address or what problems to attack, and/or where to direct time and resources

**policy assessment**   appraisal of conditions that are presumed unchangeable in existing policies and regulations

**portfolio**   a collection of student work and educator data from informal and performance assessments

**predisposing factor**   factors that are present before a behavior occurs that provide a rationale or motivation for the behavior

**prevalence**   total number of active or existing cases of a disease

**primary care**   the provision of integrated, accessible health care services by clinicians who are accountable for addressing a large majority of personal health care needs, developing a sustained partnership with patients, and practicing in the context of family and community (Murphy, 1996)

**primary prevention**   action taken to avert the occurrence of disease

**principles**   general guidelines for action

**profession**   the sociological construct for an occupation that has special status

**professional socialization**   the process by which recruits into the profession develop values, attitudes, and beliefs that support their roles as practitioners

**program goals**   broad statements of the program's intended achievements

**program objectives**   precise statements that address who will receive the program, what health benefit they will receive, how much of that benefit should be received, and by when the benefit should be achieved

**psychomotor domain**   physical skills and the aspects of learning in which the individual applies accumulated knowledge and attitudes to behavior or action

**public health agencies** community agencies created by government and funded by taxes for the purpose of protecting, improving, and maintaining the health of the citizens

**qualitative measurement**   that which attempts to provide statements describing processes or experiences resulting from exposure to a program or an activity

**quantitative measurement** that which yields numerical values such as how many, how much, or how often

**reciprocal determinism**   a foundation of social learning theory; the interaction occurring among a person, the person's behavior, and the environment within which the behavior is performed

**registration**   placement of the individual's name on a list of those who perform certain tasks

**reinforcing factor**   factors that are present after the behavior has occurred that can encourage repetition or abandonment of it

**reliability**   the ability of a measurement instrument to yield consistent results each time it is used

**risk conditions**   factors that influence health, either through risk factors or by operating directly on human biology over time, and that are unlikely to be under the control of the individuals at risk

**risk factors**   aspects of human behavior that put one at risk for disease or injury

**school health coordinating council**   body of concerned community members that serves as a liaison with the outside environment, ensuring support and establishing links between the school health program and outside community

**school health coordinator**   the professional responsible for the management and coordination of all health education policies, activities, and resources within a school

**school health services**   all procedures to promote, appraise, and protect the health of every child in school

**scope**   the total range of subject areas or health topics selected to represent the body of knowledge of the discipline

**screening**   preliminary appraisal technique that identifies health problems or deviations from the average

**secondary prevention** action taken to identify diseases at their earliest stages and to apply appropriate treatments to limit their consequences and severity

**self-control** the condition in which the individual can gain control of his or her own behavior and controlling reinforcers

**self-efficacy** the internal condition of experiencing competence to perform desired tasks that will influence the eventual outcome

**sensitivity** the ability of a measurement instrument to reflect changes in the state or amount of the phenomenon being measured

**sequence** order of the organizing elements to be taught in a curriculum

**skills** the abilities to do or to apply something in order to carry out activities

**social assessment** the application, through broad participation, of multiple sources of information designed to expand people's understanding of their own quality of life and aspirations for the common good

**social capital** a sense of trust and long-term reciprocity among individuals and community organizations

**social ecology** the health perspective that takes into account the social, political, and economic milieu in which people exist

**social engineering phase** the period of time between 1960 and 1975, when legislation and policy prioritized equal access to health services

**social health** ability to perform the expectations of our roles effectively, comfortably, with pleasure, without harming other people; the ability to interact effectively with others and the social environment

**social marketing** the planning and implementation of programs to bring about social change using concepts from commercial marketing

**specificity** the ability of a test to correctly rule out those who do not have the characteristic of interest

**spiritual health** a high level of faith, hope, and commitment in relation to a well-defined world view or belief system that provides a sense of meaning and purpose to existence in general, and that offers an ethical path to personal fulfillment that includes connectedness with self, others, and a higher power or larger reality (adapted from Hawks, 1994)

**state teacher certification** legal recognition authorizing the individual holder of the certificate to perform specific services in public schools within the state

**summative evaluation** evaluation done to ascertain if the program has met predetermined objectives

**tertiary prevention** specific interventions to assist diseased or disabled persons in limiting the effects of their diseases or disabilities; also may include activities to prevent recurrence of a disease

**type A** an action-emotion complex observed in a person aggressively involved in a long-term, ceaseless struggle to achieve more and more in less and less time, even against opposition by other things or persons

**utilitarianism** the theory that uses overall benefit to society as a standard for curtailing self-destructive behaviors

**validity** the tendency of a measurement instrument to measure what it is intended to measure

**values** the underlying constructs of right or wrong that give direction to every decision and result in the action the person takes

**variables** operational definitions of concepts that specify how the concept is to be measured

**voluntary certification** the process by which a nongovernmental agency or association grants recognition to an individual who has met certain predetermined qualifications

**wellness** the quality of life that includes physical, mental-emotional, family-social, and spiritual health

# Index